PRACTICAL PAEDIATRIC
RESPIRATORY MEDICINE

PRACTICAL PAEDIATRIC RESPIRATORY MEDICINE

EDITED BY

Michael Silverman
Professor and Head, Department of Child Health
and Institute for Lung Health, University of
Leicester, Leicester, UK

Christopher L. O'Callaghan
Professor of Paediatrics, Department of Child
Health and Institute for Lung Health, University of
Leicester, Leicester, UK

A member of the Hodder Headline Group
LONDON • NEW YORK • NEW DELHI

First published in Great Britain in 2001 by
Arnold, a member of the Hodder Headline Group,
338 Euston Road, London NW1 3BH

http://www.arnoldpublishers.com

Distributed in the United States of America by
Oxford University Press Inc.,
198 Madison Avenue, New York, NY 10016
Oxford is a registered trademark of Oxford University Press

Whilst the advice and information in this book are believed to be true and
accurate at the date of going to press, neither the authors nor the publisher
can accept any legal responsibility or liability for any errors or omissions
that may be made. In particular (but without limiting the generality of the
preceding disclaimer) every effort has been made to check drug dosages;
however it is still possible that errors have been missed. Furthermore,
dosage schedules are constantly being revised and new side-effects
recognized. For these reasons the reader is strongly urged to consult
the drug companies' printed instructions before administering any of
the drugs recommended in this book.

British Library Cataloguing in Publication Data
A catalogue record for this book is available from the British Library

Library of Congress Cataloging-in-Publication Data
A catalog record for this book is available from the Library of Congress

ISBN 0 340 74126 0

1 2 3 4 5 6 7 8 9 10

Publisher: Joanna Koster
Production Editor: James Rabson
Production Controller: Iain McWilliams
Cover Design: Terry Griffiths

Typeset in 9.5/12pt Palatino by
J&L Composition Ltd, Filey, North Yorkshire
Printed and bound in Great Britain by The Bath Press

What do you think about this book? Or any other Arnold title?
Please send your comments to feedback.arnold@hodder.co.uk

CONTENTS

CONTRIBUTORS

Dr P Barry
Honorary Senior Lecturer in Child Health
Department of Child Health
Clinical Sciences Building
Leicester Royal Infirmary
PO Box 65
Leicester LE2 7LX

Dr C Beardsmore
Lecturer in Child Health
Department of Child Health
University of Leicester
Clinical Sciences Building
Leicester Royal Infirmary
PO Box 65
Leicester LE2 7LX

Dr A Brooke
Honorary Senior Lecturer in Child Health
Consultant Community Paediatrician
Leicestershire and Rutland Healthcare Trust
Bridge Park Plaza
Bridge Park Road
Thormaston
Leicester LE4 8PQ

Dr M Browning
Senior Lecturer in Immunology
Maurice Shock Medical Sciences Building
University Road
PO Box 138
Leicester LE1 9HN

Dr E Carter
Consultant Paediatrician
Children's Hospital
Leicester Royal Infirmary
Infirmary Square
Leicester LE1 5WW

Dr M A Chilvers
Specialist Paediatric Registrar
Leicester Royal Infirmary
Infirmary Square
Leicester LE1 5WW

Dr A Custovic
Reader in Respiratory Medicine and Allergy
North West Lung Centre
Wythenshawe Hospital
Southmoor Road
Manchester M23 9LT

Dr N Dogra
Division of Child Psychiatry
University of Leicester
Greenwood Institute
Westcotes House
Westcotes Drive
Leicester LE3 0QU

Ms H Dunbar
Paediatric Advanced Nurse Practitioner
(Respiratory Diseases)
Ward 12, Leicester Royal Infirmary
Infirmary Square
Leicester LE1 5WW

Mr R K Firmin
Consultant Cardio-thoracic Surgeon
Glenfield Hospital
Groby Road
Leicester LE3 9QP

Professor I Gordon
Department of Radiology
Great Ormond Street Hospital
Great Ormond Street
London WC1N 3JH

Dr M R Green
Consultant Paediatrician
Children's Hospital
Leicester Royal Infirmary
Infirmary Square
Leicester LE1 5WW

Dr J Grigg
Senior Lecturer in Child Health
Department of Child Health
University of Leicester
Clinical Sciences Building
Leicester Royal Infirmary
PO Box 65
Leicester LE2 7LX

Dr W Hoskyns
Consultant Paediatrician
Children's Hospital
Leicester Royal Infirmary
Infirmary Square
Leicester LE1 5WW

Dr G Jones
Consultant Paediatric Anaesthetist
Leicester Royal Infirmary
Infirmary Square
Leicester LE1 5WW

Dr A Kotecha
Senior Lecturer in Child Health
Department of Child Health
University of Leicester
Clinical Sciences Building
Leicester Royal Infirmary
PO Box 65
Leicester LE2 7LX

Dr D Luyt
Consultant in Paediatric Intensive Care
Leicester Royal Infirmary
Infirmary Square
Leicester LE1 5WW

Mr A Moir
Consultant Ear, Nose and Throat Surgeon
Leicester Royal Infirmary
Infirmary Square
Leicester LE1 5WW

Dr S Nichani
Consultant in Paediatric Intensive Care
Leicester Royal Infirmary
Infirmary Square
Leicester LE1 5WW

Professor C L O'Callaghan
Professor of Paediatrics
Department of Child Health
University of Leicester
Clinical Sciences Building
Leicester Royal Infirmary
Infirmary Square
Leicester LE1 5WW

Dr J Paton
Reader in Paediatric Respiratory Disease
Department of Child Health
Royal Hospital for Sick Children
Yorkhill
Glasgow G3 8SJ

Dr G J Peek
Lecturer in Cardiac Surgery
University of Leicester
Glenfield Hospital
Groby Road
Leicester LE3 9QP

Ms G Phillips
Lecturer in Physiotherapy
King's College London
GKT School of Biomedical Sciences
Shepherd's House, Guy's Campus
London SE1 1UL

Ms S Pike
Clinical Specialist Paediatric Physiotherapist
Royal Brompton Hospital
Sydney Street
London SW3 6NP

Professor M Silverman
Head of Department of Child Health
University of Leicester
Robert Kilpatrick Clinical Sciences Building
Leicester Royal Infirmary
PO Box 65
Leicester LE2 7LX

Dr A Smyth
Consultant in Paediatric Respiratory Medicine
Department of Paediatrics
Nottingham City Hospital
Hucknall Road
Nottingham NG5 1PB

Ms S Storer
Play Services Manager
Children's Hospital
Leicester Royal Infirmary
Infirmary Square
Leicester LE1 5WW

Dr AH Thomson
Consultant in Paediatric Respiratory Medicine
Department of Paediatrics
John Radcliffe Hospital
Level 4
Headington
Oxford OX3 9DU

Dr C Wallis
Consultant in Respiratory Paediatrics
Great Ormond Street Hospital
Great Ormond Street
London WC1N 3JH

Mrs D Wensley
Respiratory Research Nurse
Department of Child Health
University of Leicester
Clinical Sciences Building
Leicester Royal Infirmary
PO Box 65
Leicester LE2 7LX

Dr M Wiselka
Consultant in Infectious Diseases
Leicester Royal Infirmary
Infirmary Square
Leicester LE1 5WW

Professor A Woodcock
Head of South Manchester Academic Group
North West Lung Centre
Wythenshawe Hospital
Southmoor Road
Manchester M23 9LT

PART ONE

CLINICAL MEASUREMENT AND CLINICAL ASSESSMENT

CHAPTER ONE

INTRODUCTION: PRACTICAL SKILLS *AND* PATIENT MANAGEMENT

M. Silverman and C. O'Callaghan

There is a striking discrepancy between the way in which clinical practice is conducted (Figure 1.1), and the way in which learning material is structured in textbooks.

- Patients seek help because of 'low level' symptoms; textbooks (in general) provide information about 'high level' diagnoses, with remarkably little on the important steps involved in reaching these diagnoses.

- Patients present with problem

  ↓

- Health professionals assess and create diagnostic hypotheses

  ↓

- 'Bedside' tests and other investigations performed to reach diagnosis, assess impact and inform management

  ↓

- Adaptive and therapeutic management plan

  ↓

- Management procedures and process carried out

  ↓

- Evaluate outcome

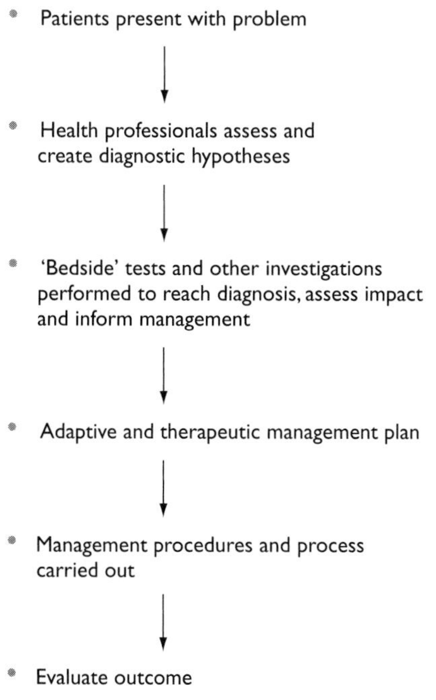

Figure 1.1: The bones of clinical practice.

- Health professionals must elicit signs and conduct or commission investigations; textbooks are usually reticent about these important steps in testing initial diagnostic hypotheses.
- Management of disease requires therapeutic skills which often require practical experience; textbooks rarely provide the background knowledge on which these skills are based, especially if those skills are not specific to a single disease (Table 1.1).

Knowledge of the practical procedures which are commonly used in diagnosis, evaluation and management is vital. Reading however, complements but does not replace doing! This book does not provide 'standard operating procedures' or protocols for the techniques described. It complements the traditional apprenticeship system whereby practical skills are usually learned in clinical practice. It is aimed at health professionals with an interest in respiratory disorders of children. It will provide paediatricians and children's nurses in training with the opportunity to compensate for ever-shortening training periods and ever-fewer opportunities to learn important special skills. Trainees should be encouraged to see and do the practical procedures described for themselves. Health professionals specializing in one field of respiratory disease may gain understanding of the way their skills integrate in practice, with those in related fields. Although not aimed at the Paediatric Pulmonologist, much of the text is relevant to trainees and to the many professions represented in the Paediatric Pulmonology

Table 1.1: Some clinical skills which cross disease boundaries

	Asthma	Cystic fibrosis	Host-defence disorders	Upper airways obstruction
Investigations				
▪ skin prick tests	++	+	+	−
▪ special radiology	−	±	++	+
▪ immune function	+	±	+++	−
Therapeutic procedures				
▪ inhalation therapy	+++	++	±	+
▪ guided self-management	+++	++	+	±
▪ physiotherapy	±	+++	+++	−

Team, whether in hospital practice, community care or primary care.

We thank our colleagues in Leicester and beyond for accepting the unusual (and difficult) task which we set them, of describing clinical practice from the 'bottom up'. Their contributions are rooted in many years of clinical practice, and seek to combine experience with knowledge. The clinical case studies (vignettes) may help to jog the reader's memories, so that they are thereby helped to assimilate the written word in clinical context – the mature approach to learning.

CHAPTER TWO

TAKING *A* HISTORY: SYMPTOMS

A. Smyth

- Background information
- Specific symptoms and their significance
- Specific questions
- Congenital syndromes

- Research issues
- References
- Further reading

BACKGROUND INFORMATION

THE GENERAL APPROACH TO HISTORY TAKING

In paediatric history taking, it is usually not the patient but the parent, or accompanying adult, who tells the story. A study which compared parents' responses to a questionnaire about respiratory illness to those given by the child, found that in many cases they did not agree.[1] The same may be true of traditional, narrative history taking and so it is important to record who has been interviewed. If you take the history from the parent, verify some points with older children (primary school age). In the case of a teenager, take the history from them, but bear in mind that they may be reticent or minimize their symptoms. It is important to take into account the effect of social and ethnic background on parental perception of the child's problems. Parents often feel disempowered when consulting a doctor.[2] Acknowledge their concerns whilst taking the history.

As you take the history and examine the child, you should be forming a hypothesis about the likely diagnosis, which you can test by further questioning, by eliciting physical signs and later by investigations. This is an active, iterative process, not passive information gathering.

WHAT IS THE PRIMARY PROBLEM?

Establish what the parents and child perceive as the problem. This may be different from the impression given by another health professional. Determine the duration of the symptoms and, if the problem is chronic, find out why the parents have brought their child now. This will lead in to a narrative 'history of presenting complaint' which should be a succinct chronology of events. For example, if the presenting complaint is cough (see below) find out when it began; how long episodes last (hours, days or weeks); what appears to trigger an episode (e.g. viral infection, food or drink, exercise); diurnal variation; response to treatment; and impact on the child's life (e.g. school absence, waking at night).

When you are reviewing a child with an established diagnosis or a chronic illness, a different set of questions are appropriate. Try to ascertain the effect of the illness on the child and their family. Establish the pattern of disease and the frequency and severity of the exacerbations (for instance, of asthma or cystic fibrosis). How often do they require 'rescue' medication (e.g. oral steroids in asthma or intravenous antibiotics in cystic fibrosis)? What degree of disability has their illness caused (e.g. the ability to participate in sport)? Do they receive disability benefit?

(Receipt of such benefits may bear no relation to the severity of their disease.)[3]

OTHER SPECIFIC ASPECTS OF THE HISTORY

This follows conventional paediatric history taking and the main points to be covered are shown in Table 2.1.

SPECIFIC SYMPTOMS AND THEIR SIGNIFICANCE

COUGH

Cough is one of the most common reasons for parents of pre-school children consulting their general practitioners[2] and this may lead to a referral to a paediatrician. Parents will vary in how much their child will cough before they consider it to be abnormal. A study of healthy primary school children found that some children had over 30 episodes of coughing per day, with a mean of 11 episodes.[4] Parental reporting of night-time symptoms may also be unreliable. Although parents can accurately report whether their child coughs at night, their reporting of whether their child wakes correlates poorly with video recordings of the sleeping child.[5]

The duration and time of onset of cough is clearly important. A short history of coughing in children may be due to upper respiratory infection or lower respiratory infection such as bronchiolitis. This may occur because viral infections strip respiratory epithelium and expose submucosal cough receptors.[6] The cough may persist for months after the infection has been cleared ('post-viral cough'). A suggested algorithm for the investigation of the child with chronic cough is given in Figure 2.1. Children with primary ciliary dyskinesia often have a history of a 'moist' cough in infancy (see Case study 2.1). Where persistent cough follows an episode of pneumonia, the problem may be persistent atelectasis, which if untreated could lead to bronchiectasis.

Pre-school children do not usually expectorate, but swallow (and may hence vomit) their sputum.

Table 2.1: Key items in the history

Pregnancy and birth: Perinatal illness may give clues to later diagnosis. Summarize this period (e.g. respiratory symptoms, need for mechanical ventilation, or supplementary oxygen).

Feeding:[27] The risk of a child having respiratory disease may be influenced by how they were fed in infancy and so this should be recorded.[24,26] Recurrent vomiting, possetting or dysphagia are important clues for recurrent pulmonary aspiration.

Immunizations: A full immunization history should be taken and confirmed by reference to the child's personal child health record. Note BCG scar.

Development: Developmental disorders may result from, or lead to chronic respiratory illness. Sleep disturbance (which can be caused by nocturnal cough or wheeze) can affect cognitive ability.[28] Developmental milestones or, in older children, school performance, should be recorded. Children with neuromuscular or developmental problems may have respiratory disease, the aetiology of which may be multifactorial, e.g. recurrent aspiration, kyphoscoliosis, weak cough.

Past medical history: Previous respiratory illnesses such as bronchiolitis may be associated with illness in children many years after the original episode.[29]

Family history: May provide important clues, e.g. of asthma, atopy, cystic fibrosis. Ask about consanguinity, e.g. primary ciliary dyskinesia.

Social history: Ask about the parent's smoking habits[30] and the physical state of the child's home.[31]

Drug history: Detailed information about medication is important. 'Two puffs' of inhaled steroid could mean a tenfold difference in effective dose, depending on the strength and nature of the device. Direct questioning of the child is more likely to elicit information about compliance.

Chronic cough

Does the child wheeze?

Yes →

No ↓

All ages, consider:

* Asthma
* Viral associated wheeze
* Gastro-oesophageal reflux (*Vomiting?*)
* Obliterative bronchiolitis (*History of adenovirus infection?*)
* Left ventricular failure
* Inhaled foreign body (*Localized wheeze?*)

Is the cough productive?

Yes ↙   **No** ↘

In infants also consider:

* Tracheobronchomalacia (*Bronchodilators and steroids ineffective?*)
* Bronchopulmonary dysplasia (*Prematurity?*)

Investigations:

Is there reversible lower airways obstruction?
* Bronchodilator response
* Peak flow diary
* Exercise testing
No? asthma unlikely

* Chest X-ray
Air-trapping? Localized–foreign body. Generalized–asthma
* pH study
* ECG and echocardiogram

Consider:

* High resolution CT
* Bronchoscopy

Consider:

Cystic fibrosis* (*Is the child thriving?*)
Bronchiectasis
(*History of severe episode of pneumonia?*)
Immune deficiency* (*SPUR?*)
Primary ciliary dyskinesia* (*Sinusitis?*)
Inhaled foreign body*

* The cough may not be productive initially

Investigations:

* Sweat test
* Chest X-ray ± High resolution CT
* Immunoglobulins, IgG subclasses, functional antibodies and T/B cell subsets
* Ciliary studies

Consider:

Cough variant asthma
Gastro-oesophageal reflux
'Post-viral cough'
Left ventricular failure
Habit/psychogenic cough
Whooping cough

Investigations:

Is there reversible lower airways obstruction?
* Bronchodilator response
* Peak flow diary
* Exercise testing
No? asthma unlikely

* Chest X-ray
* pH study
* ECG and echocardiogram

Figure 2.1: An algorithm for investigating chronic cough.

Case study 2.1: Productive cough

James, aged 11, presents with a history of daily productive cough from the age of 5 years. He is unable to do games at school. In the neonatal period he had an episode of pneumonia. His cough is temporarily relieved by antibiotics and he has never wheezed. Latterly he has complained of headache and purulent nasal discharge. On examination his weight and height are on the 90th centile. Chest examination is unremarkable. A number of chest radiographs (the earliest from age 5) show persistent right middle lobe collapse (Figure 2.2). A sweat test was normal as were immunoglobulins, IgG subclasses, and T and B-cell subsets. Ciliary studies in this child showed primary ciliary dyskinesia. Typically there is a history of cough and transient tachypnoea in early infancy and in 50% of patients a history of ear problems; glue ear is particularly common in the pre-school years. Sinusitis is a feature of this condition, as is suppurative lung disease. The sinusitis is suggested in the history by the nasal discharge and headache. In cystic fibrosis, nasal discharge may also occur due to nasal polyps and headache may occur due to CO_2 retention in the terminal stages.

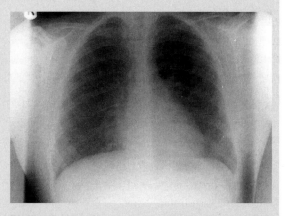

Figure 2.2: Chest radiograph of the child described in Case study 2.1.

Cough in this age group is therefore usually unproductive but may sound 'moist'. Those conditions which may lead to sputum production are listed separately in Figure 2.1.

In children with asthma there is usually a history of wheezing or dyspnoea as well as cough. There has been much debate about whether children in whom cough is the only symptom, could have asthma and whether they should be treated with anti-asthma medication. Although series of children with cough-variant asthma have been described from specialist institutions,[7] epidemiological studies have shown that a minority of children in whom cough is the only symptom, have asthma.[8] Furthermore, asthma medications are often unhelpful, although a therapeutic trial of limited duration (say 4 weeks) may be useful. A randomized controlled trial of a bronchodilator and an inhaled steroid in children with recurrent cough has shown neither to be effective.[9] The pathways mediating cough are different to those mediating bronchospasm. For example, inhaled sodium cromoglycate blocks the bronchoconstriction induced by nebulized water but not the cough. Conversely, lignocaine blocks the cough but not the bronchoconstriction.[10]

Post-nasal drip is listed in many textbooks as a cause of chronic cough in children. This is controversial. There are no cough receptors above the larynx and so the mechanism by which post-nasal drip might cause cough is not clear. A history of snoring, with disturbed sleep and arousals, suggests that the child may also have obstructive sleep apnoea. Gastro-oesophageal reflux may cause cough, irrespective of whether aspiration occurs, and may occur in an infant in the absence of vomiting. In children who have aspirated a foreign body the typical history of choking may be absent. Children who have had a repair of tracheo-oesophageal fistula in the newborn period, or who have primary tracheo-bronchomalacia have a characteristic harsh cough and usually do not present a diagnostic problem. Psychogenic cough should only be diagnosed after a thorough clinical assessment has ruled out an organic cause; the quality of the cough ('honking') is characteristic. A weak cough is suggestive of vocal cord palsy or a neuropathic condition.

WHEEZING

Although it may be clear to clinicians what is meant by the term 'wheezing', patients and parents do not always mean the same thing. One study looked at children who were believed by their parents to be wheezing and found that the doctor agreed in only 65% of cases.[11] It is best to describe the sound to the parent (e.g. *'a whistling noise in the chest when your child breathes out'*) and ask if the description fits their child's symptom. It is important to distinguish wheezing from a moist 'ruttle' in the upper airways which may be found in healthy infants.[12] The precipitants (dust, pollen, upper respiratory tract infection (URTI), bird exposure etc.), timing (diurnal variation), seasonality and severity of wheeze should be ascertained. Variation when the environment changes, for example symptom changes when away on holiday, should be asked for. Home visits may be informative in selected cases. Wheezing is a common symptom in children. In asthma, people describe 'chest tightness' and 'breathlessness' in association with wheeze in varying proportions. Recent epidemiological studies of children, in the developed world, have shown that almost half will wheeze in their first 6 years,[13] whilst a third of UK secondary school children reported an episode of wheezing in the last year.[14] Studies using a questionnaire, completed by the parents of pre-school children, have found that questions relating to wheeze (unlike cough) are highly repeatable after an interval of 6 months. Cohen's Kappa statistic for the question *'Has your child ever had attacks of wheezing?'* was 0.88 in one study.[15] The same may be true when questions relating to wheeze are asked as part of conventional history taking.

There is a wide differential diagnosis of wheezing in children (Table 2.2). There is considerable overlap with conditions causing chronic cough. There is controversy over whether non-atopic children with episodic wheeze precipitated by respiratory viral infection should be referred to as having asthma or whether another diagnostic term such as viral associated wheeze should be used.[16] Where these children are referred to as having asthma, it is important to point out to the parent that many children, who have been labelled as having asthma, will have mild or transient symptoms. Almost 20% of pre-school children in one study had wheezing

Table 2.2: Differential diagnosis of wheezing in children

Acute wheeze	Chronic wheeze
■ Asthma	■ Asthma
■ Viral wheeze	■ Gastro-oesophageal reflux
■ Acute bronchiolitis	■ Bronchopulmonary dysplasia
■ Foreign body aspiration (wheeze may be unilateral)	■ Tracheobronchomalacia
	■ Obliterative bronchiolitis (e.g. as a sequel of adenovirus pneumonia)
	■ Left ventricular failure
	■ Glottic (laryngeal) wheeze
	■ Foreign body

Conditions where wheezing may be present but may not be the predominant feature:
■ Cystic fibrosis
■ Bronchiectasis/host of defence defects

in the first 3 years of life but were symptom free by the age of 6 years.[13]

During the winter months, it may be difficult to distinguish an infant having a first asthma attack from one who is suffering from acute bronchiolitis. Infants with bronchiolitis are usually under a year, having their first attack of wheeze and have marked coryza (see Chapter 5, Acute assessment). A therapeutic trial of a nebulized bronchodilator is rarely effective.[17] A history of a poor response to previous treatment may be very helpful in evaluating children who wheeze, as it makes simple reversible airways obstruction less likely. However the most common reason for poor response to treatment is poor drug delivery due to poor inhaler technique (see Chapter 20, Aerosols).

Gastro-oesophageal reflux may account for some of the nocturnal symptoms of asthma in children and one study has shown a temporal relationship between reflux episodes and episodes of wheeze.[18] The association between gastro-oesophageal reflux and wheezing may be related to aspiration of small amounts of milk feed or other material into the airway. However wheeze can be associated with reflux in the absence of aspiration and this is thought to occur via a vagal reflex.[19] Recurrent aspiration is a major problem in children with disorders of swallowing.

OTHER NOISY BREATHING

Wheeze must be distinguished from other forms of noising breathing such as stertorous breathing and stridor. Stertorous (or 'snuffly') breathing is due to nasal obstruction and is particularly common in young infants who are preferential nose-breathers. The symptom is seen in healthy infants but is more pronounced in those with an abnormal nasal airway. Stridor is a harsh sound, originating in the trachea or upper airways. The age of onset will be important in distinguishing stridor due to a congenital abnormality from other causes. (See Table 3.2, Chapter 3, Physical examination: Signs). The accompanying symptoms may give a clue to the diagnosis. In an infant with congenital stridor ask about vomiting, which may suggest a vascular ring and consider subglottic stenosis following neonatal intubation. In acute stridor ask about accompanying fever or difficulty in swallowing. Stridor may occur during inspiration or (less commonly) expiration. Expiratory stridor (e.g. due to tracheobronchomalacia) may be difficult to distinguish from wheeze, but may be accompanied by a cough reminiscent of a cow or of the honk of a goose (a 'TOF cough').

APNOEA AND CYANOTIC SPELLS

A number of definitions of apnoea have been suggested but the definition put forward by the National Institutes of Health[21] is commonly used: 'An unexplained episode of cessation of breathing for 20 seconds or longer, or a shorter respiratory pause associated with bradycardia, cyanosis, pallor, and/or marked hypotonia.'

Case study 2.2: An infant with cough and noisy breathing

An 8-month-old baby presents with a history of cough and noisy breathing from a few weeks of age. He has had numerous admissions to hospital with chest problems and he is currently taking both a bronchodilator and regular inhaled steroids via a spacer. Despite this, his mother says he is wheezing every day, even when prescribed a short course of oral prednisolone at an appropriate dose. There is no family history of atopy and he is the first child. On examination he is thriving. There is an obvious barking cough, chest indrawing and a diffuse harsh expiratory sound, which is more consistent with expiratory stridor, but no inspiratory wheeze.

Expiratory stridor is found in abnormalities of the intrathoracic airway. Both vascular ring and tracheobronchomalacia are possible diagnoses. A flexible bronchoscopy was performed with the child breathing spontaneously and the distal trachea was found to collapse completely during expiration confirming the diagnosis of tracheobronchomalacia. There was no tracheo-oesophageal fistula. (A further useful investigation in this case would have been a barium swallow, where a vascular ring would have appeared as a posterior indentation of the oesophagus (Figure 2.3).) The management of tracheobronchomalacia is expectant with supplementary oxygen where necessary (though stenting procedures have been tried). Prognosis is good and most children are asymptomatic by school age (apart from reduced exercise tolerance).[20]

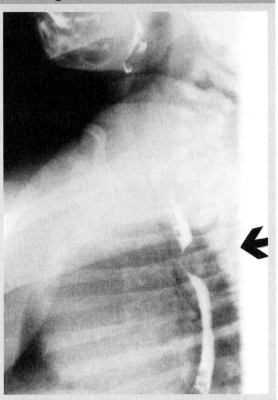

Figure 2.3: Barium swallow of an infant with a vascular ring showing a posterior indentation of the oesophagus.

An anxious parent may be unable to recall the precise duration of apnoeic episodes, but this definition is useful if the infant is admitted to hospital for monitoring. Periodic breathing may be mistaken for apnoea (Chapter 5). In some cases the apnoea and cyanosis may be prolonged accompanied by the infant becoming limp and choking, in which case the term acute life-threatening episode (ALTE) may be used. Some parents may misinterpret transient colour changes in infants or older children as cyanosis. However when a parent reports cyanosis, this should be taken seriously. In children with pneumonia, the mother's impression that the child has been 'going blue' is an important predictor of hypox-aemia.[22] Cyanosis during an acute asthma attack is a late sign, indicating impending respiratory fail-

ure. Chronic cyanosis is a feature of cyanotic congenital heart disease, Eisenmenger's syndrome and end-stage respiratory failure.

BREATHLESSNESS / DYSPNOEA

Patient's reporting of subjective symptoms such as breathlessness may be variable. However, in paediatric history taking, this symptom may be even more uncertain because you may be asking a parent whether they think their child feels breathless. In one questionnaire study this was described as feeling '... *out of breath or puffed*.'[23] This symptom had a one year prevalence of 8.5% in 7 and 11-year-old school children; however the repeatability of questions relating to breathlessness was poorer than those relating to wheeze. In a study of children attending in an emergency setting, dyspnoea was assessed by an investigator (rather than the parent) and was strongly correlated with forced expiratory volume (FEV$_1$).[24] In fact, when parents are asked whether their child has been breathless, they may base their reply on the child's appearance in a similar way to a doctor or nurse.[11] Chest 'tightness' is described by some patients with asthma (where it appears to describe dyspnoea) and with cystic fibrosis (where it seems to be related to difficulty in expectorating sputum).

POOR FEEDING

One of the first signs of dyspnoea in young infants is poor feeding. The baby may fail to finish a bottle feed or come off the breast after a short time. This may indicate respiratory or cardiac disease and may lead to significant dehydration and weight loss in a short space of time. In some cases the child may be fed nasogastrically while a full assessment is carried out, but the nasogastric tube will partially obstruct the nasal airway and may exacerbate the problem necessitating a short period of intravenous fluids.

A HISTORY OF 'RECURRENT INFECTIONS'

This history is commonly given when the child has simply had their normal quota of viral upper respiratory infections over a short space of time. However some episodes which are described by the parent (and indeed the health professional) as 'infections' may in fact be episodes of viral associated cough and wheeze. It is difficult to differentiate the two retrospectively, but ask about response to any treatment prescribed at the time such as antibiotics, bronchodilators or steroids. The 'SPUR' acronym (Severe/Persistent/Unusual/Recurrent) is a useful mnemonic for identifying those children who need investigations for host-defence problems (Table 2.3). (See also Chapter 12.)

Table 2.3: The 'SPUR' acronym for investigation of children with recurrent infection

- **Severe**
  Further investigations are indicated if a severe infection is caused by an organism of low pathogenicity e.g. chronic enterovirus encephalitis may be found in X-linked hypogammaglobulinaemia.

- **Persistent**
  Chronic discharging sinuses may be found in boys with chronic granulomatous disease, or children with ciliary dyskinesia.

- **Unusual**
  Where an infant presents with a *Pneumocystis carinii* pneumonia investigations should be performed looking for vertical transmission of human immunodeficiency virus (HIV) or other deficiency of cell mediated immunity.

- **Recurrent**
  More than one episode of serious pneumococcal infection (at any site) should lead to the search for hyposplenism or deficiency of functional pneumococcal antibodies.

SPECIFIC QUESTIONS

Experienced clinicians form working diagnostic hypotheses as soon as the consultation begins. Directed questions should follow. For example, in a child with a history of cough and wheeze, it is important to ask whether there is a personal or family history of atopy, wheezing is less likely to be transient. A history of delayed passage of meconium in the neonatal period or of loose offensive stools is suggestive of cystic fibrosis in a child with chronic cough. Recurrent severe otitis media or sinus disease (sometimes presenting as headache) may support a diagnosis of primary ciliary dyskinesia or an immune deficiency. Such children may also have a history of a 'moist' cough from infancy. A history of severe respiratory infection (e.g. pertussia or measles) in children with a productive cough may provide support for a diagnosis of bronchiectasis. Vomiting or possetting in the young child is usually (but not always) a clue to gastro-oesophageal reflux as the cause of the recurrent moist cough. It may also be seen in children with a vascular ring. Ask specifically about a history of choking or a child having a small toy in their mouth, where foreign body aspiration is a possibility. However a positive history may be obtained in only a minority of cases.[25]

CONGENITAL SYNDROMES

A number of congenital syndromes are associated with respiratory disease and their presence should alert the clinician to ask about specific respiratory problems. Children with Down syndrome often have upper airways obstruction as a result of their large tongue, crowded pharynx, floppiness and nasal infections, and a high proportion develop obstructive sleep apnoea syndrome. In children with severe cerebral palsy there may be gastro-oesophageal reflux and dysphagia with recurrent aspiration and so it is important to ask about respiratory infections. The Di George syndrome (which arises from an embryological defect of the 3rd and 4th pharyngeal pouches) comprises T-cell deficiency, hypoparathyroidism and cardiac defects. A chromosomal deletion on the long arm of chromosome 22 (the so called 'CATCH 22' syndrome) may be associated with the condition (Case study 2.3). These children are prone to recurrent respiratory infections, as are those with immunoglobin deficiencies and cystic fibrosis (CF).

RESEARCH ISSUES

Research into good history taking is difficult to do well. Qualitative research has given us an insight into parent's beliefs and expectations.[2] However basic tools to enhance history taking, such as questionnaires and symptom diaries are often drawn up on an *ad hoc* basis. A number of important points must be established with a symptom questionnaire which also apply to individual questions which may be asked during conventional history taking.

- **Validity:** This means demonstrating that the questionnaire measures what is intended. This can involve an assessment of 'face' validity (i.e. the questions seem intuitively sensible) and content validity (in comparison with a 'gold standard'). The latter requirement has proved very hard to fulfil for respiratory symptom questionnaires, particularly in young children where the use of lung function tests may not be practical. One approach has been to compare the questionnaire score with the opinion of 'expert' clinicians. Once a questionnaire has been shown to be valid in one population the process should be repeated in another group of children to establish its generalizability.
- **Repeatability:** This has been evaluated in a number of questionnaires by repeating the questionnaire in a subgroup after a short interval.[15,23] If the interval is too long then

---

Case study 2.3: A wheezing infant

George, a 6-month-old baby was admitted with his first wheezing illness. His weight had fallen from the 10th to below the 3rd centile. There was no family history of chest problems. Prior to this episode, he had received no medication. Examination revealed tachypnoea, intercostal recession and diffuse wheeze. There was fixed splitting of the 2nd heart sound. During an admission lasting several weeks the following pathogens were isolated from respiratory secretions: respiratory syncytial virus (RSV) (on two occasions, 3 weeks apart); influenza A; and echovirus B19.

Fixed splitting of the 2nd heart sound suggested an atrial septal defect. This was confirmed by echocardiogram. Three different respiratory viral infections in a few weeks and the persistent excretion of RSV are suggestive of immune deficiency (the 'SPUR' acronym, Table 2.3). Viral infection suggests a defect in cellular immunity and indeed T cell numbers were reduced. Increased susceptibility to respiratory viral infection is also seen in secretory IgA deficiency however immunoglobulins were normal in this case. The unifying diagnosis was Di George syndrome. This child also had low parathyroid hormone level and a low normal serum calcium. Fluorescent *in situ* hybridization (FISH) showed a deletion on the long arm of chromosome 22 ('Catch 22 syndrome'). This child has a mild case of Di George syndrome and the prognosis is good.

variation may be due to a genuine change in symptom severity over time.

- **Clinical relevance:** The questionnaire score should change in response to improvement in symptoms with sufficient sensitivity to allow it to be used to evaluate an intervention.
- **Sensitivity and specificity:** Even less data are available on the sensitivity and specificity of specific items in the history for determining the presence of a specific illness. In African children under 2 months, with pneumonia, a history obtained from the mother that the child has appeared blue was 100% specific but only 36% sensitive for the presence of hypoxaemia. On the other hand, mother's history of difficult respiration in her child had a specificity of only 10% but was 92% sensitive for hypoxaemia.[22] There are no similar studies for the developed world.

CHILDREN VS PARENTS AS HISTORIANS

Most questions used to assess children are directed at their parents. Pictorial versions of linear analogue scores may be suitable for use in children but care must be taken to validate these properly. Children may choose an illustration (e.g. a 'smiley face') not because it describes the way they feel but simply because they prefer one illustration to another (e.g. a sad face). Children's responses to questionnaires may differ to their parents' responses on their behalf.[1] It will therefore be an important research challenge to find the best way of allowing older children to speak for themselves about their respiratory symptoms.

REFERENCES

1. Wong TW, Yu TS, Liu JL, Wong SL. Agreement on responses to respiratory illness questionnaire. *Arch Dis Child* 1998; **78**: 379–80.

2. Kai J. What worries parents when their preschool children are acutely ill, and why: a qualitative study. *BMJ* 1996; **313**: 983–6.

3. Hunter MF, Heaf DP. Allowances for care for children with cystic fibrosis. *Arch Dis Child* 1993; **68**: 144–6.

4. Munyard P, Bush A. How much coughing is normal? *Arch Dis Child* 1996; **74**: 531–4

5. Fuller P, Picciotto A, Davies M, McKenzie SA. Cough and sleep in inner city children. *Eur Respir J* 1998; **12**: 426–31.

6. Higgenbottom T. Cough induced by changes of ionic composition of airway surface liquid. *Bull Eur Physiopathol Respir* 1984; **20**: 553–62.

7. Cloutier MM, Loughlin GM. Chronic cough in children: A manifestation of airway hyperreactivity. *Pediatrics* 1981; **67**: 6–12.

8. Ninan TK, Macdonald L, Russell G. Persistant nocturnal cough in childhood: a population based study. *Arch Dis Child* 1995; **73**: 403–7.

9. Chang AB, Phelan PD, Carlin JB, Sawyer SM, Robertson CF. A randomised, placebo controlled trial of inhaled salbutamol and beclomethasone for recurrent cough. *Arch Dis Child* 1998; **79**: 6–11.

10. Sheppard D, Rizk NW, Boushey HA, Bethel RA. Mechanism of cough and bronchoconstriction induced by distilled water aerosol. *Am Rev Respir Dis* 1983; **127**: 691–4.

11. Cane RS, Ranganathan SC, McKenzie SA. Parents understanding of 'wheeze'. *Arch Dis Child* 2000; **82**: 327–32.

12. Elphick HE, Ritson S, Rodgers H, Everard ML. When a "wheeze" is not a wheeze: acoustic analysis of breath sounds in infants. *Eur Respir J* 2000; **16**: 593–7.

13. Martinez FD, Wright AL, Taussig LM, Holdberg CJ, Halonen M, Morgan WJ. Asthma and wheezing in the first 6 years of life. *N Engl J Med* 1995; **332**: 133–8.

14. Kaur B, Anderson HR, Austin J, *et al.* Prevalence of asthma symptoms, diagnosis and treatment in 12–14 year old children across Great Britain (international study of asthma and allergies in childhood, ISAAC UK). *BMJ* 1998; **316**: 118–24.

15. Luyt DK, Burton PR, Simpson H. Epidemiological study of wheeze, doctor diagnosed asthma and cough in preschool children in Leicestershire. *BMJ* 1993; **306**: 1368–90.

16. Silverman M, Wilson N. Asthma – time for a change of name? *Arch Dis Child* 1997; **77**: 62–4.

17. Gadomski AM, Lichenstein R, Horton L, King J, Keane V, Permutt T. Efficacy of albuterol in the management of bronchiolitis. *Pediatrics* 1994; **93**: 907–12.

18. Martin ME, Grunstein MM, Larsen GL. The relationship of gastroesophageal reflux to nocturnal

wheezing in children with asthma. *Ann Allergy* 1982; **49**: 318–22.

19. Mansfield LE, Stein MR. Gastroesophageal reflux and asthma: a possible reflex mechanism. *Ann Allergy* 1978; **41**: 224–6

20. Finder JD. Primary bronchomalacia in infants and children. *J Pediatr* 1997; **130**: 59–66.

21. National Institutes of Health. Infantile apnea and home monitoring. *NIH consensus development conference consensus statement* 1986; **6**: 1–10.

22. Onyango FE, Steinhoff MC, Wafula EM, Wariua S, Musia J, Kitonyi J. Hypoxaemia in young Kenyan children with acute lower respiratory infection. *BMJ* 1993; **306**: 612–15.

23. Clifford RD, Radford M, Howell JB, Holgate ST. Prevalence of respiratory symptoms among 7 and 11 year old schoolchildren and association with asthma. *Arch Dis Child* 1989; **64**: 1118–25.

24. Kerem E, Canny G, Tibshirani R, *et al.* Clinical-physiologic correlations in acute asthma of childhood. *Pediatrics* 1991; **87**: 481–6.

25. Abdulmajid OA, Ebeid AM, Motaweh MM, Kleibo IS. Aspirated foreign bodies in the tracheobronchial tree: report of 250 cases. *Thorax* 1976; **31**: 635–40.

26. Wilson AC, Forsyth JS, Greene SA, Irvine L, Hau C, Howie PW. Relation of infant diet to childhood health: seven year follow up of cohort of children in Dundee infant feeding study. *BMJ* 1998; **316**: 21–5.

27. David TJ. Infant feeding causes all cases of asthma, eczema and hay fever. Or does it? *Arch Dis Child* 1998; **79**: 97–8.

28. Dahl RE. The impact of inadequate sleep on children's daytime cognitive function. *Semin Pediatr Neurol* 1996; **3**: 44–50.

29. Noble V, Murray M, Webb MS, Alexander J, Swarbrick AS, Milner AD. Respiratory status and allergy nine to 10 years after acute bronchiolitis. *Arch Dis Child* 1997; **76**: 315–19.

30. Cook DG, Strachan DP. Health effects of passive smoking – 10: Summary of effects of parental smoking on the respiratory health of children and implications for research. *Thorax* 1999; **54**: 357–66.

31. Paton J. 'Can I have a letter for the housing, doctor?'– Commentary. *Arch Dis Child* 1998; **78**: 506–7.

FURTHER READING

1. Dinwiddie R. *Diagnosis and management of paediatric respiratory disease.* London: Churchill Livingstone, 1997.

2. West JB. *Respiratory physiology.* Baltimore: Williams & Wilkins, 1995.

CHAPTER THREE

PHYSICAL EXAMINATION: SIGNS

A . Smyth

- Background
- Specific signs and their significance

- Clinical research issues
- References

BACKGROUND

THE GENERAL APPROACH TO EXAMINATION

The co-operation of both the parent and child are essential to a successful physical examination. Introduce yourself and establish who the accompanying adult is – he or she may not be a parent. Get down to the child's level, do not tower above them. Observation is vital. For example, you may lose the co-operation of a 2-year-old as soon as you touch them, so gather as much information as you can just by watching and taking a history. Talk to the child but do not give instructions – asking a child to 'breathe normally' usually has the opposite effect!

WHY EXAMINE THE CHILD?

When you examine a child, you are trying to establish the severity of the problem and also to test a hypothesis which will allow you to reach a diagnosis (see Chapter 2, Taking a History: Symptoms). These roles go in tandem, even when a child requires immediate resuscitation. Hypothesis testing, with the aim of rapid diagnosis, takes place at the 'secondary survey' stage, if not before. Whether a child is being assessed in an emergency department or an outpatient clinic, the investigations needed to test the hypothesis should be planned during the examination. Examination may need to be repeated many times particularly during an evolving acute illness, where signs may initially be absent or subtle. These fundamental issues, relating to every day clinical practice, are often poorly researched. The sensitivity and specificity of some of the physical signs for detecting respiratory illness are discussed later.

With improvements in the range and quality of imaging techniques, properly conducted physical examination is becoming a neglected skill. However imaging techniques may be costly, may involve radiation exposure and are not available in many parts of the developing world. Furthermore, physical examination may give more information about the diagnosis, complications and impact of a child's condition than imaging. In pneumonia, physical signs are a better predictor of the severity of the illness than radiological findings.[1]

GENERAL PHYSICAL SIGNS WITH IMPORTANCE TO THE RESPIRATORY SYSTEM

Ensure the child's weight and height are recorded (at each assessment if appropriate) and plotted on a suitable centile chart (state clearly whether allowance for prematurity has been made). Make a note of the birth weight and any other measurements available from the child's personal child health record. Failure to thrive may suggest chest disease associated with malabsorption (e.g. cystic fibrosis) increased energy requirements (e.g. bronchopulmonary dysplasia) or chronic infection (tuberculosis). Poor linear growth in asthma, for example, may suggest severe chest disease or the effects of corticosteroids. A growth velocity chart may provide early warning of declining growth velocity, but requires more than one measurement and is highly influenced by natural short-term variations in growth rate and by the accuracy with which length is measured. Late puberty in atopic children may cause 'physiological' deviation from the average, with later catch-up.

When children are acutely unwell, their state of hydration should be evaluated. Dehydration may be due to poor fluid intake, caused by dyspnoea, and it may in turn worsen airway disease such as acute asthma. Mothers rarely miss the presence of fever, when their children feel hot to touch.[2] Fever in the presence of lower respiratory signs does not always imply a bacterial chest infection. Upper respiratory tract viral infections are common triggers for acute asthma,[3] leading to both fever and wheezing, without a significant 'chest infection'. Tachypnoea must be interpreted with caution in the presence of fever. A 1°C increase in the child's temperature can produce an increase in respiratory rate of around 10 breaths per minute.[4]

SPECIFIC SIGNS AND THEIR SIGNIFICANCE

LOOKING AND LISTENING

Cyanosis

Cyanosis is a blue discolouration of the skin and mucous membranes, due to the presence of reduced haemoglobin in the capillary bed. Central cyanosis (observed on the lips or tongue) is a more reliable physical sign than peripheral cyanosis as the latter can be induced by peripheral vasoconstriction without hypoxaemia. Cyanosis is an important physical sign which is easy to miss in dark skinned children or in a poorly lit environment. Lundsgaard and Van Slyke, in a monograph written in 1923,[5] first proposed that at least 5 g/dL of reduced haemoglobin must be present in the capillary bed for cyanosis to be readily detectable. Subsequent authors, who have suggested this figure is too high, may in fact have assumed that the 5 g/dL figure referred to arterial reduced haemoglobin which is always less than that in the capillaries.[6] In an anaemic patient, cyanosis only becomes detectable with more severe hypoxaemia (Table 3.1). In young infants, concentrations of fetal haemoglobin are higher than in older children, and fetal haemoglobin binds oxygen more avidly. However, as haemoglobin concentration is also higher in the neonatal period, cyanosis is no more difficult to detect in young infants. Unfortunately the ability, even of trained observers, to detect cyanosis is poor. In a study performed on healthy volunteers breathing mixtures with a reduced oxygen concentration (FiO_2),[7] the majority of observers were unable to detect the presence of definite cyanosis until the arterial oxygen

Table 3.1: Calculated values of arterial oxygen saturation (SaO_2) and partial pressure of oxygen (PaO_2) needed to detect cyanosis at different haemoglobin concentrations[6]

Haemoglobin concentration (g/dL)	Minimum SaO_2 needed to detect cyanosis (%)	Minimum PaO_2 needed to detect cyanosis (kPa)
18	83	6.4
15	78	5.9
12	73	5.2
9	64	4.7

saturation (Sa_{O_2}) had fallen to approximately 80%. There was marked variation in the ability of the same observer to detect cyanosis in different subjects or even the same subject on different occasions. In sick children with pneumonia, cyanosis, whether observed by the parent or the doctor, is a highly specific but insensitive indicator of hypoxaemia.[1]

Respiratory distress

Children with any one of a number of acute respiratory disorders may show signs of respiratory distress (Figure 3.1). The primary muscles of inspiration are the external intercostal muscles and the diaphragm. For the 2nd to 7th ribs, contraction of the intercostal muscles during inspiration increases the antero-posterior diameter of the chest whilst in the case of the lower ribs the intercostal muscles increase the transverse diameter of the chest (the 'bucket handle' effect). The dome-shaped diaphragm attaches to the lower six ribs and costal cartilages. During inspiration, the diaphragm flattens and so increases the vertical dimension of the thoracic cavity. When a child is breathing quietly, expiration is a passive process, due to the elastic recoil of the lungs. Signs of respiratory distress arise in the presence of respiratory disease through the use of accessory muscles of respiration or because of the greater negative intra-thoracic pressure generated as a result of increased respiratory effort or because active expiratory effort is involved.

Accessory muscles include the dilators of the anterior nares which increase the calibre of the nasal airway causing nasal flaring (50% of airway resistance is due to the nose). In children with asthma the abdominal muscles contract to produce forced expiration against the resistance caused by bronchospasm. Increased inspiratory effort to overcome mechanical problems leads to greater negative intra-thoracic pressure and to recession of the soft tissues of the chest wall: the supra-clavicular space, the supra-sternal notch, and the intercostal spaces. Chest indrawing ('subcostal recession') arises because of violent diaphragmatic contraction pulling on the attachments to the lower six ribs and costal cartilage and is a sign of more severe respiratory distress, enhanced in the presence of hyperinflation. Tracheal tug also arises from vigorous contraction of the diaphragm, pulling on the mediastinum and trachea against the counter pressure of the jaw and pharynx.

Where the upper airway is partially or completely occluded, the diaphragm may contract pushing the abdominal wall outwards, but the chest wall is unable to move outwards causing paradoxical (see-saw) breathing. Paradoxical breathing is also seen in neuromuscular disorders in which the diaphragm is relatively spared in comparison with the intercostal muscles (e.g. severe spinal muscular atrophy) and in diaphragmatic weakness where the reverse is the case (e.g. some of the myopathies). In the latter situation, breathlessness is especially severe in the supine posture.

Stridor

Not all signs of respiratory distress are visual. Stridor is a coarse sound indicative of upper airway narrowing (Table 3.2). Unlike wheeze, it does not have a 'whistling' quality and is more often heard in inspiration. Stridor is usually audible without a stethoscope. Children with stridor may present in the outpatient department with classic stridor or in the emergency department with acute stridor and respiratory distress. The presence of stridor indicates some degree of upper airway obstruction but the severity of stridor does not indicate the severity of the obstruction. Expiratory stridor suggests that the cause of the airway obstruction is below the thoracic inlet. Collapse of the

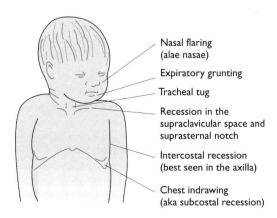

Nasal flaring (alae nasae)

Expiratory grunting

Tracheal tug

Recession in the supraclavicular space and suprasternal notch

Intercostal recession (best seen in the axilla)

Chest indrawing (aka subcostal recession)

Figure 3.1: Signs of respiratory distress in the young child.

Table 3.2: Causes of stridor

Congenital stridor	Acute stridor
Laryngomalacia	Croup
Tracheobronchomalacia	– infective (laryngotracheobronchitis)
Intraluminal obstruction	– spasmodic (atopic)
e.g. subglottic haemangioma, laryngeal	Foreign body in the larynx/upper airway
polyps	
Extrinsic compression e.g. vascular ring	Epiglottitis
Congenital vocal cord palsy	Inhalational injury
	Anaphylaxis
	Tetany

Subglottic stenosis may be congenital or acquired (due to prolonged or traumatic intubation). Severe upper airway obstruction may be precipitated in these patients by an otherwise mild episode of croup.

intra-thoracic airway is more likely in expiration when the airway is not held open by negative intra-thoracic pressure.

Other noisy breathing

Grunting is an important physical sign in infants. The noise is glottic in origin and represents expiratory braking by the infant to maintain functional residual capacity in the face of decreased compliance (e.g. consolidation).[8] Grunting is not always indicative of respiratory disease and it may be seen in infants who are septicaemic, in cardiac failure, who are cold or in pain.[9] Stertorous (or 'snuffly') breathing due to nasal obstruction has been considered in Chapter 2. A hoarse voice (dysphonia) may occur acutely due to laryngitis, or chronically as a result of drug therapy such as inhaled steroids in asthma and dornase alfa in cystic fibrosis or may indicate intrinsic laryngeal dysfunction (e.g. laryngeal palsy). Inability to produce an explosive, sharp cough is a sign of laryngeal dysfunction.

Respiratory rate

The measurement of respiratory rate is one of the most valuable observations in the examination of the respiratory system but it is often neglected. Respirations should be counted over one minute in infants below 2 months old who may show periodic breathing. This pattern of breathing is usually a normal variant at this age and comprises short periods (<10 seconds) of apnoea followed by longer periods (15 seconds) of rapid breathing.

This pattern may be exaggerated in the sick infant. Respirations may be counted over 30 seconds in older infants and children where breathing is more regular. Respiratory rate should be measured by unobtrusive observation, rather than using a stethoscope which will result in a faster respiratory rate.[10] It may be easier to watch abdominal movement in young infants. Obviously the child should not be crying.

The World Health Organization (WHO) encourages the use of respiratory rate as an important physical sign in the diagnosis of pneumonia in children (Table 3.3).[11] Tachypnoea has been shown to be a good indicator of the presence of pneumonia in developing countries (where there is a high prevalence of bacterial pneumonia), particularly in young children.[12] In infants aged 2–6 months, the WHO threshold of >50 breaths per minute for tachypnoea had a sensitivity of 91% and a specificity of 94% for predicting radiological pneumonia. Where sophisticated monitoring, such as pulse oximetry, is not available, tachypnoea is a useful clinical indicator of hypoxaemia.

Table 3.3: World Health Organization (WHO) definitions of 'fast breathing' in a child with suspected pneumonia[11]

Age range	Definition of 'fast breathing' (breaths/minute)
Up to 2 months:	>60
2–12 months:	>50
12 months–5 years:	>40

A respiratory rate of >70 had a sensitivity of 51% and a specificity of 83% for predicting an oxygen saturation of <90% in Kenyan infants.[1] However, tachypnoea is also seen in children with asthma, systemic sepsis, or simply pyrexia. In the developed world (where bacterial pneumonia is less prevalent) tachypnoea should be considered in combination with other physical signs in the diagnosis of pneumonia.

Chest expansion and chest deformity

As well as looking for acute signs of respiratory distress, thorough inspection should include an assessment of chest expansion and chest deformity (Table 3.4). First stand in front of the child to assess any asymmetry in chest movement, during quiet breathing. Then move to one side to deter-mine whether the antero-posterior chest diameter is increased. (This occurs when there is chronic airways obstruction, such as in asthma or cystic fibrosis.) Finally inspect from behind to see whether scoliosis is present. The child with lobar collapse or an effusion may have reduced expansion on the affected side which may lead to scoliosis. Conversely a scoliosis arising from a primary musculo-skeletal abnormality may lead to a restrictive pattern of ventilatory abnormality or in extreme cases to type II respiratory failure.

Harrison's sulci are concavities seen bilaterally over the lower ribs at the costochondral junction. They were first described in children with rickets, due to the action of the diaphragm leading to deformity of the abnormally soft ribs but are now more commonly seen in children with chronic upper or lower airway obstruction such as

Table 3.4: Conditions associated with chest wall deformity

Predisposing condition	Chest wall abnormality
Isolated skeletal anomaly	■ Pectus carinatum / pectus excavatum
Rickets	■ Pectus carinatum ■ Harrison's sulci
Severe airway obstruction	■ Hyperinflation
Chronic upper airways obstruction e.g. adenotonsillar hypertrophy	■ Harrison's sulci
Disorders of connective tissue e.g. Marfan's syndrome (autosomal dominant)	■ Pectus carinatum / pectus excavatum
Skeletal dysplasias e.g. achondroplasia (autosomal dominant)	■ Kyphosis
Jeune's syndrome (autosomal recessive)	■ Small thoracic cavity (Figure 3.2)
Mucopolysaccharidoses e.g. Hurler's syndrome (autosomal recessive)	■ Kyphosis
Neurocutaneous syndromes e.g. neurofibromatosis (autosomal dominant)	■ Scoliosis
Neuromuscular disorders e.g. Duchenne muscular dystrophy (X-linked)	■ Scoliosis / kyphosis
Severe cerebral palsy e.g. spastic quadriplegia	■ Scoliosis / kyphosis

adenotonsillar hypertrophy or asthma. In pectus carinatum ('pigeon chest') the sternum is abnormally prominent and in pectus excavatum ('funnel chest') the sternum is 'sunken' (meeting the vertebral column in extreme cases). An abnormally small chest may be seen in conditions such as Jeune's syndrome ('asphyxiating thoracic dystrophy') which may ultimately lead to type II respiratory failure (Figure 3.2). Before completing the inspection of the chest, make a note of the presence of any surgical scars. Surgeons try to conceal scars to make them more cosmetically acceptable so pay particular attention to concealed areas such as the axilla.

Clubbing

Finger clubbing is thought to occur due to the action of platelet derived growth factor in the capillaries of the nail bed.[13] Megakaryocytes are released in small amounts from the bone marrow and when intrapulmonary shunting occurs (such as in chronic suppurative lung disease) they bypass the pulmonary capillaries before 'shattering' into platelets and enter the systemic circulation. They pass to the finger tips in axial vascular streams and impact in the capilliaries releasing platelet derived growth factor. This causes increased capillary

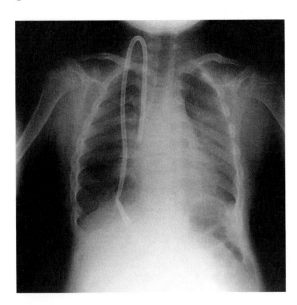

Figure 3.2: Chest radiograph of a child with Jeune's syndrome showing the small thoracic volume. (Jeune's syndrome is also associated with renal dysplasia. Note the central venous catheter for haemodialysis.)

permeability and connective tissue hypertrophy, leading to finger clubbing. Platelets may accumulate in the capillaries of the nail bed in a similar way in conditions characterized by thrombocytosis (e.g. inflammatory bowel disease) or platelet clumping (e.g. infective endocarditis). There are many causes of clubbing (Table 3.5).

To identify finger clubbing look at the fingers in profile and establish whether the angle between the nail and the nail bed has been lost (Figure 3.3). Later the ends of the fingers become swollen and the curvature of the nail increases. Try to avoid using terms like 'early clubbing'; clubbing is either absent or present, and (if present) moderate or severe.

PALPATION

Having gained as much clinical information as possible by observation, you may now touch the child. Palpate the trachea to evaluate tracheal displacement, indicating mediastinal shift. The mediastinum may be 'pulled' to the side affected by lobar collapse or 'pushed' away from the side affected by an effusion or by unilateral hyperinflation due to air trapping. Whilst palpating the neck, look for cervical lymph node enlargement. Great enlargement of the deep cervical nodes may accompany glandular fever and bacterial tonsillitis. Cervical lymph node enlargement may be a manifestation of extrapulmonary tuberculosis,

Table 3.5: Causes of finger clubbing

Pulmonary causes:
Suppurative lung disease, e.g. cystic fibrosis, bronchiectasis
Interstitial lung disease, e.g. fibrosing alveolitis
(In adults carcinoma of the bronchus is a common cause)

Cardiac causes:
Cyanotic congenital heart disease, e.g. uncorrected transposition of the great vessels
Eisenmenger's syndrome
Infective endocarditis

Other causes:
Inflammatory bowel disease
Benign congenital clubbing

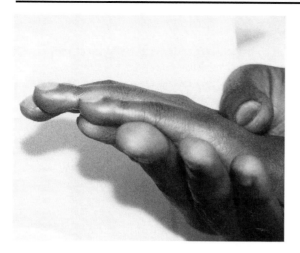

Figure 3.3: Examination of the fingers to detect clubbing.

though this is rare in the developed world. Palpation of the apex beat may confirm mediastinal displacement or, where the apex is difficult to palpate, may suggest hyperinflation of the chest. Rarely the apex may be palpated on the right side of the chest, e.g. in dextrocardia accompanying Kartagener's syndrome.

Evaluate the pulse volume. In patients with hypercapnia or patent ductus arteriosus the pulse volume is increased although inter-observer variability in detecting an increased pulse volume is high.[14] Pulsus paradoxus is the observation that the peripheral pulse volume diminishes during inspiration. This is caused by pooling of blood in the pulmonary capillaries during inspiration, reducing venous return to the left side of the heart. Pulsus paradoxus is seen in conditions where a greater negative intra-thoracic pressure is generated as a result of increased respiratory effort, most commonly in acute asthma. The difference in pulse pressure between inspiration and expiration may be measured, although it is unhelpful in determining the severity of asthma as significant paradoxus is absent in one third of patients with severe airways obstruction.[15]

PERCUSSION

Percussion may be omitted in the very young infant with a small chest but is a useful procedure in older infants and children. Your hands will

be warmer and less intimidating than your stethoscope. It is unnecessary to percuss each intercostal space or to strike the clavicles vigorously in children. Where the percussion note is dull, try to quantify this: is the note stony dull (suggestive of an effusion, Case study 3.1) or is it simply diminished (suggestive of underlying consolidation)? Where there is dullness to percussion, evaluate this further in the older, co-operative child by asking them to say 'ninety nine' to elicit transmitted vocal fremitus. ('Fremitus' simply means vibration. Vibration due to speech is readily transmitted by consolidated lung but poorly transmitted by effusion fluid.) Do not attempt to elicit vocal fremitus if you have not demonstrated dullness to percussion or auscultatory signs.

Auscultation

After gaining as much information as possible by observation and after gaining the child's confidence, use your stethoscope. Auscultate anteriorly, in the axillae and at the back. In a child who is relatively immobile (e.g. in intensive care) it may be more practical to perform steps prior to auscultation on the front of the chest before asking the child to roll on to their side or to sit up. First establish whether breath sounds are normal in quality (inspiration louder than expiration) and if there is a pause between the two. In bronchial breathing inspiration and expiration are equal in volume and the pause is absent. In addition the breath sounds have a harsh, high pitched, grating quality. (Listen to the chest of a healthy individual anteriorly, over the upper sternum to hear an approximation to bronchial breathing.) Breath sounds may also be diminished in volume. This effect can be focal, for instance as an early sign in pneumonia or due to poor air entry associated with mucus plugging or a foreign body (see below), or generalized throughout the lung fields e.g. the 'silent chest' in severe asthma. Now listen for added sounds such as crackles and wheezes. (These were referred to as crepitations and ronchi respectively.)

Crackles

These are generated by the explosive opening of airways in parts of the lung which are deflated to

Case study 3.1: A toddler with cough and fever

Louise, a 2-year-old girl, was admitted to hospital with a 5-day history of fever and cough. She had received antibiotics prior to admission for what was assumed to be a chest infection. *Inspection* revealed she was not cyanosed, but was tachypnoeic with a respiratory rate of 60 breaths per minute. Intercostal recession was seen on the right but not on the left side of the chest. By *palpation* the trachea was shifted to the right. The percussion note was dull at the left base and axilla. On auscultation, transmitted vocal fremitus was diminished and breath sounds were reduced, again over the left base and axilla.

A chest radiograph (Figure 3.4A) showed a left-sided effusion. Ultrasound confirmed the presence of a loculated effusion. A pleural tap was performed and purulent fluid obtained, which was sent for Gram staining and culture (which was negative). A small 'pigtail' catheter was inserted under sedation and local anaesthetic and the fibrinolytic agent urokinase was infused. Intravenous antibiotics were given (for a total of one week). After 4 days of this treatment significant resolution of the effusion had occurred (Figure 3.4B).

This case illustrates the importance of a structured examination in formulating a diagnostic 'hypothesis' which can then be tested by appropriately focused investigations (chest radiograph, ultrasound and pleural tap). This allowed the least invasive method to be chosen for drainage, with rapid resolution of this little girl's empyema.

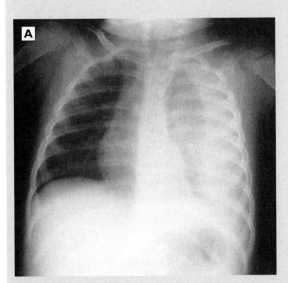 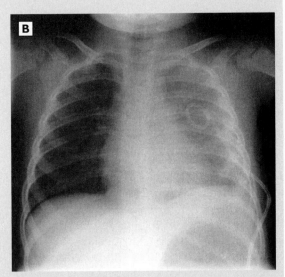

Figure 3.4: Chest radiograph of the child in Case study 3.1: (A) before and (B) after intercostal tube drainage with a pigtail catheter.

residual volume.[16] There is a sudden equalizing of pressure up stream and down stream of a closed section of airway during inspiration. Crackles commonly occur at the lung bases and they change with posture. They are indicative of reduced pulmonary compliance due to inflammatory fluid (as in pneumonia); oedema (fine crackles in left ventricular failure) or fibrosis (as in fibrosing alveolitis). Focal crackles exaggerated by voluntary coughing are suggestive of bronchiectasis.

Wheeze

Wheeze is thought to be produced when air flows at high velocity through an airway narrowed to the point of closure.[16] Bronchospasm does not produce wheezing directly, because the combined cross sectional area of the small airways is large, meaning that high velocity flow does not take place. Instead, children with bronchospasm generate a positive intra-thoracic pressure, during forced expiration, which causes dynamic compression of large airways (probably lobar bronchi).[17] Each airway generates its own musical note and so the wheezing is 'polyphonic.' This is seen in children with acute asthma. When airway narrowing is so severe as to prevent high velocity airflow, this is described as 'the paradoxical absence of wheezing' or 'the silent chest'.[17] A child with this physical sign is in incipient respiratory failure. Monophonic wheeze suggests narrowing of a single airway and may be seen with an inhaled foreign body or focal stricture. In this case turbulent, high velocity flow occurs during inspiration and expiration and so the wheezing is present during both phases of the respiratory cycle. Wheezing may also be localized to the affected side and accompanied by signs of mediastinal shift (see Case study 3.2). It is important to distinguish wheeze from expiratory stridor such as that found in children with tracheobronchomalacia. In some patients with apparent 'wheeze,' a noise is produced during both inspiration and expiration by paradoxical adduction of the vocal cords. This is termed the vocal cord dysfunction syndrome or glottic wheeze and patients may also show apparently low peak flow readings. However they are usually unable to perform spirometric tests reproducibly.[18]

EXAMINATION OF OTHER SYSTEMS RELEVANT TO RESPIRATORY DISEASE

Examination of the respiratory system should be accompanied by a thorough cardiovascular examination in most cases. In children with cardiac disease, the history may be identical to that obtained in a primary respiratory problem. Severe respiratory or systemic infection may be accompanied by signs of cardiac failure. Abdominal examination should also be performed (Case study 3.3). The upper border of the liver can usually be percussed to the level of the 6th rib in the midclavicular line.

Case study 3.2: Sudden onset of cough and unilateral wheeze

Tara, an 18-month-old girl was seen in the accident and emergency department with a history of coughing and wheezing for 24 hours. The onset was sudden and there had been no previous episodes. On examination she was afebrile, the respiratory rate was 40 breaths per minute and there was some intercostal recession, but no chest indrawing. She was not cyanosed and her oxygen saturation was 96%. The trachea appeared deviated to the right (tracheal palpation is difficult in young children: if not obvious do not persist). There was unilateral wheezing, audible only on the left. Breath sounds on the right were normal. The unilateral wheezing was still present after administration of a bronchodilator. A chest radiograph (Figure 3.5) revealed hyperinflation of the left lung with mediastinal shift to the right. A peanut was removed from the left main bronchus, under general anaesthetic, using a rigid bronchoscope.

In this case it is important to put together the findings on palpation (tracheal displacement) with the auscultatory findings (unilateral wheeze). There is no history of choking to suggest a foreign body, but this history is not always present.[19] Although wheezing may be unilateral in acute asthma, this diagnosis was less likely as the wheezing remained unilateral after a bronchodilator was administered.

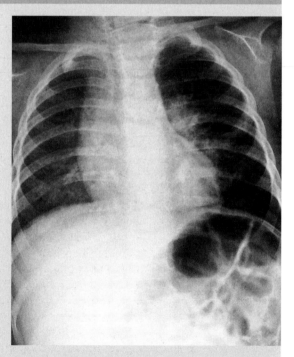

Figure 3.5: Chest radiograph of the child in Case study 3.2, showing overinflation of the left lung due to an inhaled foreign body.

If it is lower than this the liver may be pushed down, due to hyperinflation of the chest, or enlarged.

Respiratory examination is not complete without inspection of the upper airway. Examine the nose for the presence of nasal polyps. These are very uncommon in children under 10 and their finding should look to a sweat test to exclude cystic fibrosis (CF). Primary ciliary dyskinesia is another rare cause. Look at the throat to establish whether the tonsils are enlarged. Ensure that the palate is normal and assess any abnormalities of the jaw such as micrognathia.

Examine the skin looking for signs of eczema, and specific eruptions such as erythema multiforme (found in mycoplasma infection or as an idiosyncratic reaction to medication such as antibiotics) or erythema nodosum (seen in tuberculosis and streptococcal infection). Neurological examination may also be helpful, particularly assessment of conscious level in children with incipient respiratory failure.

Sometimes it is helpful to go back and observe the child during other activities such as feeding or sleeping. In the young infant, look for choking or nasal regurgitation during feeding (which may suggest aspiration of milk feeds during swallowing). Direct observation of the sleeping child can be of great value in assessing possible diagnoses such as the obstructive sleep apnoea syndrome. The recording of overnight video studies, in the child's home, allows clinical examination to be performed outside the artificial surroundings of the hospital ward or consulting room.[20]

CLINICAL RESEARCH ISSUES

Unfortunately there are few well designed research studies, with adequate patient numbers, examining the value of specific physical signs in diagnosing respiratory disease in children. Paediatricians in every specialty perform physical examinations every day of their working lives. It is wasteful to spend time eliciting a useless physical sign just as it is wasteful to spend money on a useless drug and yet drug trials far outnumber careful studies of physical signs in the literature.

REPEATABILITY

Clearly it is important that the same clinical observation, made by more than one observer, should give the same value. This allows criteria for

---

Case Study 3.3

A 2 year-old boy called Jerry was seen at the request of the paediatric surgeons. He was due to be admitted electively for repair of a rectal prolapse. The surgeons were concerned that he might represent an anaesthetic risk. He has a history of episodes of coughing and wheezing since infancy when he had bronchiolitis due to respiratory syncytial virus. He was taking inhaled budesonide and terbutaline (both given using a metered dose aerosol and spacer). On examination he was a thin child (weight on the 0.4 centile and height on the 2nd centile – Figure 3.6). There were bilateral Harrison's sulci but no other abnormal physical signs. The rectal prolapse was not present at the time of the examination.

The diagnosis of cystic fibrosis was confirmed by a sweat test (sweat chloride = 160 mmol/L; sweat sodium = 114 mmol/L; 320 mg of sweat). Genetic testing revealed he was homozygous for the G553X mutation (and hence was missed by the neonatal screening service operating in his region).

It is clearly important to integrate the general examination (proper documentation of height and weight – even if only one measurement is available) with the chest findings (Harrison's sulci) and the findings in other systems (rectal prolapse). Rapid diagnosis in this case required all these factors to be considered.

Once pancreatic enzyme supplements were started, Jerry showed a rapid gain in weight to the above 9th centile (figure 3.6). In addition chest physiotherapy and continuous anti-staphylococcal antibiotic prophylaxis were given.

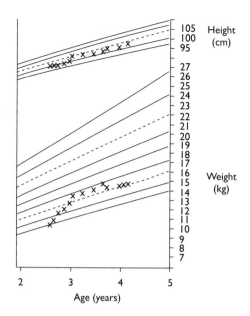

Figure 3.6: Growth chart for the boy described in Case study 3.3, showing weight gain following diagnosis.

PATHOPHYSIOLOGY

Studies of physical signs in acutely ill children may lead to new avenues of investigation into the pathophysiology of the condition. One recent example is a study of prognostic factors in children with malaria performed in Kenya,[22] which showed increased mortality in children with severe respiratory distress. This was defined as abnormally deep breathing with recession and was found to be associated, not with anaemia and heart failure as was previously thought, but with metabolic acidosis. This has important implications for the management of these children as children with severe anaemia and heart failure are managed by slow transfusion, whilst children with acidosis should have rapid fluid resuscitation. Simple bedside observations in these children could identify over 80% of children who had a fatal outcome.

NEW TECHNOLOGY

Some aspects of physical examination may be refined by computer. Computerized breath sounds analysis allows wheeze to be reliably identified by its spectral pattern. It has been found that bronchospasm induced by histamine may be detected more readily by this method than by conventional lung function testing.[23] This technique may also allow physical signs such as wheeze and 'ruttles' (which are readily confused by parents and by paediatricians) to be distinguished.[24]

admission or drug intervention to be applied consistently by a number of clinicians. However, as has been pointed out in the discussion of cyanosis (see above), inter-observer variability may be high. Similar variability has been found in the recording of physical signs such as retractions. Cohen's Kappa varied from 0.05–1.0 in one study of infants with bronchiolitis.[21] Further work is needed, looking at ways of reducing inter-observer variability. Video recordings of physical signs may provide useful reference points.

SENSITIVITY AND SPECIFICITY

Combining a number of observations into an overall score will be considered in Chapter 4, (Acute assessment). The sensitivity and specificity of individual observations such as respiratory rate, cyanosis and crepitations, in determining hypoxaemia, have been studied in the developing world.[1] Less information is available about the performance of these signs in developed countries. Indeed signs such as pulsus paradoxus, which discriminate poorly between those with mild and severe respiratory disease continue to be advocated in many textbooks and protocols.[15]

REFERENCES

1. Onyango FE, Steinhoff MC, Wafula EM, Wariua S, Musia J, Kitonyi J. Hypoxaemia in young Kenyan children with acute lower respiratory infection. *BMJ* 1993; **306**: 612–15.

2. Whybrew K, Murray M, Morley C. Diagnosing fever by touch: observational study. *BMJ* 1998; **317**: 321.

3. Johnston SL, Pattemore PK, Sanderson G, *et al.* Community study of role of viral infections in exacerbations of asthma in 9–11 year old children. *BMJ* 1995; **310**: 1225–9.

4. Gadomski AM, Permutt T, Stanton B. Correcting respiratory rate for the presence of fever. *J Clin Epidemiol* 1994; **47**: 1043–9.

5. Lundsgaard C, Van Slyke DD. Cyanosis. *Medicine* 1923; **2**: 1–76.

6. Martin L, Khalil H. How much reduced hemoglobin is necessary to generate central cyanosis? *Chest* 1990; **97**: 182–5.

7. Comroe JH, Butelho S. The unreliability of cyanosis in the recognition of arterial hypoxaemia. *Am J Med Sci* 1947; **214**: 1–6.

8. Knelson JH, Howatt WF, DeMuth GR. The physiologic significance of grunting respiration. *Pediatrics* 1969; **44**: 393–400.

9. Poole SR, Chetham M, Anderson M. Grunting respirations in infants and children. *Pediatr Emerg Care* 1995; **11**: 158–61.

10. Rusconi F, Castagneto M, Gagliardi L, *et al*. Reference values for respiratory rate in the first 3 years of life. *Pediatrics* 1994; **94**: 350–5.

11. World Health Organization. *Acute respiratory infections in children: Case management in small hospitals in developing countries*. Geneva: WHO, 1990.

12. Singh S, Dhawan A, Kataria S, Walia BN. Validity of clinical signs for the identification of pneumonia in children. *Ann Trop Paediatr* 1994; **14**: 53–8.

13. Dickinson CJ, Martin JF. Megakaryocytes and platelet clumps as the cause of finger clubbing. *Lancet* 1987; **2**: 1434–5.

14. Davis P, Turner-Gomes S, Cunningham K, Way C, Roberts R, Schmidt B. Precision and accuracy of clinical and radiological signs in premature infants at risk of patent ductus arteriosus. *Arch Pediatr Adolesc Med* 1995; **149**: 1136–41.

15. Pearson MG, Spence DP, Ryland I, Harrison BD. Value of pulsus paradoxus in assessing acute severe asthma. *BMJ* 1993; **307**: 659.

16. Forgacs P. Crackles and wheezes. *Lancet* 1967; **2**: 203–5.

17. Forgacs P. The functional significance of clinical signs in diffuse airway obstruction. *Br J Dis Chest* 1971; **65**: 170–7.

18. Thomas PS, Geddes DM, Barnes PJ. Pseudo-steroid resistant asthma. *Thorax* 1999; **54**: 352–6.

19. Abdulmajid OA, Ebeid AM, Motaweh MM, Kleibo IS. Aspirated foreign bodies in the tracheobronchial tree: report of 250 cases. *Thorax* 1976; **31**: 635–40.

20. Fuller P, Picciotto A, Davies M, McKenzie SA. Cough and sleep in inner city children. *Eur Respir J* 1998; **12**: 426–31.

21. Wang EE, Law BJ, Stephens D, *et al*. Study of interobserver reliability in clinical assessment of RSV lower respiratory illness: a Pediatric Investigators' Collaborative Network for Infections in Canada (PICNIC) study. *Ped Pulm* 1996; **22**: 23–7.

22. Marsh K, Forster D, Waruiru C, *et al*. Indicators of life-threatening malaria in African children. *N Engl J Med* 1995; **332**: 1399–404.

23. Beck R, Dickson U, Montgomery MD, Mitchell I. Histamine challenge in young children using computerized lung sounds analysis. *Chest* 1992; **102**: 759–63.

24. Elphick HE, Ritson S, Rodgers H, Everard ML. When a "wheeze" is not a wheeze: acoustic analysis of breath sounds in infants. *Eur Respir J* 2000; **16**: 593–7.

CHAPTER FOUR

EVALUATION *IN* EMERGENCY SETTINGS

E . Carter

- Background
- How to do it
- Interpretation of results

- Organization of care: research issues
- Appendix
- References

BACKGROUND

Respiratory illnesses account for a large proportion of acute secondary care, paediatric referrals in the UK (30–50%, depending on season, in Leicester). Many are self-limiting or respond rapidly to treatment without admission. It is preferable to treat children at home wherever possible, avoiding family disruption and reducing health costs.[1,2]

An accurate assessment is needed to provide effective emergency treatment, plan investigation and management, and to decide where the child should be cared for: the children's ward, intensive care unit, short-stay unit, or his or her own home.

The rate of referral for acute secondary care is increasing in the UK by 5% per annum. Many hospitals have responded by providing specialist units dedicated to acute referrals.[2–5] In such a unit the initial triage assessment and treatment can take place under the care of dedicated staff.

Facilities for short stay observation are very important. For instance a baby with mild bronchiolitis can be observed for a few hours to ensure adequate oral fluid intake and oxygen saturation, or a child with asthma or croup can be monitored to ensure a sustained response to emergency therapy. This enables more children to be discharged home. The provision of an overnight stay

area with facilities for overnight observation and discharge next morning, is more controversial.

Whether assessment takes place in a dedicated Assessment or Admissions Unit, or in the Accident and Emergency Department, the environment should be child and family friendly, with space and privacy for parents, while providing toys, play and comfort for the child. Unpleasant tests and treatment must be made as pain free as possible by use of local anaesthetic cream for cannulation, by undertaking unpleasant procedures in a separate treatment room, away from the bedside (perceived by the child as a safe area) and by the use of preparation and distraction therapy by play leaders.

Modern information technology and trained clerks are essential to provide medical records rapidly and to process paperwork. Direct contact with the labs is helpful to ensure specimens can be sent quickly (e.g. by shute) and results received back promptly by local computer network. Likewise rapid access to radiology is necessary. Nursing, medical and clerical activity can take place concurrently to reducing waiting time.

A five-bed Children's Assessment and Admissions Unit has been set up in Leicester on the principles discussed above, and it deals with up to 1000 medical referrals per month (Figure 4.1A and B). It has resulted in a more efficient and rational delivery of care, and enabled over 40% of children referred for admission by the Primary Care Team

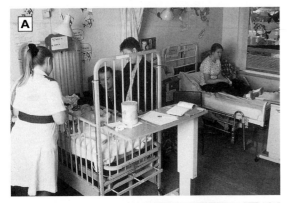

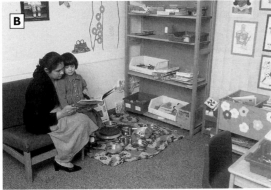

Figure 4.1: Children's Assessment and Admissions Unit, Leicester Royal Infirmary: (A) the main ward and (B) the play room.

(General Practitioner) or the Emergency Department to be discharged home the same day. It is supported by a system of 'rapid access clinics' to review children discharged early, and by a daily general practitioners' helpline to enable GPs to speak to a senior paediatrician about specific cases.[2,3]

A comprehensive set of equipment for examination, investigation and emergency treatment is needed (see Appendix, p.39).

HOW TO DO IT

Assessment of respiratory illness in the acute setting should be *objective* rather than *subjective* wherever possible. The child should be made as comfortable as possible and careful attention paid to observable physical signs (Box 4.1).

Firstly, what is the severity of the illness? Simple observation can help decide (Table 4.1).

Box 4.1: Principles of emergency evaluation

- Keep the child calm during the examination, on the parent's knee if appropriate.
- Observation is more helpful in reaching a diagnosis in children than auscultation and percussion.
- If a child is unco-operative, examine what is easiest first, and not necessarily in the 'correct' order, but do not omit any of the examination.
- Count what can be counted, as this gives hard, baseline data.

Table 4.1: Assessing severity of illness: features of concern in a young ill child

General behaviour	Irritable: starts easily Crying and inconsolable Not smiling Unusual cry Unhappy
Wakefulness/state of arousal	Excessive sleepiness Difficult to wake Not very responsive Unarousable
Tone	Poor or floppy
Activity	Not playful Poor interaction
Fever	Persistent Variable
Heart rate	Raised (see Table 4.7)
Respiratory rate	Raised (see Table 4.7)

NB: LEARN TO OBSERVE
- Observe parents playing with the child
- Most of the above assessments can be made by observing the child from a distance
- Handle and play with the child
- Reassess when fever settles

The mildly unwell child is likely to be able to go home, while the moderately unwell will require admission. If the child is severely unwell, resuscitation is the first priority. This is the basis for setting priorities (triage).

RESUSCITATION[6]

The International Liaison Committee On Resuscitation (ILCOR) Advisory Statements, 1997 provide current resuscitation guidelines[7] which have been adopted worldwide. They are reviewed on a 4-yearly basis, and form the basis for the Paediatric Advanced Life Support (PALS), Advanced Paediatric Life Support (APLS) and Advanced Life Support (ALS) courses.

If the child is seriously ill, the first priority is resuscitation.[6] The method follows the rules of 'A, B, C, D' (Table 4.2). If the child is seriously injured, the same basic rules are followed as above with notable additions (Table 4.3).

If there is cardio-respiratory arrest the same format applies i.e. A, B, C.[6] First shout for help, as resuscitation always needs more than one person. Ensure you do not put yourself in danger during resuscitation and ensure further harm to the child is avoided (Table 4.4). Then assess A, B, C.

In a choking child, attempts should be made to remove the foreign body, by manoeuvres described in Figures 4.5 and 4.6.

Table 4.2: The seriously ill child (Figures 4.2 and 4.3)

	Assessment	Management
Airway	If the child is able to speak or cry, the airway is patent *Look, listen and feel:* ■ look – for rise and fall of the chest ■ listen – for sounds of breathing ■ feel – for breath coming from the nose and mouth	If airway is inadequate, improve it: (a) using manual methods – lift the chin and tilt the head back. (b) using artificial methods – insert an airway/intubate
Breathing	Check for adequate ventilation Assess work of breathing – presence of recession, use of accessory muscles, respiratory rate, grunting, nasal flaring, stridor or wheeze Assess adequacy of breathing – chest wall movement, air entry, cyanosis, oxygen saturation Assess effects of inadequate breathing – poor perfusion, tachycardia	(a) Oxygen: if needed, give maximum concentration, i.e. O_2 supply turned up to full, and using a non-rebreathing bag with reservoir. This gives up to 80% oxygen (cf. 30% with no reservoir) (b) If self-ventilation inadequate, use bag and mask or intubate and bag, using a reservoir to give 99% O_2 (cf. 50% without a reservoir)
Circulation	Pulse rate, pulse volume, colour, temperature of skin and capillary refill time – should be <2 seconds	Give volume expander – (colloid or crystalloid) if needed
Disability A child in respiratory failure may have reduced conscious level. As failure becomes worse, the score reduces. This must therefore be assessed as well as the respiratory system	Glasgow coma score (GCS)[22] or AVPU score AVPU is quicker than GCS: A – alert V – response to verbal command P – responds to pain; corresponds to 8 by GCS U – unconscious; corresponds to 3 by GCS	GCS of 8 or less is an indication for intubation to control airway and respiration

Table 4.3: The seriously injured child (Figures 4.2 and 4.3)

	Assessment	Management
Airway and cervical spine	Cervical spine injury should be assumed to be present until proven otherwise	Head tilt-chin lift manoeuvre is contra-indicated following trauma, as it could turn a fractured cervical spine into a transected cervical cord Jaw thrust is recommended – 3 fingers placed behind the jaw lifting it gently forwards, with minimal angulation of the head The head must be maintained in a straight line with the body at all times. A hard collar must be applied as soon as possible (Figure 4.4). Sandbags and tape can then hold the position. Only when cervical spine X-rays and neurological examination are known to be normal, may the collar be removed
Breathing – as above		
Circulation and haemorrhage control		Good vascular access is required at two sites If peripheral lines impossible due to shock, use femoral vein cannulation, long saphenous cut-down or intra-osseous needle in tibia. Avoid use of neck veins as they are more liable to complications. Boluses of fluid are given if shock is present: 20 mL/kg of colloid or crystalloid. If poor response – further 20mL/kg colloid. Poor response – 20mL/kg blood. Use 0-Negative or type-specific, as cross-matching takes time. Poor response – urgent surgical opinion to look for intra-abdominal bleeding
Disability – as above		
Expose	Look for other injuries	Remove the child's clothes Remember this may cool the child, who should be kept warm with blankets, and the time of exposure should be kept to a minimum

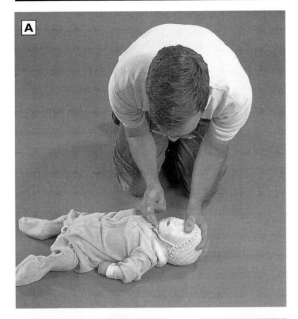

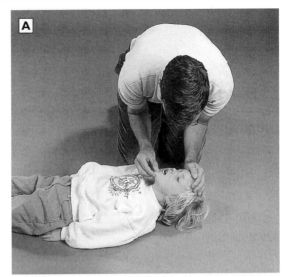

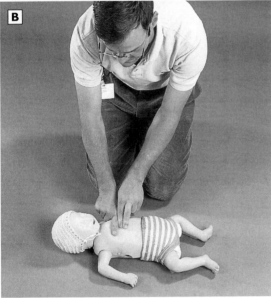

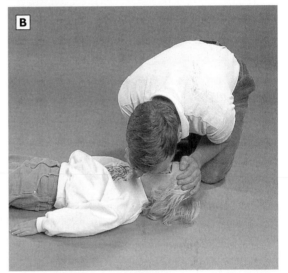

Figure 4.2: Resuscitation of an infant.
(A) Airway – head tilt and chin lift manoeuvre;
(B) Cardiac – external cardiac massage.

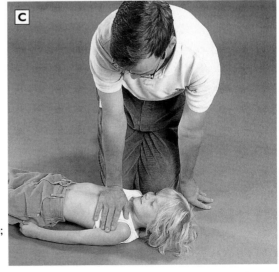

Figure 4.3: Resuscitation of a child.
(A) Airway – head tilt and chin lift manoeuvre;
(B) Breathing – mouth to mouth;
(C) Cardiac – external cardiac massage.

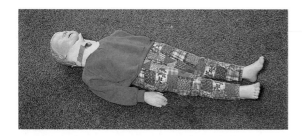

Figure 4.4: Immobilized head and neck after a road traffic accident.

Assessing specific disorders

Use objective assessments or scores for specific illnesses where these are available. Most have been poorly evaluated.

Croup[8]

The diagnosis of croup (acute laryngo-tracheo-bronchitis) is a clinical one, and there is no need for any investigation. Alternative important diagnoses (such as inhaled foreign body or epiglottitis),

Table 4.4: Summary of basic life support in cardio-respiratory arrest

	Assessment	Management
Adopt the SAFE approach:	**S** – Shout for help **A** – Approach with care **F** – Free from danger **E** – Evaluate: A, B, C, D	
Ask	Are you alright?	
Airway	Airway opening manoeuvres	
Breathing	Look, listen and feel	If breathing is absent – give 5 rescue breaths. Each should be of good volume, lasting about a second each Ensure the chest rises with each breath. If it does not, adjust the position of the airway
Circulation	Feel the pulse for 5 seconds – brachial in an infant, carotid in an older child	Absent pulse in child, or <60 in infant - institute cardiac massage **Infant** – 1 finger breadth below inter-nipple line. Use 2 fingers in centre of sternum. Compress at 100 per minute to a depth of about ⅓ anterior-posterior chest diameter. **Child** – heel of the hand placed 1 finger breadth above the xiphi-sternum. Compress at 100 per minute and to a depth of about ⅓ AP chest diameter. Continue with 20 breaths per minute and 100 compressions per minute, i.e. ratio of 5:1. Basic life support must not be interrupted unless the child takes a breath or in order to summon help
Call emergency services		

Open ──────→ Breathe
airway

Check mouth   5 back
and clear   blows (Figure 4.6A)

                5 chest
                thrusts
                (infant or
                older child)
                (Figure 4.6B)

                5 abdominal
                thrusts
                (>1 year old only)
                (Figure 4.6C)

Figure 4.5: The choking child.

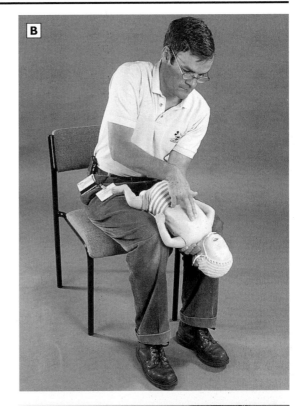

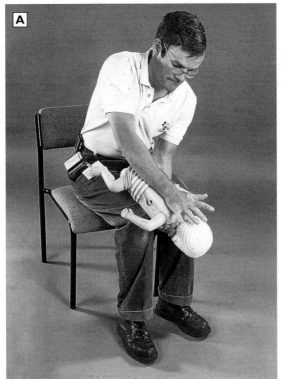

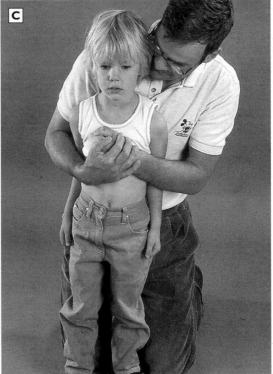

Figure 4.6: Removing a foreign body in the airway of a choking child. (A) Back blows in a baby;
(B) Chest thrusts in a baby; (C) Heimlich manoeuvre in a child.

should be borne in mind; a few well directed questions will usually suffice.

It is helpful to use a scoring system, which can help to guide management (Table 4.5). Use of this 'Score' enables a rapid, accurate and objective assessment of the severity of the croup, and enables rapid management decisions to be taken.

Asthma[9]

A similar score has been devised for asthma, enabling rapid action to be taken in a systematic way (Table 4.6).

Acute anaphylaxis

There are no formal scoring systems for acute anaphylaxis; perhaps because of its variable features. With regard to the airway, it is most important to recognize early features (pharyngeal itching, for example and facial, lip or tongue swelling) to take account of any previous episodes and to monitor closely for progression to major airway oedema while initiating emergency therapy (Table 4.8).

Table 4.5: Grading of croup (from Reference 8)

	Mild	Moderate	Severe	Very severe
Inspiratory stridor	+	+	+	+
Expiratory stridor	−	+	+	+
Palpable paradox	−	−	+	+
Severe features*	−	−	−	+

ACTIONS:	
■ Mild:	home; steroids (oral).
■ Moderate:	steroids (nebulized or oral); monitor and observe; admit.
■ Severe:	oxygen; steroids; epinephrine nebulizer; IV fluids; if no reversion to moderate in 2 hours, refer to Children's Intensive Care Unit (CICU).
■ Very severe:	CICU; 100% O_2; steroids; repeated epinephrine nebulizer until intubation performed.

* Severe features include: marked retractions, sternal recession, any cyanosis, confusion, drowsiness, SaO_2<92% when stable.

Table 4.6: Severity of asthma score

	Mild	Moderate	Severe
Respiratory rate	<40	>40	>40
Recession	Absent	Present	Marked
Accessory muscle use	Absent	Present	Marked
Able to talk/count to 10	Yes	No	No
PEF (% best or predicted)	50–75%	30–50%	<30%
Hypoxia (in air)	SaO_2 >92%	SaO_2 <92%	SaO_2 <85%

ACTION:	
■ Mild:	β_2 agonist by MDI/ spacer, oral prednisolone; home if good response; GP follow-up in primary care.
■ Moderate:	admit; regular nebulized β_2 agonist; daily prednisolone; monitor, including O_2 saturation; teaching for parents.
■ Severe	continuous nebulized or intravenous β_2 agonist; 6-hourly ipratropium neb; IV hydrocortisone; improves – to ward; no improvement – to CICU; CXR to exclude pneumothorax; blood gas analysis; ventilate if rising CO_2, falling O_2 or reduced conscious level or other deterioration.

Pneumonia

The WHO programme to control acute respiratory infections uses simple clinical signs to identify pneumonia and assess its severity.[10] The programme reflects the high mortality from acute respiratory infection (ARI): 3 million children under 5 years of age die annually worldwide from ARI. Deaths of infants under 2 months of age are 20–30% of total deaths from ARI under 5 years of age.[11–13] WHO respiratory rate thresholds (upper limit of normal) are given in Table 3.3 (Chapter 3). These figures are based on studies of healthy children. A project in Swaziland to assess current WHO guidelines on respiratory rate and radiological evidence of pneumonia, found the WHO criteria predicted X-ray documented pneumonia with a specificity of 72% and a sensitivity of 85%.[10] The WHO guidelines thus appear to predict pneumonia with reasonable accuracy in the developing countries, but more research is needed for infants under 2 months of age (Case study 4.1).

FURTHER ASSESSMENT AND MANAGEMENT

After immediate assessment and resuscitation have been carried out, a full history and examination are necessary.

History

Chapter 2 deals in detail with history-taking. In the emergency setting, there are several important points. The onset of illness, its duration and precipitating factors are particularly important diagnostic clues, especially in obstructive airway disorders (Case studies 4.2 and 4.3). Neonatal lung disease of prematurity, meconium aspiration or transient tachypnoea are important precursors. Vaccination history and past medical history (bronchiolitis, previous respiratory or ear, nose and throat (ENT) disease, episodes of cyanosis or lost consciousness) may raise diagnostic possibilities for the first time. Systems review should seek to answer the question 'Why now?' with regard to the crisis: is there a second, complicating diagnosis (for example sickle cell disease presenting as pneumonia)? Drug history and travel history are vital.

Examination

Chapter 3 considers general aspects of the physical examination. A knowledge of cardiorespiratory values for children is essential (Table 4.7). Pay special regard to: general features such as cyanosis, pallor, respiratory distress, agitation (occurs in hypoxia), clubbing, fever and drooling. Noises may be present including stridor, grunting

---

Case study 4.1: Acute pneumonia

A 3-year-old girl called Donna presented with a temperature of 40°C, lethargy, vomiting and abdominal pain. Examination revealed a respiratory rate of 45, but no other abnormal sign. SaO_2 was 92% by oximetry. Her abdomen was soft and urine dipstick was negative.

Investigation indicated infection with a peripheral blood white count of 33,000 × 10^9/L and neutrophilia. A CXR confirmed left lower lobe pneumonia. The antibiotic of choice is penicillin, and in view of the vomiting, the level of illness and her age this was given intravenously. She also needed intravenous fluid maintenance as she could not drink and had a fever. Oxygen was given by nasal cannulae until oxygen saturation improved.

24 hours later Donna was much improved and her temperature was back to normal. Oral amoxycillin was substituted and she went home one day later. Blood culture results later confirmed *Streptococcus pneumoniae* as the organism.

NB
- If there had been clinical signs of pneumonia, then one would treat even in the absence of radiological changes, which may lag by a day or so.
- A positive bacterial culture is uncommon in pneumonia.

Case Study 4.2: A wheezy infant

Tracey, an 18-month-old girl presented with her first episode of wheeze and persistent cough. She had a normal neonatal history, no previous illnesses, her parents were non-smokers, and there was a strong family history of asthma.

Examination revealed widespread wheeze, with recession and tachypnoea, but oxygen saturation was normal. She had no evidence of an upper respiratory tract infection. She received two doses of nebulized salbutamol, but there was no improvement, raising the suspicion that asthma was not the cause. A further history was therefore taken, which revealed that she had been eating nuts while playing the previous evening, and her symptoms began immediately after this. The possibility of a foreign body was raised, and she had a bronchoscopy which revealed fragments of nuts in her airway. These were removed, with complete resolution of her symptoms.

Without the history of possible inhalation of nut fragments, a first episode of asthma may have been suspected. Asthma, triggered by a viral URTI, is by far the commonest cause of wheeze in this age-group but other causes must be considered, especially in the first episode.

Case study 4.3: Anaphylactic shock (Table 4.8)

Archie, a 3-year-old boy with known peanut allergy attended his friend's birthday party.

Fifteen minutes after a meal, he developed generalized itching, a swollen mouth and tongue, a rash and then difficulty in breathing. He was taken to the Accident and Emergency Department, where he was found to be cyanosed and confused and with marked stridor. He was intubated immediately and given epinephrine (adrenaline) intramuscularly. His condition improved, with adequate ventilation and oxygen saturation, but his capillary refill remained poor at 4 seconds. He received 20mL/kg colloid, and 30 minutes later his perfusion had returned to normal. Intravenous hydrocortisone was given, and he was transferred to CICU. Four hours later, there was an airleak round his ET tube, indicating that the swelling had reduced, and he was successfully extubated.

Although the hosts had tried to ensure a nut-free party, it was later discovered that there were small amounts of nuts in some of the biscuits.

He had taken his Epi-pen to the party, but no-one there felt confident to administer it. In future, he will take his own provisions and his parents will ensure that an adult is able to administer epinephrine via his Epi-pen.

Table 4.7: Normal values for children (rates per minute)

Age	Heart rate	Respiratory rate
0–1	120–160	30–40
2–4	100–120	25–30
5–12	80–100	20–25
> 12	60–80	15–20

Blood pressure. There are various centile charts and formulae in existence for normal values of blood pressure. A simple one is given below:
Systolic blood pressure = 70+(age × 2) mmHg
There are more sophisticated data available.[23]

or wheeze. Observe respiratory rate, intercostal recession, use of accessory muscles, hyperinflation, flaring of alae nasae. Finally, auscultate and percuss. The upper respiratory tract must be included – ear, nose and throat and cervical glands. It is important to review the child repeatedly to ensure a satisfactory response, or to detect deterioration. If the symptoms do not fit the initial diagnosis, *always reconsider the diagnosis or suspect a second diagnosis* (Case study 4.4).

Case study 4.4: Deteriorating upper airway obstruction

Karl, a 9-year-old boy had upper respiratory symptoms for a week then showed the classic triad of barking cough, inspiratory stridor and a hoarse voice. He had a temperature of 39°C and mild recession and seemed generally unwell. Sao$_2$ was 96%.

An assessment was made of the degree of upper airway obstruction, and a cause sought. A diagnosis of croup was made, as he showed the classic symptoms. However, he is older than the average age for croup (pre-school age), and more 'toxic' than would be expected, so other causes were considered. The most likely alternative would be acute bacterial tracheitis: toxic; tracheal (central chest) pain; painful cough with or without purulent sputum; a raised white count with neutrophilia and raised level of c-reactive protein (CRP) would be expected. Epiglottitis was unlikely as there was no drooling or shock and he had received Hib vaccine. There was no history of foreign body. Other rarer causes of upper airways obstruction were considered: inhalation of smoke; diphtheria (no foreign travel, e.g. to Russia) and a rapidly expanding mediastinal tumour (CXR was not performed).

Croup was the likeliest diagnosis: his airway obstruction was assessed as moderate, so he was treated with oral dexamethasone, but deteriorated rapidly with increased recession, distress and arterial desaturation to 90%. He was now at risk of severe respiratory failure, so was given nebulized epinephrine (adrenaline) with temporary relief, 100% oxygen, transferred to CICU and intubated and given intravenous antibiotics. At intubation, there was marked inflammation of his larynx and trachea, with pus from which *Staphylococcus aureus* was seen on Gram-stained film and subsequently isolated.

The diagnosis staphylococcal tracheitis, which can mimic croup, and has physical signs similar to epiglottitis is a well-recognized cause of upper airway obstruction and inflammation in school-age children.

Table 4.8: Anaphylactic shock

	Assessment	Management
Airway	If no problem	Go to breathing
	If total obstruction	Intubate
	Incomplete obstruction	Get help
		epinephrine nebulizer
		epinephrine IM
		reassess
Breathing	If no problem	Go to circulation
	If no breathing	5 rescue breaths and continue with basic life support
	If wheeze	Give epinephrine IM if not already given and salbutamol nebulizer
Circulation	If no problem	Expose patient
	If shock	Give IM epinephrine if not already given and 20 mL/kg volume expander
	Reassess A, B, C	Consider hydrocortisone IV and aminophyeline IV for on-going wheeze
Remember: remove the allergen if possible!		

Medical guidelines

Guidelines should be provided for common acute respiratory disorders and emergencies. They must be regularly up-dated in line with changing evidence, and agree with the consensus of opinion in the department. Rapid assessment scores should be used where possible. They should be based on sound evidence, and be fully referenced. Teaching programmes, run by the Acute Admissions Team, should be provided to encourage their use and provide for discussion.

Information and training for families

A range of leaflets for parents on common respiratory disorders, inhalers and their use and maintenance is essential. Parents are more likely to remember advice if they have written material to refer to when they get home, as well as verbal advice given in context. Up to 25% of referrals for admission are asthma related. A brief period spent with the family teaching about asthma and training on use of inhalers can reduce re-admissions significantly.[14]

INTERPRETATION OF RESULTS

Investigations should be kept to a minimum, and performed with a view to aiding diagnosis, estimating severity of the illness and hence deciding on therapy and the appropriate place for management.

Evidence of infection can be sought by throat swab for bacterial (especially streptococcal) infection, nasopharyngeal aspirate for viruses (especially respiratory syncitial virus) and per nasal swab for *Bordettella pertussis*. A raised white blood count with neutrophilia may indicate bacterial infection but has low specificity, while monospot and cold agglutinins can provide a rapid and specific diagnosis of Epstein–Barr virus (EBV) and mycoplasma infection, but with poor sensitivity and specificity. While not providing an immediate diagnosis, acute phase serology is useful in cases where the diagnosis is obscure: a second specimen 10–14 days later may provide an accurate diagnosis.

Infection may cause raised plasma viscosity or c-reactive protein (CRP). Specific investigations such as Mantoux test or immunoglobulin levels (with IgG subsets) may assist diagnosis of chronic or recurrent productive cough or pneumonia. Urgent bronchoscopy is necessary in cases of suspected foreign body inhalation.

Outpatient investigations can be arranged if indicated for chronic symptoms, including barium swallow, oesophageal pH study or sweat test, once the immediate emergency has been resolved.

Severity of the illness must be monitored by simple, accurate tests. Peak expiratory flow (PEF) is a rapid and effective method of assessing degree of lower airway obstruction in asthma, and is useful in assessing response to treatment. Blood gas analysis and oxygen saturation monitoring helps identify impending respiratory failure, and provides a baseline to assess progress. Remember to view all results with caution. For example a saturation monitor will not give an accurate reading in an under-perfused child.

Chest X-ray (CXR) is indicated in suspected pneumonia and occasionally in asthma (but only in the first attack, presence of focal or assymetrical signs, or failure to respond to standard therapy).[15] It is not necessary to perform follow-up CXR in uncomplicated pneumonia, if there is complete clinical resolution.[16]

Many children with respiratory complaints do not need investigations and in some it is indeed dangerous to do any. For example upper respiratory tract infections should be managed by reassurance and as little intervention as possible. X-rays and painful procedures are contraindicated until the airway is secure. These guidelines are especially important if acute epiglottitis is suspected.

ORGANIZATION OF CARE: RESEARCH ISSUES

The number of childhood admissions with respiratory illness increases annually, and this, together with the recognition that children are best cared for at home where possible, has led to alternative methods of management in a semi-outpatient manner. A review of admissions in Nottingham,

UK, showed that most children were discharged within 24 hours.[17] Many hospitals have responded by creating 'assessment units' where a child can be assessed, treated, and observed for a short period without being admitted to an in-patient bed.[5] The experience of a unit opened in Leicester in 1994 has shown that the number of admissions can be substantially reduced by having an assessment unit,[2,3] while another found a similar reduction in admission rate, and also reduced costs of the service.[4] There are now many assessment units in the country, but still wide variations in admission rate and length of stay between regions. Research is needed to find the optimum method of organization of such care.

An American model, suitable to a managed care system, uses primary care paediatricians in a community setting, away from the hospital, reducing referral rate to hospital. The service was especially effective at nights and weekends, when children could be seen near to home.[18] With the advent of Primary Care Groups this may well be a model for the future in the British system.

There are other ways of reducing acute respiratory admissions, especially for asthma. Phelan found several preventable factors in his study of admitted asthmatics.[19] A 'home intervention plan' was developed by Lieu and colleagues which gave parents a plan of early intervention at the onset of an asthma attack, and the results showed the children were less likely to need admission.[20] The provision of a structured nurse-led home management and teaching plan at discharge reduced the readmission rate of children with asthma.[14]

Admission protocols have been developed and used in the USA for over 20 years. These provide guidelines to aid the decision as to whether to admit a sick child or not, aiming to limit costs and improve efficiency in emergency care. The appropriateness of such a tool was recently evaluated for use in British hospitals, but the idea must be viewed with caution as the UK Health Service is very different from that of the USA.[21] The involvement of GPs and practice nurses in local asthma clinics, together with health education by school nurses are further areas to help prevent asthma admissions. All these areas require audit and standardization to ensure the best practice.

The change in emphasis in paediatric practice to a more preventative and community-based approach has training implications for future paediatricians. The former emphasis on training in medical schools, on the rare and serious, has given way to a more appropriate focus on generic skills and common paediatric problems which might best be taught in a community setting.

ACKNOWLEDGEMENT

The help of Mr Ian Buck-Barrett, Resuscitation Officer, University Hospital of Leicester, is gratefully acknowledged.

APPENDIX: EQUIPMENT REQUIRED FOR EFFECTIVE MANAGEMENT IN THE EMERGENCY SETTING

INTUBATION EQUIPMENT (FIGURE 4.7)

Suction with Yankauer sucker.
Pharyngeal airways – a range of sizes is required.
Laryngoscopes – two blades are needed – straight for an infant and curved for a child.

ET tubes – sizes from 2.5 to 8 mm internal diameter.

To calculate size - preterm neonate – 2.5mm
term neonate – 3.0mm
6 months old – 3.5mm
older child – 4+ (age/4)mm
adult – 7.0–8.0mm.

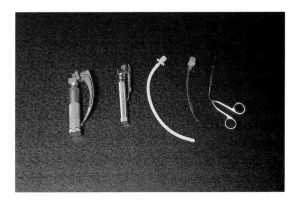

Figure 4.7: Intubation equipment – ETT, laryngoscopes, Magills forceps, introducer, Yankauer suction.

Magills forceps.

Tracheal suction catheters – in a range of diameters to fit inside ET tubes.

Cricothyroidotomy cannulae.

WALL OXYGEN

Flowmeter able to supply at 15L/min.

Bags should be self-inflating – two sizes needed – 1600 mL for children and 500 mL for infants. Reservoirs are needed to ensure 99% oxygen is delivered (Figure 4.8).

Masks – a range is needed to fit all ages. The mask should fit from the bridge of the nose to the groove between the chin and lower lip.

Masks should be colourless to enable visualization of the airway in case of vomit or other obstruction.

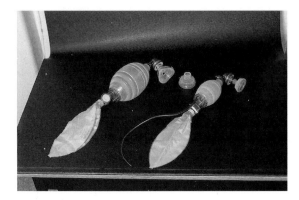

Figure 4.8: Bag and masks for resuscitation – 500 mL and 1600 mL, with reservoirs.

DRUGS ON CARDIAC ARREST TROLLEY

Epinephrine: 1 in 10,000 – 0.1 mL/kg for first dose
1 in 1000 – 0.1 mL/kg for second and subsequent doses

Atropine: 0.02 mg/kg

Adenosine: 0.05mg/kg

Sodium bicarbonate: 4.2% – 1 mL/kg

10% glucose: 5 mL/kg

Colloid: 20 mL/kg

Crystalloid: 20 mL/kg

DRUGS IN THE EMERGENCY CUPBOARD

Salbutamol and ipratropium bromide for nebulization

Hydrocortisone

Aminophylline

Range of antibiotics for IV and PO use

Budesonide for nebulization

Prednisolone

Dexamethasone

Epinephrine for nebulization and IV/IM use

Chlorpheniramine – IV and PO.

REFERENCES

1. Department of Health. Welfare of children and young people in hospital. London: HMSO, 1991.

2. Carter EP, Hall SA, Hartley S, Houtman PH. Reducing in-patient paediatric admissions. *Family Med* 1997; **1**: 7–11.

3. Hall AS, Carter EP. Keeping children out of hospital. *Family Med* 1997; **1**: 28–9.

4. Beverley DW, Ball RJ, Smith RA, *et al.* Planning for the future: the experience of implementing a children's day assessment unit in a district general hospital. *Arch Dis Child* 1997; **77**: 287–92.

5. Meates M. Ambulatory paediatrics – making a difference. *Arch Dis Child* 1997; **76**: 468–73.

6. Advanced Life Support Group: Advanced paediatric life support. The practical approach. Mackway-Jones K, Molyneux E, Phillips B, Wieteska S (eds). London: BMJ Publishing Group, 1996.

7. 1997 Resuscitation guidelines for the UK. ILCOR Advisory statements, 1997.

8. Klein M. Respiratory disorders. In: Heese H de V (ed): Handbook of paediatrics. Cape Town: Oxford University Press, 1995: 507–29.

9. The British guidelines on asthma management. *Thorax* 1997; **52** (suppl. 1): 13–19.

10. World Health Organization. Fourth programme report, 1988–89, ARI. Programme for control of acute respiratory infections. Geneva: WHO, 1990; **7**: 31.

11. Berman S, Simoes EA, Lanata C. Respiratory rate and pneumonia in infancy. *Arch Dis Child* 1991; **66**: 81–4.

12. Singhi S, Dhawan A, Kataria S, Walia BN. Clinical signs of pneumonia in infants under 2 months. *Arch Dis Child* 1994; **70**: 413–17.

13. Rusconi F, Castagneto M, Gagliardi L, *et al.* Reference values for respiratory rates in the first 3 years of life. *Pediatrics* 1994; **94**: 350–5.

14. Wesseldine LJ, McCarthy P, Silverman M, Structured discharge procedure for children admitted to hospital with acute asthma: a randomised controlled trial of nursing practice. *Arch Dis Child* 1999; **80**: 110–14.

15. Canny GJ, Reisman J, Healy R, *et al.* Acute asthma: observations regarding the management of a pediatric emergency room. *Pediatrics* 1989; **83**: 507–12.

16. Gibson NA, Hollman AS, Paton, JY, Value of radiological follow-up of childhood pneumonia. *BMJ* 1993; **307**: 1117.

17. Stevenson T. Paediatrics in the year 2010, a document of the RCPCH, 1998.

18. Shanon A, Reisner S, Paswell J, *et al.* The role of a secondary pediatric ambulatory care service within the community. *Pediatr Emerg Care* 1997; **13**: 50–3.

19. Ordonez GA, Phelan P, Olinsky A, Robertson CF. Preventable factors in hospital admissions for asthma. *Arch Dis Child* 1998; **78**: 143–7.

20. Lieu T, Ouesen CP, Capra AM, *et al.* Out-patient management practices associated with reduced risk of pediatric asthma hospitalization and emergency department visits. *Pediatrics* 1997; **100**: 334–41.

21. Werneke U, Smith H, Smith IJ, *et al.* Validation of the paediatric appropriateness: evaluation protocol in British practice. *Arch Dis Child* 1997; **77**: 294–8.

22. Gemke RJ, Tasker RC. Clinical assessment of acute coma in children. *Lancet* 1998; **351**: 926–7.

23. Report of the Task Force on blood pressure control in children. From the National Heart, Lung and Blood Institute, Bethesda, Maryland. *Pediatrics* 1987; **79**: 1–25.

CHAPTER FIVE

MONITORING ACUTE DISEASE *IN* HOSPITAL

W. Hoskyns

- Introduction
- Classification of admissions
- Why monitor
- How to monitor

- Interpretation
- How to integrate results into management
- Clinical research issues
- References

INTRODUCTION

Respiratory illness is the commonest cause of admission to hospital in childhood. Review of our local experience in Leicester, from a relatively unselected population, shows that in the quieter summer months 31% of referrals to hospital have a primary respiratory diagnosis (range 6–50% each day). In the winter when admissions increase by 2 to 3-fold, this rises to 47% (range 33–63%) (unpublished data). In the last 30 years, paediatric consultations in primary care[1] and admissions to hospital in the UK have increased, and this is particularly noticeable in relation to asthma.[2] The cause is not known but might be explained by changes in referral patterns, increased recognition of morbidity in primary care settings, increased prevalence of disease, increased severity of disease or a combination of any of the above. There certainly seems to be an increase in use of asthma as a diagnostic label and it is possible that this has increased awareness of morbidity and expectations of treatment, which in turn has increased referral rates. There is also some evidence that asthma prevalence has shown a true increase[3] but evidence of increased severity is hard to find.[4] In the future it is possible that improved primary care respiratory management (mainly based around asthma treatment) will help reduce hospital admissions (see Chapter 24).

CLASSIFICATION OF ADMISSIONS

Successful outcome of a hospital admission may be difficult to define. Many acute admissions are for self-limiting illnesses where treatment is supportive and discharge from hospital may be considered evidence of a good outcome. However, reasons for admission are dependent on many factors other than the disease and a small number of children have disproportionately high use of hospital services. It is important that the monitoring during a hospital admission is appropriate and used as an opportunity to educate the child and the family in disease control and prevention of re-admission.

Respiratory problems in hospital can broadly be divided into three groups (Table 5.1). The emphasis of monitoring in acute respiratory illness is to follow the natural history of the disease and treatment. This will alert the clinician to deviation from the expected course which may indicate disease severity or complications (see Case study 5.1). In exacerbations of chronic disease there is the additional need to document longer term measures of wellbeing such as nutritional status, treatment side effects and lung function (see Case study 5.2). Although respiratory paediatricians are primarily concerned with the respiratory outcome it is clear that there are other potential outcomes (neurodevelopmental, social,

Table 5.1: Types of illness and appropriate monitoring

	Examples of disease	Monitoring required
Acute	Upper respiratory infection Bronchiolitis Croup Pneumonia	Respiratory parameters Systemic effects
Chronic respiratory with exacerbation	Asthma Cystic fibrosis Tracheostomy	Respiratory parameters Systemic effects Long-term well-being (e.g. growth) Lung function
Complicating other disease	Neuromuscular Neurological Gastro-intestinal Scoliosis	Respiratory parameters Specific features (e.g. sleep and oesophageal pH) Lung function

financial etc.) which will influence the respiratory management. The overall management of the child must take precedence over any of the individual organs.

WHY MONITOR

Children are admitted to hospital because they have symptoms and a decision is made that they need investigations or therapeutic intervention not available at home. Alternatively, the child's condition suggests that intervention may be necessary in the near future. In either case, there is an obligation to monitor the child's condition to show the progress of the illness and the effectiveness of any treatment. Clinical decisions are usually based not so much on the severity of illness as on the perceived rate of change of symptoms and signs. To know rates of change implies repeated observations of parameters, which ideally should be objective, repeatable (by different observers) and reflect the severity of the illness (i.e. valid).

In addition to helping management of individual patients, monitoring allows comparisons to be made between individuals and groups. This, of course, is the basis of the application of science to medicine – defining populations, auditing current practice and testing management hypotheses.

HOW TO MONITOR

A number of common measurable parameters are listed in Table 5.2 and discussed below.

RESPIRATORY RATE

The respiratory rate is an easy reproducible measurement of respiratory function if measured over 30 seconds (or more in infants). Over a shorter period, it may be more variable, particularly in babies with periodic breathing and self-conscious older children.

The respiratory rate varies with age, which may make interpretation more difficult, but as a trend monitor in combination with the pulse rate it is extremely valuable (Case study 5.1).

RESPIRATORY DISTRESS

Clinical studies support the contention that respiratory distress is the most important single clinical sign of respiratory illness.[5] The drawback of using it for monitoring progress or in research is that it is very subjective. The observer has to take a number of diverse signs (cough, stridor, wheeze, grunting, intercostal recession, subcostal recession, sternal recession, tracheal tug, tachypnoea, chest and abdominal movement and flaring nostrils) and esti-

Table 5.2: Usefulness of monitoring tools

Parameter	Reproducibility	Applications	Drawbacks
1. Primary respiratory signs			
Respiratory rate	Fair	All illness	Short-term variations
Respiratory distress	Poor	All illness	Subjective
Chest X-ray	Good	Diagnostic rather than monitoring	Changes may lag behind other features
Oxygen saturation	Excellent	All illness	Movement artefact
Blood gases	Excellent	Serious illness	Invasive
Peak flow/ spirometry	Excellent if patient co-operation	Chronic illness	Not possible in under 5's Reflects large airway more than small airway function
Requirement for β_2 agonist	Fair	Asthma	Subjective
2. Secondary effects of respiratory disease			
Pulse rate	Good	All respiratory disease as measure of circulatory effects	Minute to minute variability
Blood pressure (cuff inflation method) and 'pulsus paradoxus'	Fair	Obstructive lung disease (pulsus paradoxus) Serious infective illness	Needs good technique and equipment Often difficult to obtain in smaller children
Temperature	Excellent	Infective illnesses	Variation with site of reading
3. General effects of disease			
Nutritional status	Excellent (weight + height measurement)	For all chronic problems	Height measurement very operator dependent
Nutritional intake	Fair	Acute and chronic illness	May be difficult to assess in ward setting

mate the degree of difficulty to breathing that this represents. Given the variation in patterns of breathing of different children, quantifying respiratory distress is difficult even for a single observer.

CHEST X-RAY

The chest X-ray is a helpful diagnostic investigation but for monitoring the progression of disease it is of limited value. It also has limitations in monitoring of chronic conditions. For instance, CXR is normal in 50% of bronchographically proven bronchiectasis. It may be helpful in an acute deterioration to exclude lung collapse or pneumothorax, and in pneumonia, a repeat X-ray if fever persists or recrudesces may confirm development of a pleural effusion (Case study 5.1).

OXYGEN SATURATION

Non-invasive oxygen saturation monitoring has made a huge contribution to assessment and monitoring of children with respiratory problems. It is useful because it measures the most important function of the lungs, namely gas exchange. Because of the shape of the oxygen dissociation curve it is not a very sensitive measure of high oxygen tensions. In practice one is only concerned about low Sao_2. High Pao_2 is only relevant in pre-term infants where hyperoxia is a factor in retinopathy of prematurity.

The alveolar gas equation (Figure 5.1) shows the relationship of O_2 to CO_2 in the alveolus (and consequently in arterial blood). If the subject is breathing air (Fio_2 = 0.21) any rise in the level of CO_2 must be accompanied by a corresponding fall in O_2. In other words, if the Sao_2 is normal in air (over 96–97%), CO_2 can be assumed to be near normal.

Blood gases

Arterial blood gases provide a direct measure of gas exchange in the lungs and represent the gold standard for assessing respiration. The invasive-ness of arterial puncture or an indwelling arterial line means that sampling is only appropriate for sick patients who need, or may need, intensive care treatment. Skilled nursing care is needed to reduce the risk of complications of arterial cannu-lae. Single puncture of the radial artery using a small gauge butterfly needle carries little risk, but is painful and multiple puncture is not usually jus-

$$Pao_2 = Pio_2 - Paco_2/R$$

Pao_2 is the alveolar oxygen concentration which equates to arterial oxygen (Pao_2)

Pio_2 is the partial pressure of inspired oxygen (assumed to be saturated with water vapour and at body temperature); this is: (barometric pressure − water vapour pressure)× Fio_2 (where Fio_2 is the fractional inspired oxygen concentration).

$Paco_2$ is the alveolar carbon dioxide concentration which equates to the arterial CO_2 for practical purposes.

R is the respiratory quotient which depends on diet and is usually 0.8.

If the inspired oxygen is constant, any change in the CO_2 level is mirrored by a reciprocal change in O_2.

Figure 5.1: The alveolar gas equation in its simplest form.

tified. Venous and capillary blood gases can be measured but are influenced by tissue perfusion and the effects of tissue respiration. This makes the Po_2 results uninterpretable. The pH and CO_2 tension are difficult to interpret in children with poor peripheral perfusion, but for the majority of cases a lower limit estimate of the pH (and upper limit of CO_2 for capillary samples) is useful for making clinical decisions, although trends are often more useful than snapshots.

Apnoea monitoring

There are several relatively cheap devices designed to sense breathing movements, and to raise an alarm when movements cease for a pre-determined period (normally 10–20 seconds). They are useful in infants at high risk of apnoea or sudden death. The rationale for their use is that they may prevent death from apnoea.

To be effective the apnoea alarm needs to :

1   alert the parent or nurse to the lack of airflow in the baby;
2   have an acceptable level of false alarms;
3   provide sufficient warning for intervention to be successful.

There is little good evidence that they can achieve any of these goals, but they are still widely used on neonatal units, paediatric wards and in the home in the hope that they may prevent a death.

The apnoea alarms in common use work by sensing breathing movements either through a mattress laid under the baby or a pressure sensi-tive capsule sited on the baby's upper abdomen. Because they measure body movement rather than airflow, they will not alarm during 'obstruc-tive apnoea', where respiratory movements con-tinue despite lack of airflow.

There has always been a division of opinion amongst paediatricians as to their usefulness. These concerns are less of an issue in the hospital setting where easy access to heart rate and Sao_2 monitoring makes their use less critical.

Lung function tests

The peak flow meter is the most useful clinical tool in the acute setting as it is robust, portable, cheap and gives reproducible results. It cannot be relied upon in children less than 5 years of age (and older if breathless) as it requires co-operation with a forced expiration. In older children with reversible obstructive airways disease (asthma) who have been trained to use it, it can be used to monitor recovery although it is not very sensitive to mild disease. Plotting pre- and post-bronchodilator peak flow, 4–6 hourly gives information about the overall trend of lung function, diurnal variation, and response to therapy. All of these may be useful in predicting recovery and targeting treatment (Figure 5.2).

Spirometry has similar drawbacks to peak flow but provides a more comprehensive picture of lung function (Chapter 7), and is the best method of examining small airway disease but is impractical for monitoring changes in individuals with severe breathlessness.

Full recovery of lung function may take up to 14 days following admission for acute severe asthma. It is not useful to provide a precise target value before allowing a child to go home. The trend and clinical status are more useful.

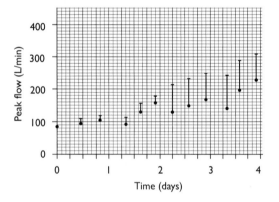

Figure 5.2: Peak flow (PF) chart of recovery in hospital from an asthma attack. Pre-bronchodilator PF is shown as a filled circle, each connected to its post-bronchodilator result. The normal range for the patient's height (150 cm) is 280–450 L/min. The initial PF is 20% of expected for height with no bronchodilator response. The baseline PF improves gradually with improved bronchodilator response and development of a marked diurnal pattern.

REQUIREMENT FOR DRUGS

Medication for acute relief of symptoms (such as bronchodilators for asthma) can be monitored and will reflect to some extent the severity of the illness. The child, the family, medical and nursing staff may all be involved in making decisions about medication, making this a subjective parameter unless the local hospital has pre-defined criteria for drug administration.

PULSE RATE

The pulse rate is an easy, reproducible measurement usually reflecting the metabolic influence of respiratory disease. It is usually raised in acute respiratory disease and falls as the condition improves (Case study 5.1). It is a rather non-specific measurement as it is influenced by physiological factors (such as state of activity) and by many others including pyrexia, anxiety, pain and cardiac failure.

BLOOD PRESSURE

Blood pressure changes are important in severe illness and continuous intra-arterial monitoring is standard practice in the intensive care unit. However, for most admissions it is not a sensitive measure of the patient's condition as there are potent physiological mechanisms for maintaining blood pressure. In addition, measurement using the correct cuff size and good technique without disturbing the child may present problems in the ward setting. In obstructive lung disease, the degree of pulsus paradoxus (decline in blood pressure on tidal inspiration) gives an indication of the severity of the lung disease. It represents the huge swings in intrathoracic pressure associated with the mechanical load imposed by severe lung disease. The sign is very unreliable and has been dropped from current management guidelines.

TEMPERATURE

Because so many children have an infective component to their symptoms, temperature is an important measure of well being and response to treatment (Case study 5.1). It is also highly reproducible. Rise in temperature generally implies infection, but discriminates poorly between viral and bacterial disease. Hypothermia may be a feature of overwhelming bacterial infection in a young infant.

COMPLIANCE WITH TREATMENT

In acute severe respiratory illness in hospital, compliance with treatment tends to be good as it is administered by ward staff and the patient and family have a strong incentive to try to improve the child's condition. When parent(s) fail to comply with appropriate treatment requests it is possible that there is poor understanding of the child's situation, poor parental skills, poor coping strategies, neglect or, in extreme cases, factitious illness by

Case study 5.1: Unresolved pneumonia

Paula, a 5-year-old child was admitted to hospital with a 4-day history of high fever with delirium. Her respiratory rate was 80 with a pneumonic breathing pattern and lobar pneumonia was diagnosed on chest X-ray. Figure 5.3 shows her progress on intravenous antibiotics. Paula was afebrile by day 8 of her illness (after 4 days in hospital), but had a re-crudescence of fever 3 days later. Further chest X-ray was performed on day 7 of admission which showed a pleural effusion.

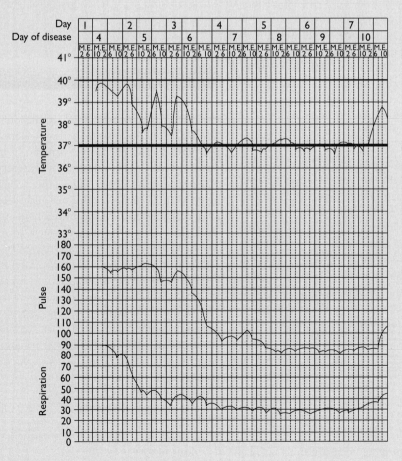

Figure 5.3: Pneumonia: progress on antibiotics.

Case study 5.2: Deterioration in a young person with cystic fibrosis

Jo, a 16-year-old child with cystic fibrosis was admitted to hospital for a 2-week course of antibiotics. She had become more breathless with increase in sputum production. She was colonized with *Pseudomonas* and had had overnight home oxygen for the previous 6 months.

Respiratory monitoring in hospital included: temperature, pulse and respiration, continuous pulse oximetry, sputum volume and daily FEV_1.

Other monitoring considered important in the longer term included weight, dietary intake, FEV_1, compliance with treatment and cardiac function.

She improved subjectively and on objective respiratory measurements over the 2 weeks. Her FEV_1 improved from 25% to 60% of that expected for her height (her normal level when well). She regained some weight but her intake remained sub-optimal and contributed to the decision to insert a gastrostomy tube for nutritional support a few months later. Compliance with treatment had always been an issue for the patient and it was felt that it had contributed to her deterioration over the years. This problem was addressed (but not solved) by continued education and clinical psychology input. Her cardiac function showed good right ventricular function with minimally raised pulmonary pressure.

proxy. More commonly, poor compliance is a problem in older children with chronic disease (Chapter 22). Although hospital is a very different environment to home, monitoring compliance in patients who are old enough to have some control over their treatment may be useful in planning longer term management.

NUTRITIONAL STATUS

This is most simply measured by weight and height although there are more sophisticated methods (upper arm circumference, skinfold thickness). Weight loss caused by anorexia and increased metabolic demands is a feature of virtually all acute illness. Failure to thrive may be precipitated or exacerbated by acute illness in those children with chronic symptoms and marginal calorie intake. Repeated measurements are helpful to monitor children who have prolonged hospital stays or repeated admissions. In susceptible children, monitoring of weight during the stay in hospital is indicated and the need for nutritional support should be anticipated.

NUTRITIONAL INTAKE

Anorexia is the norm in acute respiratory admissions and recovery of appetite is a marker of improvement. Food intake is recorded routinely for most admissions but is somewhat subjective. Drug treatment (particularly oral steroids) may stimulate hunger.

INTERPRETATION

For the three commonest admission diagnoses (croup, bronchiolitis and asthma) there have been numerous attempts to make scoring systems for illness severity. The number of different systems used highlights, firstly, the need for objective measurement of these conditions and, secondly, the lack of agreement on the components of the score and the relative weighting for each. To some extent the need for scoring systems is driven by the lack of other measures or their inappropriateness, e.g. use of lung function tests such as peak flow in preschool children. However, it is also the case that they are used to portray a more global view of the illness related to clinical practice. As such they are attempts to validate clinical examination and our concept of illness. The latter can be seen from a variety of perspectives so it is unlikely that a one-dimensional score can fully satisfy our wishes.

The scores have been used in two main ways:

- to evaluate the effect of treatment (i.e. trend monitoring);
- to assess severity and predict outcome (e.g. does the patient need admission, intensive care etc.).

Although the scores of a group of children may show changes reflecting other measures of outcome, the use of a scoring system to document change in an individual is more difficult. It is common practice in many hospitals to use scores on individuals in this way but there is very little data to justify it.

CROUP

In addition to the standard components that have been used in croup scores (Table 5.3), heart rate, respiratory rate and temperature are usually recorded but not incorporated as part of the score. Published croup scores are fairly consistent in their component parts. This is because upper airway obstruction is a relatively circumscribed entity. However, there is variation in the relative importance of usual features of the syndrome[6] versus rare but important features like level of consciousness.[7] Few correlations of scores or their component parts to other measures of severity or outcome are available to validate them. Kristjanson et al.[8] reported no correlation of the score with SaO_2 but this is not surprising as gas exchange is only affected with severe degrees of upper airway obstruction.

BRONCHIOLITIS

Of the components for bronchiolitis scores (Table 5.4), heart rate, respiratory rate and SaO_2 were measured in virtually all publications but not used as part of the scoring system. Recession (i.e. work of breathing) and severity of wheeze are the key features identified by the scores but measured in different ways. Recession is measured as a single item in some studies[9] and divided into supraclavicular retraction, intercostal retraction and chest indrawing by others.[10] In one study[11] the overall score was correlated with the need for further treatment with a correlation co-efficient of 0.647. The individual components of the score with the best correlations were; wheeze (0.69), intercostal recession (0.67) and chest indrawing (0.59). There was only a weak correlation with respiratory rate (0.39) and SaO_2 (-0.29). In addition Sanchez et al.[12] found no correlation between the bronchiolitis score and total airway resistance. Crepitations, although a frequent clinical sign of acute bronchiolitis, do not normally contribute to scores.

The populations used in the different studies varied which may affect the generalizability of the results but it is clear that the scores do measure something which correlates with other measures of outcome although they are by nature subjective.

ASTHMA

The factors measured in published studies of asthma scores are given in Table 5.5. These are particularly relevant in younger children (<6 years) where there is no possibility of measuring peak flow (or other tests of lung function). They are widely reported in papers evaluating effects of treatment on groups of subjects.[13,14]

All scores recorded wheeze (and/or breath sounds) and some measure of respiratory distress (e.g. use of accessory muscles, retraction, dyspnoea) but the weighting of these items varied.

Table 5.3: Croup scores[6,7,8]

Item	Recommended
SaO_2 /colour	+++
Stridor	+++
Cough	+++
Recession	+++
Respiratory distress	++
Air entry	+
Level of consciousness	+

+++ = in virtually all scores
 ++ = in the majority
  + = occasionally

Table 5.4: Bronchiolitis scores[9–12,14]

Item	Recommended
Signs of recession	+++
Wheeze	+++
Grunting	+
Respiratory rate	+
Air entry	+
Air hunger	+
General appearance	+
Cyanosis	+

+++ = in virtually all scores
 ++ = in the majority
  + = occasionally

Table 5.5: Asthma scores[13, 14]

Item	Recommended
Wheeze/breath sounds	+++
Respiratory distress	+++
Respiratory rate	++
Mental state	++
Pulse rate	++
Cyanosis	+
Pulsus paradoxus	+
I:E ratio	+
Speech impairment	+

+++ = in virtually all scores
 ++ = in the majority
  + = occasionally

Most scores included respiratory rate and decreasing numbers used mental state assessment (anxiety, fatigue), pulse rate, pulsus paradoxus, inspiratory:expiratory breathing ratio, and speech impairment. Scores used for evaluative purposes (i.e. trend over a period of time) tended to place more emphasis on respiratory rate and pulse rate. In general, asthma scores showed some correlation with other measures of asthma severity and to that extent have some validity. However, the degree of correlation varied from study to study and in many studies was reported as being consistent with other measures but not statistically analysed. It is clear that radiological changes bear no relation to asthma scores.

In general asthma scores are more sensitive than specific in predicting the requirement for hospital treatment. Scores may have some value in monitoring change in clinical condition and response to treatment in individuals but the evidence base for this is lacking.

HOW TO INTEGRATE RESULTS INTO MANAGEMENT

The plethora of respiratory scoring systems in paediatrics gives two messages to clinicians. Firstly, there is a need both clinically and for research purposes to accurately measure severity of disease and secondly, there is a lack of agreement on the best way of doing this. For monitoring individual children there is also a balance between tests/observations that have a poor predictive power but are easy and reproducible and those that have better predictive power but are invasive or very subjective.

In measuring illness we are trying to put a value on how ill a child is. This begs the question of what we mean by 'ill'. Some scoring systems for croup, for instance, put a high weighting on the rare but serious adverse events of cyanosis and loss of consciousness. These scores are designed to predict need for intubation or high dependency monitoring in hospital which is very different from using a croup score to monitor the resolution of the illness or response to steroid or nebulized adrenaline treatment. In other words, the observations need to be tailored to a purpose.

For common respiratory illnesses the most important single observation is the degree of respiratory distress which has a consistently high correlation with other measures of severity. The problem has always been the subjective nature of the measurements. Anyone with experience of trying to observe the effect of bronchodilators on an infant wheezer will know how difficult it is to define. In addition, a few children do not display signs of respiratory distress when they 'should'. Children with neurological or neuromuscular disease may not be capable of responding to a respiratory stress and children with chronic respiratory disease may have patho-physiological or behavioural adaptations to reduce their perceived distress. In these groups, blood gas measurements are necessary.

The widespread use of oxygen saturation monitoring has been a great advance for the care of children in hospital and is recommended for all children admitted with a respiratory problem. For high risk patients and those on supplementary oxygen, continuous SaO_2 monitoring is appropriate. It will be abnormal in both type 1 and type 2 respiratory failure but is unsatisfactory as an early marker of upper airway obstruction. In fact, a fall in SaO_2 in obstructive disease (whether due to laryngeal obstruction in croup, or pharyngeal obstruction in obstructive sleep apnoea) should ring warning bells, as it implies probable under-ventilation with hypercapnia and respiratory acidosis.

Hypoxaemia in acute respiratory disease is a measure of disease severity and resolves as the disease improves. Recovery of a normal SaO_2 is not critical to discharge home provided the overall clinical progress is good. For chronic disease the picture is different. Chronic hypoxaemia eventually leads to pulmonary hypertension and cor pulmonale. In children at risk, SaO_2 levels should be kept near normal (> 94% is an arbitrary limit often used) and this may delay discharge or lead to consideration of home oxygen treatment.

CLINICAL RESEARCH ISSUES

One approach to progress in monitoring respiratory disease is to use the parameters available to us now and develop more appropriate scoring systems. The objective is to emulate what the experienced clinician would do and assumes that their decision making is the standard to be aimed at. This is more difficult than it sounds as, how ill a child is at one point in time is not measured on a single scale. It is influenced by (amongst others) the degree of functional impairment seen, the projected natural history of the illness with or without treatment, the risk of an adverse event and the subjective experience of the child (or, more commonly, the projection of the clinician of what the child may be experiencing). There may be some merit in asking how the clinical decision making process is influenced, but a comprehensive answer is likely to be too complex for hospital ward application. Alternatively, scoring systems with more circumscribed objectives could be developed which would, for instance, predict the need for assisted ventilation, or need for admission to hospital.

Alternatively, there are avenues for exploring new ways of monitoring illness. There is a need for objective, non-invasive measurements, which correlate with outcome measures and a number of possibilities are mentioned below. Standard lung function testing is difficult in young children where co-operation is not possible. Modifications, such as the respiratory jacket to produce forced expiratory flow volume loops and occlusion techniques, have extended lung function testing to infants but the techniques are useful for research rather than clinical management. End-tidal CO_2 measurement is used in ventilated patients but the application to spontaneously breathing children is technically difficult. Development of non-invasive arterial pH and CO_2 estimation would make blood gas estimation accessible outside the intensive care and acute resuscitation environments. It is possible that research into breath sound analysis will lead to a system for monitoring severity in croup and possibly asthma and bronchiolitis. If respiratory distress is such an important sign there would be great value in a test that could give a numerical value to respiratory effort. Unfortunately measurement of respiratory effort is difficult and the values are very dependent on the pattern of breathing which changes from minute to minute. Finally, the elucidation of the inflammatory process may lead to inflammatory markers, patterns of markers or cells which predict particular outcomes or which can be used serially to measure progress.

REFERENCES

1. Platt MJ. Trends in childhood disease. *Curr Paediatr* 1998; **8**: 167–72.

2. Strachan DP, Anderson HR. Trends in hospital admission rates for asthma in children. *BMJ* 1992; **304**: 819–20.

3. Ninan T, Russell G. Respiratory symptoms and atopy in Aberdeen schoolchildren: evidence from two surveys 25 years apart. *BMJ* 1992; **304**: 873–5.

4. Anderson HR, Butland BK, Strachan DP. Trends in prevalence and severity of childhood asthma. *BMJ* 1994; **308**: 1600–4.

5. Morley C. Identification of infants at risk of acute illness. *Paediat Respir Med* 1994; **2**: 31–5.

6. Godden CW, Campbell MJ, Hussey M, Cogswell JJ. Double blind placebo controlled trial of nebulised budesonide for croup. *Arch Dis Child* 1997; **76**: 155–8

7. Cruz MN, Stewart G, Rosenberg N. Use of dexamethasone in the outpatient management of acute laryngotracheitis. *Pediatrics* 1995; **96**: 220–3

8. Kristjansson S, Berg-Kelly K, Winso E. Inhalation of racemic adrenaline in the treatment of mild and moderately severe croup. Clinical symptom score and oxygen saturation measurements for evaluation of treatment effects. *Acta Paediat* 1994; **83**: 1156–60.

9. Schuh S, Canny G, Reisman JJ, Kerem E, Bentur L, Petric M, Levison H. Nebulised albuterol in acute bronchiolitis. *J Pediat* 1990; **117**: 633–7.

10. Klassen TP, Rowe PC, Sutcliffe T, Ropp LJ, McDowell IW, Li MM. Randomised trial of salbutamol in acute bronchiolitis. *J Pediat* 1991; **118**: 807–11

11. Gadomski AM, Aref GH, El Din OB, El Sawy IH, Khallaf N, Black RE. Oral versus nebulised albuterol in the management of bronchiolitis in Egypt. *J Pediat* 1994; **124**: 131–8.

12. Sanchez I, De Koster J, Powell RE, Wolstein R, Chernick V. Effect of racemic epinephrine and salbutamol on clinical score and pulmonary mechanics in infants with bronchiolitis. *J Pediatr* 1993; **122**: 145–51.

13. van der Windt DA, Nagelkerke AF, Bouter LM, Dankert-Roelse JE, Veerman AJP. Clinical scores for acute asthma in pre-school children. A review of the literature. *J Clin Epidemiol* 1994; **47**: 635–46.

14. de Blic J, Thomson A. Short-term clinical measurement: acute severe episodes. *Eur Respir J* 1996; **9** (Suppl. 21): 4s–7s.

CHAPTER SIX

MEASURING CHRONIC ILLNESS AT HOME AND AT SCHOOL

A . B r o o k e

- Background information
- Symptoms
- Lung function

- Areas for future study
- References
- Further reading

BACKGROUND INFORMATION

The effective management of any medical condition depends upon the ability of the clinician to gauge accurately the level of severity of illness in the individual patient. In respiratory disease the clinician can use symptoms as subjective markers of illness severity whilst physiological measurements provide objective data. The relative contribution of these two streams of data will depend on the condition, the availability of applicable physiological measurement tools, the age of the child and finally the interrogative and integrative skills of the clinician. It is the integration of symptomatic information with physiological data that allows accurate and relevant assessment of the child's level of illness. In this way the most suitable options for both short- and long-term treatment may be decided. The appropriate education of the child with regard to the perception and control of their illness can be guided and useful insight can be gained into the functioning of the child and the family and the functional impact of disease. All these factors serve to optimize treatment and to inform guided self-management.

SYMPTOMS

SUBJECTIVE MARKERS OF RESPIRATORY ILLNESS

The symptoms of respiratory illness are well known (Box 6.1) and have been dealt with in Chapter 2. The information on symptoms may come from the child or the child's carers. The severity of symptoms may change depending on the setting in which the child is seen, leading to apparent contradictions. For example, the parents of asthmatic children often deny exercise limitation at home whilst the children themselves complain of severe activity-limiting symptoms at school. Others will be said by their parents to be only moderately affected and yet frequent school absence is attributed directly to the burden of their respiratory symptoms. Some respiratory symptoms appear to be better recalled by patients/carers than others.[1] Using symptoms as a method of assessing disease severity is hampered by the poor correlation in some individuals between symptoms and measured physiological disturbance.[2] Given the perceptual vagaries of symptoms, as well as the need for technical and physiological interpretation of many lung function tests, it is not always clear which means of assessment is 'best'. Information

---

Box 6.1: Symptoms of respiratory illness

Cough ± sputum (volume and colour)[*]

Wheeze, chest tightness

Shortness of breath

Stridor or noisy breathing

Exercise limitation

Symptoms of chronic respiratory failure or sleep disruption – morning headache, sleep disturbance and excessive day-time somnolence

Going grey or blue (cyanosis[†])

Changes in pattern of breathing: pauses or rapid breathing

---

[*] In young children, a moist cough ('like a smoker') is equivalent to a productive cough in an older subject.

[†] Whilst this is strictly speaking a sign, it is often reported by the parents and as such is used as a symptomatic marker.

from both, where available, should be integrated into management.

The pattern, severity and trend of respiratory symptoms may be important. For example, the child with episodic wheeze that occurs only with intercurrent respiratory tract infections may be distinguished from a child of a similar age with persistent wheeze made worse by a variety of triggers. Whilst both children wheeze, they may have a very different long-term prognosis.[3] The character of intermittent episodes of barking cough for example, put together with other associated respiratory symptoms may allow the child with recurrent spasmodic croup (a putative atopic condition) to be discriminated from another with cough secondary to chronic upper respiratory tract disease. The symptomatic trend may be important; cough which follows an acute episode of lower respiratory tract infection and shows no sign of abating may lead the clinician to suspect an underlying structural or host-defence problem. The association of cough with sleep disturbance may prove informative in the absence of asthma; it may suggest gastro-oesophageal reflux. In children with chronic

neuromuscular weakness, sleep disturbance accompanied by daytime somnolence and difficult behaviour may suggest sleep apnoea syndrome, while early morning headache may lead the clinician to suspect respiratory failure. Teachers may be the first to notice these symptoms. Children with cerebral palsy may experience cough during feeding due to incoordinate swallowing leading to aspiration; others may exhibit periodic stridor secondary to bulbar spasticity. An informative and often clear relationship between these symptoms and feeding can be elicited by talking to carers at home or at school.

QUANTIFYING SYMPTOMS: DIARY CARDS

The severity of symptoms can be quantified by using symptom diaries; the best examples being those used for asthma. These tools allow the daily logging of various respiratory symptoms and, for school children, are often recorded in conjunction with objective measures of lung function (usually peak flow), the frequency and amount of any prescribed treatments and other significant events in the patient's daily life (Figure 6.1). Their use is a good example of the integrative process alluded to above and allows children, their carers and the clinician to gauge current state of disease, current control, and response to treatment. This can be extremely useful in some patients: pre-school children are unable to reliably use tools to objectively measure lung function and therefore diary cards may be the only way of quantifying symptomatology which, in this age group, probably best defines disease severity (Case study 6.1). Unfortunately the evidence to validate and standardize these instruments is lacking. Many symptom scales have been developed for clinical use or for research in surveys or therapeutic trials. They may not be interchangeable and it could be argued that only diary instruments sensitive to changes in respiratory symptomatology should be used in management. Only one such instrument (Figure 6.2), for use in asthmatics, has been validated in this way,[4] but is appropriate only in the context of a clinical trial.

Case study 6.1: Monitoring symptoms in a wheezy child

Dion, a 4-year-old child with wheezing in response to various triggers since 1 year old and with multiple food allergies presented to his general practitioner with worsening nocturnal cough over a 2 month period. His parents were unable to identify any changes to the child's environment or any specific triggers for the cough. Treatment at the time consisted of inhaled corticosteroids and β_2 agonists delivered using a metered dose inhaled via a spacer device. Clinical examination of the chest was normal.

Dion's parents were asked to log cough, exercise limitation and wheeze daily for a fortnight before doubling the dose of inhaled steroid, after which the symptom diary was to be continued for a further month.

At follow-up, the diary showed that the cough was unresponsive to the increase in inhaled steroids, although the amount of recorded wheeze had decreased and exercise tolerance had improved. His chest remained clear on examination, but enlarged tonsils were noted; direct questioning of the parents elicited a history of nocturnal snoring and restlessness. Referral to an otolaryngologist resulted in the child undergoing tonsillectomy and adenoidectomy with complete resolution of the cough.

The child's cough was not due to asthma. A diary helped to quantify the response of both the wheeze and cough to changes in inhaled therapy and allowed this conclusion to be drawn. The importance of further questioning and reassessment is emphasized.

PREDICTIVE POWER OF SYMPTOM SCORES AND RELATIONSHIP WITH OBJECTIVE MEASURES OF LUNG FUNCTION

Single studies looking at physiological measurements in younger school age children show that for wheeze, symptom severity is reflected closely by reduced measures of lung function and increased levels of bronchial responsiveness.[1] The long-term epidemiological evidence available from both single and longitudinal studies suggests that wheeze severity in young children correlates with poor physiological and symptomatic outcomes in later childhood and adult life[5]; thus quantifying wheezing severity as objectively as possible and using it to guide management seems robust. The effect on prognosis of gaining control of the disease early after its onset has yet to be demonstrated.

When cough is the sole respiratory complaint it is less strongly related to reduced lung function recorded at the time. It also relates poorly in the longer term to symptomatic outcome. Whilst data generated from the clinic populations of children with chronic cough show a high proportion with poor symptomatic and physiological outcome, the epidemiological evidence does not support this. Population-based data suggest that chronic cough in young children is a poor predictor of reduced lung function or adverse long-term symptomatic outcome when compared to wheezy children. On the other hand, productive cough in children with chronic pulmonary sepsis is highly correlated to changes in lung function and the importance of early recognition of this symptom in order to commence appropriate therapy cannot be overstated. Quantification of the respiratory symptoms of cystic fibrosis can be achieved by administering standardized questionnaires or management sheets within the cystic fibrosis clinic, although the correlation between symptomatic and spirometric changes is weak.[6] Monitoring of respiratory illness in which chronic pulmonary sepsis is the main feature is probably best focused during the early stages upon early recognition of infective exacerbations. Later on in the natural history of the disease symptomatic and spirometric changes may be more important in deciding the timing of definitive procedures such as transplantation.

The effectiveness of diary keeping however is limited by the motivation of the patient to maintain the record accurately and of the clinician to demonstrate its usefulness to the diarist. The data obtained from epidemiological studies has been of limited accuracy and therefore may reduce the effectiveness of this tool for the purposes of disease monitoring.[7,8] Intervention studies have shown that the use of symptom-based diary cards to drive self-management of asthma is as effective as using peak flow monitoring,[9] and that in childhood asthma, routine peak flow monitoring contributes little to management.[10] It should be reserved for specific situations: 'brittle' asthma, changes in maintenance therapy or for 'poor perceivers'.

LUNG FUNCTION

OBJECTIVE MEASURES OF RESPIRATORY DISEASE

A wealth of research data exists to demonstrate the relationship between indices of lung function and symptomatic and prognostic outcomes. Whilst the laboratory has many different methods of measuring lung function, those available for ambulatory use are limited. Devices must be cheap, accurate, reliable, reproducible, easy for the patient to use and appropriate for the age of the child. Finally the changes in lung function must bear some relationship to the course of the child's illness. The devices most commonly used are peak flow meters. Increasingly miniature electronic spirometers are becoming available to measure other indices derived from forced expiratory manoeuvres such as the FEV_1, FVC and mid-expiratory flow (MEF_{50}). Recording spirometers (which can be downloaded via a computer) obviate the need for a written record. Using these tools at home can potentially provide more useful data on the degree of physiological disturbance from day to day than can be obtained from a single set of readings in clinic. In children with chronic pulmonary sepsis their use has the theoretical advantage of reduced risk of microbial cross-contamination compared with devices used at a clinic by many patients. The daily recording and integration of the objective data on lung function with symptomatic information affords the clinician, and the patient, insight into the degree of disease control. It can further allow (in conditions such as asthma) the identification of specific triggers that exacerbate the illness and can provide early warnings of impending deterioration; this in turn allows early treatment to commence and hence results in reduced morbidity. Where the use of integrated lung function and symptom diary proves successful, comprehensive self-management plans can be formulated on the basis of pre-determined changes in lung function (Chapter 24).

PEAK FLOW

The peak flow meter remains the most widely used tool for monitoring lung function. Many different types are available although accuracy varies between models,[11] mainly because most have 'non-linear' scales. In the United Kingdom they can be issued free to children. The accuracy with which these meters reflect the level of lung function[11] and more importantly clinically relevant changes in disease severity[12] has been questioned recently. The robustness and ease of use of the peak expiratory flow meter lends itself to use in ambulatory monitoring in childhood. The absolute value of peak flow in relation to reference data[13] is of limited use, because of the wide normal range. Its main usefulness lies in detecting changes in airway calibre and time-based changes in airflow limitation. Airway lability has been shown to be increased in adult asthmatics,[14] and in children.[15] The airway undergoes diurnal variation in calibre and is lower in the morning than in the afternoon. In asthma this variability is exaggerated and can be seen on a diary record as morning dipping (Case study 6.2). The degree of morning dipping has been correlated to the presence of nocturnal symptoms[16] and morning chest tightness in adults. Summary measures of peak flow variability have been used by some to diagnose asthma (an index of 'diurnal variation'). The unimodal distribution of this variable and its large overlap between asthmatic and non-asthmatic populations (particularly in children) preclude its use (i.e. it is neither sensitive nor specific for asthma diagnosis or management). In clinical practice, the integrative skill of assessing the degree of variability and its relation to symptoms from a peak flow/symptom diary card provides the most clinically useful data. The same integrative skills allow the interpretation of changes in the underlying base line (mean peak flow rate) around which the record varies (Case study 6.2) in relation to symptomatic data. Sometimes the absence of variability of PEF can be as important as its presence (Case study 6.3).

Despite the undoubted usefulness of peak flow meters, the relation between changes in peak flow

Case study 6.2: Peak flow monitoring

Nisha, a 12-year-old girl with spina bifida and asthma treated with inhaled corticosteroids and ß₂ agonists presented with a history of increasing cough and chest tightness, particularly in the morning. Twice daily peak flow monitoring (Figure 6.1) was agreed and a follow-up 2 weeks later showed morning dipping and excessive peak flow variability on a depressed baseline (her previous best score had been 380 L/min). She was advised to add a long-acting ß₂ agonist whilst continuing to keep a record of her peak flow readings. Her symptoms quickly settled and reinspection of the diary record at follow-up showed a higher mean peak flow with less diurnal variation and much less marked morning dipping.

Interpretation

The subject had symptoms of poorly controlled asthma, although her skeletal problems served to confuse the clinical picture. Confirmation that the symptoms were indeed attributable to asthma was gained from the peak flow data showing excessive variability. Further evidence was obtained from the patient's response to treatment.

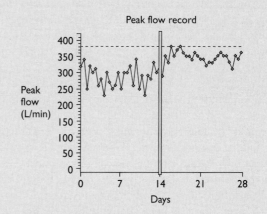

Figure 6.1: Peak flow record.

and meaningful changes in disease severity is not close in every individual.[9] The clinician needs to be aware of invented results: one study showed that up to one quarter of recorded daily readings had been invented by the diarist.[17] Careful comparison of the symptom diary and of the changes in peak flow may provide clues to the accuracy and reliability of the record. Their use in children should only be commissioned when the results are likely to be useful in predicting changes in disease state or in helping guide therapy.

FORCED EXPIRATORY MANOEUVRES

The forced vital capacity manoeuvre has been shown to have acceptable reproducibility in children of 7 years or over.[18] Hand held devices that record this data are available. In addition to giving the information to the subject, they have the ability to store records that can be downloaded onto a computer and to compute the measured indices in relation to sex-height related reference data. In this way it is possible to present relatively complicated data in a meaningful way to the patient; initial studies of adults using spirometry to track changes in lung function have demonstrated its feasibility. Although theoretically more accurate than peak flow monitoring, the added expense and complexity of the information obtained means that the devices are currently rarely used, and indeed their superiority has not been demonstrated for domiciliary use.

Case study 6.3: Isolated cough

Colin, a 6-year-old presented to clinic with a four month history of persistent cough without wheeze. The cough was worse in the day time and on exercise. Examination was uninformative, as was spirometry in the clinic. He was instructed in the use of a peak flow device and given a diary card to record symptoms and peak flow. At follow-up 4 weeks later, the symptoms had improved and the peak flow record revealed virtually no PEF variability around a mean value within the normal range for this height.

Here a 'negative' result effectively ruled out asthma. As in most cases such as this,[19] spontaneous recovery occurred.

OXIMETRY

Chronic lung disease of prematurity, is the commonest paediatric indication for domiciliary and portable oxygen therapy. Oxygen therapy can be monitored most effectively by pulse oximetry in the home. Monitoring is usually carried out intermittently at home under the supervision of a paediatric respiratory nurse specialist. Monitors store the data which can then be analysed later. Overnight recordings provide two pieces of information. Firstly, the mean level of oxygen saturation can be used to determine a child's need for, and amount of additional inspired oxygen. Secondly, episodes of nocturnal hypoxaemia can be identified allowing appropriate investigation and treatment. Because of the shape of the oxyhaemoglobin dissociation curve, small changes in arterial oxygen saturation may belie relatively large changes in the arterial partial pressure of oxygen (Chapter 21, p. 237). It is also informative to record a sleep–feed–awake cycle, to judge the overall state of oxygenation, in assessing infants with oxygen-dependent (or recently weaned) chronic lung disease, using a motion-compensated oximeter.

Overnight oximetry at home can be clinically useful in the investigation of children with sleep disruption of unknown cause and possible obstructive sleep apnoea and in the management of neuromuscular or skeletal disorders associated with hypoventilation during sleep (Case study 6.4). In these groups of patients, the solution to nocturnal hypoxaemia or hypoxic spells rarely lies in the provision of oxygen therapy!

GROWTH

Both respiratory illnesses and their treatments can have an effect on growth. Untreated asthma, poorly controlled chronic pulmonary sepsis (bronchiectasis) and chronic lung disease of prematurity with inadequate oxygenation may all hamper normal growth. However the number of patients with these clinical problems is small compared with the larger number of patients taking inhaled steroids to treat their respiratory disease. Whilst growth suppression is unlikely in children taking less than 400 micrograms per day of inhaled steroid (beclomethasone dipropionate equivalent), vigilance is required in all children taking steroids and hence routine measurement of attained height and weight are recommended (Case study 6.5).

Case study 6.4: Noisy breathing during sleep

Tim was a 4-month-old infant who had snored during sleep since a few days after birth. His sleep was described as 'restless' and he awoke almost every hour, sweaty and irritable. His weight gain was poor. During the day, he had snuffly breathing most of the time. On examination when quiet, he had snuffles and mild chest recession on inspiration. When crying, his chest was normal. Upper airway obstruction was suspected. Urgent overnight oximetry was arranged to assess the severity of the problem, while imaging and endoscopy were set up (Figure 6.2).

Periods of quiet sleep with mean SaO_2 of 95–98% alternated with brief episodic hypoxaemic spells (SaO_2 down to 60%) and arousals. During these episodes, the alarm was triggered and his parents noted snoring and irregular pauses in breathing.

Interpretation

These simple observations indicated the life-threatening severity of the condition. Choanal stenosis was the cause.

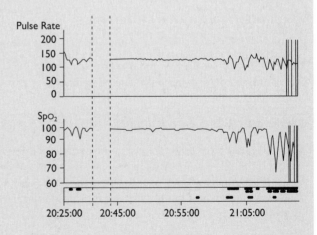

Figure 6.2: Overnight oximetry.

AREAS FOR THE FUTURE STUDY

Despite the received wisdom that monitoring of diseases such as asthma is best managed using symptom and peak flow diary cards, the literature pertaining to children with asthma provides little supporting evidence. The relative merits of using symptoms, lung function measurements, or both modalities could be relatively easily and robustly tested in a suitable population. The use of ambulatory spirometry in the management of the entire range of respiratory conditions and its superiority over simpler measurement techniques is yet to be fully demonstrated. The place of monitoring lung function in younger children using minimally invasive techniques such as the interrupter resistance (Rint) technique is becoming established (Chapter 7). Once the validity of the various monitoring techniques

described above has been established, their use can be turned to optimizing management in individual patients using well designed *n* of 1 trials.

REFERENCES

1. Brooke AM, Lambert PC, Burton PR, Clarke C, Luyt DK, Simpson H. The natural history of respiratory symptoms in preschool children. *Am J Respir Crit Care Med* 1995; **152**: 1872–8.

2. Couriel JM, Dennis T, Olinsky A. The perception of asthma. *Aust Paediat J* 1986; **22**: 45–7.

3. Godden DJ, Ross S, Abdalla M, *et al.* Outcome of wheeze in childhood: symptoms and pulmonary function 25 years later. *Am J Respir Crit Care Med* 1994; **149**: 106–12.

Case study 6.5: Stunted growth

A 10-year-old boy, Alan, was diagnosed as having asthma at the age of 3. From 6 months of life he had recurrent symptoms of intermittent cough, and persistent wheeze with associated mild breathlessness on exertion. There was a strong family history of atopy in both parents who had asthma. His symptoms remained troublesome despite early treatment with nebulized β_2 agonists initially, followed by inhaled steroids and bronchodilator. The dose of inhaled steroids had been increased over a period of two years until he was reviewed in the Paediatric Respiratory Clinic at the age of 5 where he continued to have symptoms of persistent breathlessness and cough, which was by then productive. On examination he had marked overinflation, widespread rattles and wheeze but no clubbing.

His growth chart at presentation (arrow) showed slowing of linear growth, which may have been partly the result of therapy (Figure 6.3). Growth pattern subsequently improved on lower doses of inhaled steroids.

Interpretation

High-dose inhaled steroids had probably slowed his growth velocity and as he remained symptomatic further investigations were performed, which revealed that he had a normal

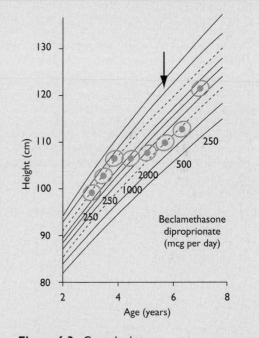

Figure 6.3: Growth chart.

sweat test, but co-existing IgG$_2$ deficiency with low functional antibodies for capsulated bacteria, and gastro-oesophageal reflux. His reflux was treated with H$_2$ receptor antagonists and antacids, and he was commenced on antibiotic prophylaxis, which resulted in an improvement in his symptoms and appetite and allowed his dose of inhaled steroid to be reduced with consequent acceleration in his height velocity.

4. Santanello NC, Davies G, Galant SP, *et al.* Validation of an asthma symptom diary for interventional studies. *Arch Dis Child* 1999; **80**: 414–20.

5. Roorda RJ. Prognostic factors for the outcome of childhood asthma in adolescence. *Thorax* 1996; **51** (Suppl. 1):S7–12.

6. Wall MA, LaGesse PC, Istvan JA. The 'worth' of routine spirometry in a cystic fibrosis clinic. *Pediat Pulmonol* 1998; **25**: 231–7.

7. Brooke AM, Lambert PC, Burton PR, Clarke C, Luyt DK, Simpson H. Night cough in a population-based sample of children: characteristics, relation to symptoms and associations with measures of asthma severity. *Eur Respir J* 1996; **9**: 65–71.

8. Archer LN, Simpson H. Night cough counts and diary card scores in asthma. *Arch Dis Child* 1985; **60**: 473–4.

9. Turner MO, Taylor D, Bennett R, Fitzgerald JM. A randomized trial comparing peak expiratory flow and symptom self-management plans for patients with asthma attending a primary care clinic. *Am J Respir Crit Care Med* 1998; **157**: 540–6.

10. Uwyyed K, Springer C, Avital A, Bar-Yishay E, Godfrey S. Home recording of PEF in young asthmatics: does it contribute to management? *Eur Respir J* 1996; **9**: 872–9.

11. Miller MR, Dickinson SA, Hitchings DJ. The accuracy of portable peak flow meters. *Thorax* 1992; **47**: 904–9.

12. Sly PD, Cahill P, Willet K, Burton P. Accuracy of mini peak flow meters in indicating changes in lung function in children with asthma. *BMJ* 1994; **308**: 572–4.

13. Wille S, Svensson K. Peak flow in children aged 4–16 years. Normal values for Vitalograph peak flow monitor, Wright and Mini Wright peak flow meters. *Acta Paediat Scand* 1989; **78**: 544–8.

14. Higgins B, Britton J, Chinn S, Jones T, Burney P, Tattersfield A. Relationship of peak flow variability to symptoms of asthma. *Thorax* 1998; **43**: P220.

15. Jamison JP, McKinley RK. Validity of peak expiratory flow rate variability for the diagnosis of asthma. *Clin Sci* 1993; **85**: 367–71.

16. Bellia V, Visconti A, Insalaco G, Cuttitta G, Ferrara G, Bonsignore G. Validation of morning dip of peak expiratory flow as an indicator of the severity of nocturnal asthma. *Chest* 1988; **94**: 108–10.

17. Verschelden P, Cartier A, L'Archeveque J, Trudeau C, Malo JL. Compliance with and accuracy of daily self-assessment of peak expiratory flows (PEF) in asthmatic subjects over a three month period. *Eur Respir J* 1996; **9**: 880–5.

18. Strachan DP. Repeatability of ventilatory function measurements in a population survey of 7 year old children. *Thorax* 1989; **44**: 474–9.

19. Fuller P, Picciotta A, Davies M, McKenzie SA. Cough and sleep in inner city children. *Eur Respir J* 1998; **12**: 426–31.

FURTHER READING

1. Silverman M, Pedersen S. Outcome measures in early childhood asthma and other wheezing disorders. *Eur Respir J* 1996; **9** (Suppl. 21): 1s–49s.

CHAPTER SEVEN

MEASURING LUNG FUNCTION

C. Beardsmore and M. Silverman

- Background
- Why perform lung function tests?
- How?
- Research issues

- Case studies
- References
- Further reading

BACKGROUND

APPLICATIONS

More than 25 years have elapsed since the publication of the first standard textbook on pulmonary function testing in children of school age by Polgar and Promadhat.[1] Studies in infants were being performed by the 1950s and 1960s, and have become more widespread over the past 15 years.[2] Whereas infants up to the age of approximately 18 months are generally studied during sleep or after sedation, the limited co-operation of pre-school children provides a challenge to the investigator and has restricted studies in this group. However, recent developments in technology and development of new tests have begun to close the gap in knowledge between infancy and school-age.

There are many facets to lung function testing (Figure 7.1). Blood gas analysis and oximetry constitute assessment of lung function, since normal values indicate adequate pulmonary function. However, the ability of the cardiorespiratory system to compensate means that blood gases can be normal in the presence of quite extensive disease. Such disease may commonly be assessed by measurements of lung mechanics, including assessment of maximal flows and distribution of lung volumes. Measures of ventilatory function can be complemented by those of pulmonary

blood flow and of the matching of ventilation and perfusion. Transfer of carbon monoxide from lung to blood can be measured in order to show whether there is limitation of diffusion across the alveolar wall. The lung is also metabolically active, and the cilia lining the respiratory tract have a role in mucus clearance. All these processes can be assessed. Finally, the rhythmicity and adequacy of breathing and its perception are controlled by the brain: control of breathing can be measured, most commonly during sleep. However, it is the measurements of lung mechanics and gas exchange which are more generally considered to constitute 'lung function', and it is these which will be mainly considered below.

DEVELOPMENTAL PHYSIOLOGY: REFERENCE VALUES

Changes in structure and function with age affect lung function, its measurement and interpretation. The greatest rate of change occurs in the period of adaptation of the neonate to extrauterine life, when failure to establish effective pulmonary perfusion, aeration of the lungs and regular tidal breathing can have lifelong adverse consequences. Mechanical function stabilizes over hours, vascular changes over days or weeks, and control of breathing over months, giving way to orderly growth (Table 7.1), although airways and

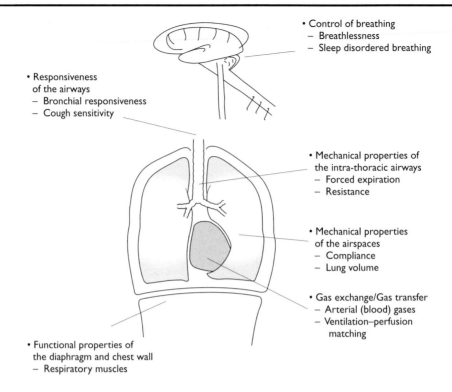

- Control of breathing
  - Breathlessness
  - Sleep disordered breathing

- Responsiveness
  of the airways
  - Bronchial responsiveness
  - Cough sensitivity

- Mechanical properties of
  the intra-thoracic airways
  - Forced expiration
  - Resistance

- Mechanical properties
  of the airspaces
  - Compliance
  - Lung volume

- Gas exchange/Gas transfer
  - Arterial (blood) gases
  - Ventilation–perfusion
    matching

- Functional properties of
  the diaphragm and chest wall
  - Respiratory muscles

Figure 7.1: What can be measured?

airspaces do not grow in proportion (i.e. growth is dysanaptic) in young children. Physiological differences important to an understanding of lung function measurement distinguish infants and older children (Box 7.1).

As well as having a feel for the normal, the clinician needs up-to-date sources of reference values for the relevant age groups and techniques (see Further Reading). Almost all are based on cross sectional studies and should not be interpreted 'as if' longitudinal. Pubertal state influences lung

Table 7.1: Lung function in healthy individuals

	Pre-term	Newborn	I year	7 years	Adult
Body weight (kg)	I	3	I0	25	70
Crown–heel length (cm)	35	50	75	I20	I75
Breathing frequency (per min)	60	45	30	20	I5
Tidal volume (mL)	7	21	70	I80	500
Anatomic dead space (mL)	3	6	20	50	I50
Maximal flow at FRC (or MEF$_{25}$) (mL/s)	80	50	300	950	2500
FEV$_1$ (mL)	–	–	–	I300	4200
FRC (mL)	25	85	250	750	2100
Lung compliance (mL/cmH$_2$O)	I.5	5	15	50	200
Airway resistance (cmH$_2$O/L/s)	80	40	15	4	2

Multiply compliance by 10 to obtain values in SI units (mL/kPa), divide resistance by 10 to obtain values as kPa/L/s.

Box 7.1: Physiological differences between infants and schoolchildren, which are important in lung function testing

- Nose breathing, the preferred route in infants, has several consequences:
  - increasing overall airway resistance
  - upper airway disorders limit most measurements of lung function
  - aerosols are preferentially deposited in the nose.

- Chest wall is more compliant (floppier) in infants:
  - lower relaxed end-expiratory lung volume therefore dynamic elevation of FRC and unstable end-expiratory lung volume
  - airway closure at end-tidal expiration
  - paradoxical (asynchronous) breathing common in disease (and normal pre-term infants) and in active sleep (REM sleep).

- Respiratory reflexes such as the Hering–Breuer reflex are stronger in infants, facilitating some measurements of passive mechanics.

Box 7.2: Applications of lung function tests

- Diagnosis
  - single observations rarely diagnostic, but occasionally confirmatory (Case study 7.1), or startling (Case studies 7.2 and 7.3)
  - sequential measurements may be more useful (Case study 7.4).

- Measuring morbidity
  - as guide to management (Case study 7.5)
  - baseline value for comparisons
  - disease progression.

- Assessing response to therapy
  - very short-term (e.g. bronchodilator responses)
  - acute therapy (e.g. in severe asthma, bronchiolitis)
  - long-term (e.g. monitoring CF or asthma).

- Teaching health professionals

- Research
  - developmental physiology
  - mechanisms of disease
  - epidemiology
  - therapeutic trials.

function, but its assessment may be inappropriate in the respiratory laboratory, so the clinician may need to use his judgement in selecting which set of predicted values to use.

The greatest developmental constraints apply to the performance of lung function tests. The need for sedation and for specialized equipment for most tests in infants, a playful environment for toddlers and an awareness of the self-consciousness of many teenagers are prerequisites to success in even the simplest procedures.

WHY PERFORM LUNG FUNCTION TESTS?

Lung function measurements are rarely diagnostic by themselves, but results can be taken together with history and clinical examination to point towards likely diagnoses. Clinical assessment is the most likely reason for testing children (Box 7.2). As with adults, repeat tests are often needed, perhaps on a single occasion for infants who are usually sedated for testing[3] or more often and over longer periods of time.[4]

Individual lung function tests may be used to measure complex lung functions. Bronchial responsiveness, for example, requires multiple measurements of (usually) FEV_1 or PEF, the results of which are integrated to provide an index of response to a challenge stimulus.

In clinical practice, as with any other investigation, the reason for performing a lung function test should be explicit: what question or problem will be resolved by this test? Whatever the reason, the results will contribute to management only after integration into a range of other clinical observations, measurements and investigations.

Finally, although most research projects are set up to answer clinical questions, there is an increasing emphasis on studying the healthy infant or child. This adds to our knowledge and understanding of growth and development of the respiratory system, and the epidemiological factors which control these.[5, 6]

How?

SCHOOLCHILDREN

Measurement conditions (Table 7.2)

Children over 6 or 7 years of age can be expected to participate fully in testing/using equipment designed for adults, given encouragement and positive feedback. In practice, most data in this group will be collected in the home, on electronic spirometers or peak flow meters. Compliance with the demands of home monitoring, and hence the amount of valid data recorded, is moderate at best.[7,8]

Children with neuromuscular disease may have difficulty with mouthpieces. In those with scoliosis, the appropriate reference values should be determined from arm span, which is normally equal to height.

AIRWAY FUNCTION: FORCED EXPIRATION

These include measurements of peak flow and electronic spirometry, which can readily be made in the home, the clinic or outpatient department, and at the bedside. The advantages of a portable test are (i) that serial measurements can be taken for an individual without the need for repeated visits to hospital, and (ii) many individuals can be tested at a single location, such as a school. Both peak flow meters and electronic spirometers can be purchased with integral data recording, dispensing with the need for paper records. Alternatively, some spirometers incorporate a printer so that results can be added to patient or subject notes.

Peak flow measurements

Peak expiratory flow (PEF) is defined as the maximum flow achieved during an expiration delivered with maximal force starting from the level of maximal lung inflation (total lung capacity: TLC). The value obtained may differ depending on the instrument used to measure it.[9] Most sets of predicted values for PEF have been obtained using Wright peak flow meters and are not suitable for use with measurements obtained from portable spirometers because the two types of instrument are not interchangeable.[10]

Most hand-held peak flow meters employ the principle of a variable orifice to measure airflow directly. The pressure exerted by a forced expiration causes a diaphragm or vane to move and, in so doing, to open a progressively larger area of the orifice. The point at which no further movement of the diaphragm occurs depends on the maximal

Table 7.2: Measurement conditions

	Infants	Toddlers	Schoolchildren
Where?	Dedicated lab (and bedside)	Any playful environment (and bedside)	Standard lab Outpatient clinic Home
Co-operation	Most lab-based studies need (sedated) sleep	Allow for measurements in unorthodox situations; on the floor or a parent's knee	Electronic monitors useful for domiciliary recordings Discreet facilities for teenagers
Equipment	Miniaturized Specific for nasal breathing (generally via facemask) and supine posture Suitable response for fast breathing (up to 100) Raw data available in real time and for analysis and quality control	Innovative and indestructible Capable of providing results during brief attention spans of toddlers Capable of displaying raw data for quality control if necessary Low range devices may be useful	Standard equipment appropriate Scales should be adaptable to expand display of graphical data for young children

pressure and hence on the peak expiratory flow which has been generated.[11] Portable peak flow meters have been available since 1976, primarily for single patient use at home in the management of asthma. The life of such a meter is usually stated as 3 years, but will depend on frequency and conditions of use and treatment. For clinical, single patient use, the most important feature is intra-instrument repeatability and consistency. For accuracy, the devices need to correlate with an accepted 'gold standard', for which the Wright peak flow meter was chosen.

There are various methods of calibrating peak flow meters and assessing their accuracy, linearity and reproducibility.[9, 11,12] For most instruments in everyday clinical use, such as the mini-Wright peak flow meter, the manufacturer's calibration will suffice, but for research purposes PEF meters should be calibrated directly.[9, 12]

HOW TO MEASURE PEAK FLOW

It is good practice to demonstrate the manoeuvre for a novice patient, ensuring that you inspire fully and use maximal effort. Ensure that the child is standing upright. The child should inspire fully, place lips around the mouthpiece and blow sharply and as hard as possible. It is not necessary to empty the lungs or sustain expiration. Note the reading, and praise the child. If the manoeuvre was unsatisfactory, demonstrate it again. Repeat the measurements until three satisfactory readings have been obtained, and record the highest. If no satisfactory readings are obtained after eight attempts, stop the measurements. It is unnecessary to use a noseclip, unless there is an oropharyngeal abnormality or muscle weakness.

Table 7.3: The adult oxygen dissociation curve (reduced)

Sao$_2$ (%)	Pao$_2$ (mmHg)	Pao$_2$ (kPa)
97.5	100	13.3
96	80	10.7
89	60	8.0
75	40	5.3
50	27	3.6

INTERPRETATION

Although it is generally easy to determine peak flow as the highest reading out of three satisfactory manoeuvres, possible reasons for variable results or apparently low readings within a single testing session include the introduction of the tongue into the mouthpiece, glottic closure (detected as grunting), blocking the orifice of the meter or impeding of the pointer, inadequate inspiratory effort (either failure to reach TLC, or slow start to expiration), or wheezing induced by repeated forced respiratory manoeuvres. When a technically satisfactory measurement has been achieved, the result should be compared with the predicted value and (where appropriate) previous measurements from the child.

The advent of the electronic spirometer has relegated PEF to three roles:

1 *diagnostic* and therapeutic home monitoring in asthma (Chapter 6);
2 as an adjunct to guided self-management for some children with difficult asthma, severe asthma or poor symptom perception (Chapter 24);
3 for speedy bronchodilator testing in the clinic or office; given the inherent repeatability of PEF (within-subject coefficient of variation 4.5%) a rise in PEF of over 10% is significant.

The forced vital capacity manoeuvre

PRINCIPLES

The era of the electronic spirometer has made the forced vital capacity manoeuvre and the maximum expiratory (and inspiratory) flow volume curve available to all. The technique is deceptively easy, but when carried out properly, provides sufficient physiological information for managing all but the rarest lung disorders in schoolchildren – the exceptions being disorders of gas exchange and control of (or sleep disordered) breathing. Because of its importance, the physiological basis of maximum flow will be briefly described and illustrated in Figure 7.2 (see Hughes and Pride 1999, Further Reading).

Following maximum inspiration, before expiration commences, the pressure throughout the airways and airspaces is atmospheric, and the maximally negative pleural pressure distends

(a) Tidal expiration

(b) Maximum forced expiration

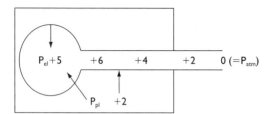
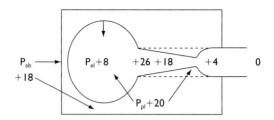

Figure 7.2: The concept of expiratory flow limitation (figures in cmH_2O). See text for explanation; P_{el} is elastic recoil pressure of the airspaces; P_{pl} is pleural pressure; P_{ab} is abdominal pressure; P_{atm} is atmospheric pressure.

the intra-pleural airways. During tidal expiration, pleural pressure becomes positive, and the summed elastic recoil of the lungs (P_{el}) and pleural pressure (P_{pl}) expel air, causing an intra-luminal pressure gradient (Figure 7.2a). The intra-luminal pressure is always greater than pleural pressure. During forced expiration, (Figure 7.2b) the airways are actually compressed distal to the equal pressure point (EPP) at which intra-luminal and pleural pressures are equal. Increased effort raises the pleural and intra-luminal pressures equally, producing no change in flow at the mouth. The properties of the airway wall at this point (its area and compliance) determine the value of flow. The smaller and floppier the airway, the lower the maximum flow at any particular lung volume.

Flow limitation probably occurs at all parts in the descending limb of the maximum expiratory flow-volume curve (including PEF). The flow limiting segment migrates from larger airways (the

trachea in normal subjects) to the periphery in the course of an expiration. Hence, flows close to TLC are said to reflect relatively large airway function and those closer to residual volume (RV), smaller airways. The reduction in airway calibre during forced expiration is sometimes referred to as dynamic airway narrowing.

The relationship between the traditional volume–time spirogram and the maximum expiratory flow–volume (MEFV) curve is shown in Figure 7.3; volume is the time integral of flow. Much more useful detail is discernible on the MEFV curve than the spirogram, but the dimension of time is missing!

Forced inspiration is limited only by effort, under normal circumstances, since the intra-thoracic airways are 'stretched' by respiratory effort (negative pleural pressure). Dynamic narrowing may occur, however, in the extra-thoracic airway.

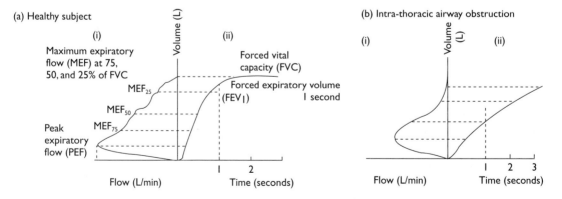

Figure 7.3: Maximum expiration: forced vital capacity (FVC). (i) Maximum expiratory flow–volume (MEFV) curve. (ii) Forced expiratory spirogram.

EQUIPMENT

Many different portable spirometers are available, ranging from simple, hand-held devices which give a digital readout of FVC, FEV_1 and PEF, to benchtop models which can display graphics and provide printouts of results. Most spirometers use either a pneumotachograph or a turbine to measure flow or volume, respectively. Flow is then integrated or volume differentiated to provide a complete portfolio of flow–volume measurements. More sophisticated devices will require the subject to inhale and exhale to provide inspiratory flows and volumes: simpler devices will record forced expiratory manoeuvres only. As with peak flow meters, some devices supplied for monitoring may function without regular calibration by the user, but others may permit or indeed require calibration. Calibration may be performed by hand using an accurate syringe, or by a pump connected to a waveform generator.[12]

Measurements made with a portable spirometer may be close to those made with a conventional, volume-displacement spirometer, but they are not identical and so the two types of instrument should not be used interchangeably.[13]

HOW TO PERFORM SPIROMETRY

As with other measurements, begin by explaining to the child what is required and demonstrate the manoeuvre, ensuring that you inspire fully and use maximal effort. The posture can be seated or standing, provided that consistency is maintained. If seated, the child should be sitting straight but comfortably. A noseclip is recommended for consistency, but if the child refuses to wear one it is not essential if pharyngeal function is normal, since positive mouth pressure closes the palatal 'valve'.

Follow manufacturer's guidelines for respiratory manoeuvres, noting whether a period of quiet breathing through the device should precede maximal inspiration and full forced expiration. Some devices allow full inspiration immediately after full forced expiration without a break, for calculation of inspiratory flows and volumes. This is important if you suspect central or extra-thoracic obstruction. Examine the reading, and praise the child. If the manoeuvre was unsatisfactory, demonstrate it again. Allow two practice blows and up to five definitive blows until three satisfactory readings have been obtained and record the best. If no satisfactory readings are obtained after

eight attempts, stop the measurement. The American Thoracic Society criteria for an acceptable value are: two best blows of FVC or FEV_1 within 5% or 200mL, whichever is the greater.[12]

The competence of the technician or other operator is fundamental to obtaining reliable data.[14] S/he must be able to coach children vigorously during forced expiratory manoeuvres, ensuring rapid inspiration to TLC followed swiftly by forceful expiration, sustained to residual volume and (where appropriate) a final forced inspiratory manoeuvre. The technician must remain sensitive to the requirements of the child since even suboptimal manoeuvres may be tiring or (if repeated in rapid succession) lead to light-headedness. Furthermore, s/he must be able to judge whether respiratory manoeuvres are technically acceptable.

INTERPRETATION

A device which can display graphics or print a flow–volume curve greatly facilitates interpretation of spirometry and is to be particularly recommended with children. Except in rare cases of fixed obstruction, a technically acceptable manoeuvre will result in a sharply defined peak flow occurring early in the breath (during the first 15% of vital capacity [VC]). If peak flow occurs later than this, the most usual explanation is submaximal effort at the outset of the manoeuvre (Figure 7.4). The terminal portion of the expiratory

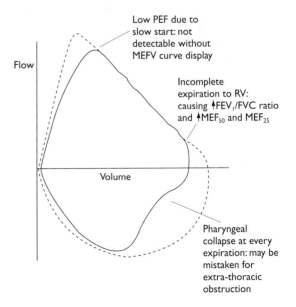

Low PEF due to slow start: not detectable without MEFV curve display

Incomplete expiration to RV: causing ↓FEV_1/FVC ratio and ↑MEF_{50} and MEF_{25}

Pharyngeal collapse at every expiration: may be mistaken for extra-thoracic obstruction

Figure 7.4: Common flow–volume artefacts.

flow–volume curve will approach residual volume smoothly: a sudden change in curve indicates either glottic closure or early onset of inspiration. Although repeated forced respiratory manoeuvres can invoke bronchoconstriction and attendant progressive changes in spirometry in a few asthmatics, repeatability is in general a good indicator of satisfactory respiratory manoeuvres. The inspiratory curve should be smooth; pharyngeal collapse may take a bite out of it (Figure 7.4). Practice may make perfect.

Repeat measurements of FVC and FEV_1 would normally be within 5%, although repeatability may be less good in the presence of disease and will certainly be worse in young children. In addition to FVC and FEV_1, maximum expiratory flows (MEF) at 75, 50, and 25% expired vital capacity are commonly reported. Where the forced inspiratory vital capacity is measured, both the peak inspiratory flow and the mid-inspiratory flow may be reported.

The absolute values of FEV_1 and FVC are important in interpretation, but both are reduced by differing degrees in obstructive disease (FEV_1/FVC <75–80%), restrictive disease (usually > 90%), or neuromuscular disease (variable). The normal FEV_1/FVC ratio in middle childhood is approximately 84% (range 79–92%). High values are more likely to result from incomplete expiration than restrictive disease and this should be checked. Small healthy children may complete forced expiration in less than one second, and in these individuals FEV_1/FVC will be 1.

The shape of the flow–volume loop provides as much information to the trained observer as the computed values (Figure 7.5). A flow–volume loop from a healthy child (Figure 7.5a) will have a fairly straight descending expiratory portion from

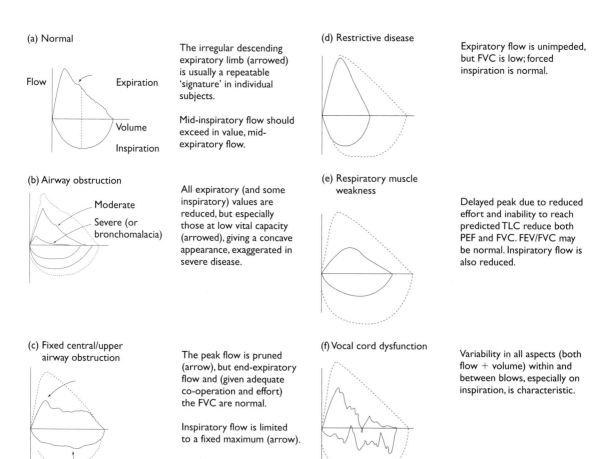

Figure 7.5: Characteristic maximum expiratory and inspiratory flow–volume curves.

peak flow to residual volume, with a rounded inspiratory section in which peak inspiratory flow occurs during the first half of the manoeuvre. The inspiratory flow at mid volume is slightly greater than mid-expiratory flow. In contrast, a child with asthma or other obstructive disease will have an expiratory flow–volume curve which is concave (Figure 7.5b). Flows measured late in vital capacity (e.g. MEF_{25}) will be proportionally reduced to a much greater extent than peak flow, which may remain within normal limits.

In severe obstructive airway disease the high positive pressures applied during forced expiration may enhance airway narrowing so that flow is even lower at a given lung volume than during tidal breathing (Figure 7.5b). This is called negative effort dependency of flow. Tracheo-broncho-malacia may result in airway collapse, usually towards end-expiration, which can give an irregular (and poorly reproducible) pattern to the expiratory flow–volume curve. This may be worsened following administration of β_2 agonists, which render the airway wall more floppy and prone to collapse.

Extra-thoracic obstruction is best detected by inspection of the inspiratory flow–volume curve (Figure 7.5c). The inspiratory flow–volume loop will show a characteristic flattened appearance which is mirrored in the expiratory loop if the cause is fixed (as opposed to dynamic) upper airway obstruction.

Fixed tracheal airway obstruction gives a characteristic truncated pattern during both expiration and inspiration which does not vary with broncho-dilators or exercise (Case study 7.3).

Restrictive patterns vary from the relatively normally shaped curves with reduced vital capacity (Figure 7.5d) to those associated with muscle weakness, which are blunted as well as reduced in capacity (Figure 7.5e).

The condition of vocal cord dysfunction can mimic (or accompany) asthma or upper airway disease (Case study 7.2). It may be episodic, but when active, may produce irregular and poorly repeatable expiratory and/or inspiratory flow–volume curves, often accompanied by exaggerated effort or difficulty breathing (Figure 7.5f).

MECHANICAL PROPERTIES OF THE LUNGS AND LUNG VOLUME

Lung volume

Vital capacity (VC) is the most commonly measured index of lung volume. However, it is a 'dynamic' volume (the maximum amount which can be breathed in or out from a position of full expiration or inspiration), and gives little indication of the absolute volume of air within the lungs at any time. The measurement of absolute lung volume which is most usually made is functional residual capacity (FRC), from which other divisions of lung volume can be derived. FRC is the volume of the lungs at the end of a tidal expiration, and under conditions of relaxation, and is determined by the balance of forces between the elastic recoil of the lungs and the chest wall. The lung volume following maximum inspiration is known as total lung capacity (TLC). Residual volume (RV) is the term used for the volume remaining in the lungs at the end of a maximum expiration (Figure 7.6).

Vital capacity is measured by spirometry, usually during forced expiration (forced vital capacity FVC); in continental Europe it is measured during inspiration from RV (inspiratory vital capacity IVC), avoiding dynamic airway narrowing, and giving a slightly greater value. A true reduction in vital capacity is important, but needs interpretation (Figure 7.7). In addition to their occasional role elucidating the cause of a reduced FVC, lung volume measurements are useful in monitoring the course of chronic progressive disorders such as CF or severe scoliosis, in order to decide the timing of a major intervention (such as lung transplantation or spinal corrective surgery, respectively) (Case study 7.4).

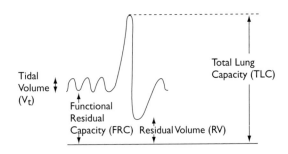

Figure 7.6: The divisions of lung volume.

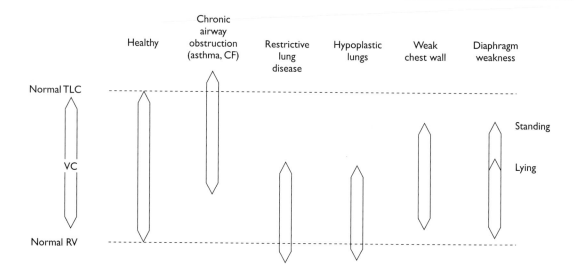

Figure 7.7: Causes of reduced vital capacity (VC).

Measurements of FRC are most commonly made by either gas dilution techniques or by plethysmography. Nitrogen washout is less commonly employed. Gas dilution techniques measure that airspace which is in communication with the airway opening and which is ventilated during tidal breathing: trapped gas is not measured. In contrast, the plethysmographic measurements include the volume of trapped gas. In healthy adults the two measurements will be close: in conditions such as advanced cystic fibrosis where there is a substantial degree of hyperinflation and trapped gas the two measurements will be discrepant.

HOW TO MEASURE LUNG VOLUME BY GAS DILUTION

The commonest gas used for this technique is a mixture of approximately 69% nitrogen, 21% oxygen, and 10% helium, which is inert and virtually insoluble. A closed spirometer (water-filled, bellows or rolling seal) is flushed with the gas mix and filled to a pre-set and known volume. The subject breathes through a mouthpiece and valve, breathing room air initially until respiratory pattern is stable. The operator switches the subject to rebreathing from the spirometer at the end of expiration. Over the next few minutes the concentration of helium will fall as air from the lungs and spirometer equilibrate, and the final, stable concentration of helium is recorded. The final

volume (spirometer plus lungs) can be calculated from the following equation:

$$\text{Final volume} = V_1 C_1 / C_2$$

where V_1 is the starting volume of the spirometer and C_1 and C_2 are the initial and final concentrations of helium, respectively. FRC can then be simply computed by subtracting the (known) spirometer volume from the final volume.

In practice, especially in obstructive airway disease, there is rarely an absolute cut-off between ventilated and non-ventilated regions of the lung: some regions may be slowly ventilated and the volume of these will be measured if sufficient time is allowed during the course of measurement.

HOW TO MEASURE LUNG VOLUME BY PLETHYSMOGRAPHY

In whole-body plethysmography the subject is seated within a sealed cabin, breathing through a pneumotachograph to record respiratory flow and volume, and an external airway which contains an occluding valve (Figure 7.8). During a short period when the valve is closed, the mass of gas within the chest remains fixed. The subject makes respiratory efforts against the closed airway and the pressure changes within the respiratory system are measured directly at the mouth. The volume changes are derived from the changes in

(a)

(b)

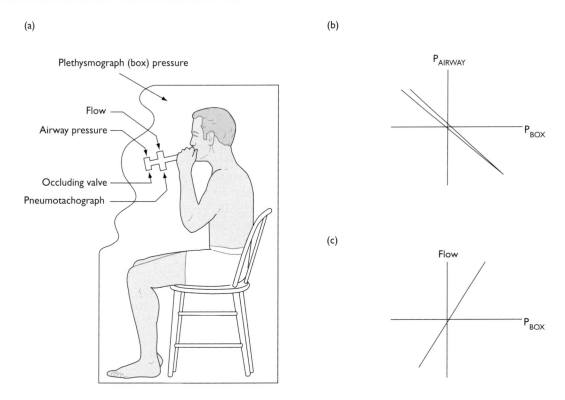

Figure 7.8: Whole body plethysmograph. (a) The equipment. (b) The slope of the relationship between airway (mouth) and box (plethysmograph) pressure during occlusion for FRC measurement is a function of lung volume. (c) The slope of the relationship between flow and box pressure during tidal breathing for resistance measurement is a function of airway resistance.

cabin pressure. The computation of lung volume (or, more accurately, thoracic gas volume) is achieved by the application of Boyle's law.[15] The method is quick and simple, and can be combined with measurements of airway resistance.

The technique assumes that pressure changes within the lung are evenly distributed and accurately transmitted to the airway opening. This assumption may not be valid in patients with severe airway obstruction, so that the measurement is inaccurate.[16] The effect is generally an overestimation of lung volume.[16, 17, 18] Errors in the technique can also be caused if the cheeks are flaccid and therefore get sucked in or blown outwards during the manoeuvre: for this reason the subject generally supports the cheeks with the hands during airway occlusion.

INTERPRETATION

In cases of restrictive disease, measurements of lung volume are essential for assessing severity and monitoring progress (Case study 7.4). Between plethysmographic measurements, vital capacity can be used to monitor more frequently. In this example the patient had a progressive scoliosis which required surgical intervention: serial measurements assisted in planning the timing of surgery, which is particularly important in paediatric patients who are still growing. In other cases, such as pectus excavatum, measurements of lung volume may reassure the clinician and the patient that the deficit is of no physiological consequence and surgery is not required (although in some cases it may be indicated on psychological grounds).

Plethysmographic measurements of FRC will indicate the degree of hyperinflation in patients with an obstructive condition. In the short term, this may be useful in asthmatic patients, where measurements before and after treatment can indicate whether the lung volume has normalized or not. Over longer periods extending into several years, measurements expressed in relation to predicted values can be useful in monitoring progress in conditions such as cystic fibrosis.

Resistance and compliance

Some techniques measure the airway resistance (R_{aw}) and others the respiratory system resistance as a whole (R_{rs}), including tissue resistance. Unlike spirometry, they do not require a full forced respiratory manoeuvre so have particular application in children with limited co-operation, or individuals with particularly sensitive airways in whom respiratory manoeuvres can provoke bronchoconstriction. Compliance is a measure of stiffness or distensibility of the respiratory system as a whole (C_{rs}) or of either of its components, the lungs (C_L) and the chest wall (C_w).

HOW TO MEASURE AIRWAY RESISTANCE

Plethysmographic method Resistance is calculated by dividing the pressure drop across the airways by the flow passing through (i.e., R = P/F). Flow is generally measured by a pneumotachograph attached to a mouthpiece. Since alveolar pressure cannot be measured directly, the measurement is made with the subject inside the whole body plethysmograph (Figure 7.8) so that changes in plethysmograph pressure during breathing can be used as a surrogate for alveolar pressure.

The relationship between pressure and flow is usually displayed on a screen, and in a healthy person this approximates a straight line with some curvature at either end at points of maximal flow. Resistance is usually reported at flows of 0.5 or 1.0 L/second, or a value approximating to the linear portion of the pressure–flow relationship is taken. The reciprocal of resistance, conductance, may be reported instead. This is because the relationship between resistance and lung volume is parabolic whereas that between conductance and volume is a straight line, facilitating calculation of specific conductance which is independent of lung volume.

Plethysmographic resistance is useful in the occasional patient who cannot perform forced manoeuvres (such as a sensitive asthmatic). Complex airway disease is better investigated by imaging (CT or MRI) or bronchoscopy than by plethysmography.

Interrupter method Flow is measured directly, usually with a pneumotachograph, during quiet breathing. A rapidly-closing valve is incorporated into the breathing apparatus which is triggered to close either at set points in the cycle or at random. The duration of closure is about 100 milliseconds. Pressure at the airway opening is measured during the period of valve closure. This shows an initial rapid rise with some transient oscillations, followed by a slow rise to a plateau which equates to alveolar pressure (Figure 7.9). Resistance is calculated by dividing this pressure (extrapolated back to the point of valve closure) by flow at the point of interruption to give the interrupter resistance (R_{int}).

This deceptively simple technique has several potential drawbacks. Because much of the change of airway pressure during occlusion is dissipated across the compliant upper airway (especially the cheeks), changes in R_{int} after an intervention are likely to be underestimated. The error is greater when true airway resistance is high. In addition, changes in glottic narrowing during the procedure will directly affect the value of R_{int}, adding variability, especially for younger children. Nevertheless, in practice, this portable technique is a valuable addition, since it allows speedy measurements during tidal breathing.[19]

Total resistance method with oesophageal catheter This technique was more commonly used with infants than adults or older children. An oesophageal catheter (either liquid-filled or covered with a small balloon) is passed through the mouth and detects changes in pleural pressure, which are assumed to equate to changes in pleural pressure. Flow and volume are recorded during tidal breathing with a pneumotachograph. At points of equal volume (usually mid-tidal volume), the recorded pressure change is divided by the difference in flow. The resistance so measured includes that of the airways and the tissue resistance of the lung. This technique is not appropriate for routine clinical investigation.

HOW TO MEASURE COMPLIANCE

Compliance (C) is a measure of distensibility and is expressed in terms of volume change per unit change in pressure: compliance = $\Delta V / \Delta P$. The compliance of the respiratory system (C_{rs}) comprises that of the two components, lung and chest

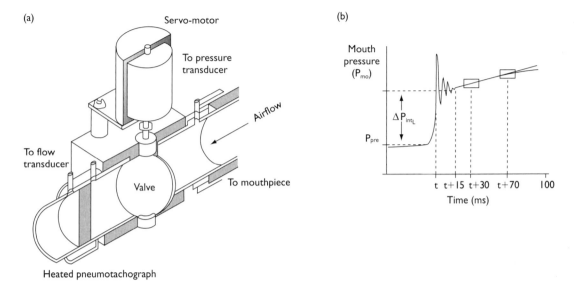

Figure 7.9: Interrupter resistance (R_{int}). (a) The apparatus consists of a breathing tube which can be rapidly occluded by a valve, and in which pressure at the subject's airway opening, and flow through the tube can be measured. (b) The analysis of the pressure/time curve over time 100 ms occlusion can be performed in one of several ways, to allow the pressure at the point of interruption (P_{int}) to be related to the flow at that moment, in order to calculate the interrupter resistance (R_{int}). The figure shows the form of the pressure curve (a rise in pressure, with early oscillations) after an expiratory occlusion. A linear, 2-point back extrapolation is used in the currently available commercial device (Micro Medical, Rochester, UK) to obtain P_{int}.

wall. The use of an oesophageal catheter (see above) enables the two components to be separated, but total compliance is most commonly measured in paediatric practice. In young children this can be done using a weighted spirometer, in which the child breathes quietly from a mechanical spirometer until a stable end-expiratory level is obtained. A weight is placed on the spirometer bell which pressurizes the system and the child will breathe at an elevated lung volume. The shift in lung volume can be measured from the change in end-expiratory level, and the applied pressure can be determined separately by measuring the pressure within the sealed spirometer when the weight is applied.[20] Repeated measurements using different weights will extend the range of the pressure–volume curve under investigation. This technique has been used experimentally, for young children. There are no published clinical applications.

GAS MIXING AND TRANSFER

Gas mixing

The uniformity of ventilation can be assessed by various gas mixing efficiency indices. Most rely on the measurement, breath by breath, of the elimination of resident nitrogen from the lungs, during 100% oxygen breathing. Efficiency is determined in relation to an 'ideal' lung model. The technique has been used experimentally in children to assess pre-symptomatic infants with cystic fibrosis, for example, but there are no routine applications in practice.

Ventilation/perfusion mismatch can be studied experimentally using inert gases and mass spectrometry, (but is more usually performed as part of a functional imaging procedure (Chapter 10)).

Gas transfer

Abnormalities in diffusion of gas across the alveolar membrane are uncommon in the paediatric age group, although oncology patients treated with bleomycin may develop thickening of the membrane and reduced gas transfer. The assessment of transfer[21] is the same as in adults where single-breath carbon monoxide diffusing capacity is measured. The basis of the test is that the patient first expires to residual volume, then inspires to total lung capacity from a gas mix containing 0.3% carbon monoxide. The breath is held for 10 seconds before the subject expires fully and a sample of alveolar gas is analysed. Carbon monoxide is chosen because its extreme affinity for haemoglobin means that once it has diffused across the lung it is immediately taken up, so that the gradient across the lung is not reduced. The fall in carbon monoxide is therefore directly proportional to the diffusing capacity of the lung. However, the manoeuvre requires considerable co-operation and only children above the age 8–10 years are usually able to perform it successfully. A steady-state method suitable for younger children and infants has been described[22] and used in research applications.

Arterial oxygenation and 'blood gases'

With the widespread use of pulse oximetry, clinicians dealing with sick children are in danger of omitting measurement of arterial P_{CO_2} and pH. Hypoxia resulting from inadequate alveolar ventilation or moderate degrees of ventilation perfusion imbalance may be reassuringly corrected by oxygen therapy, but hypercapnia (hypercarbia) and respiratory acidosis cannot. The main indication for arterial blood (or arterialized capillary blood) sampling beyond the neonatal period is to assess the adequacy of alveolar ventilation in obstructive airway diseases (asthma, severe croup) or neuromuscular disorders. Hypercapnia can of course accompany any of the other major clinical causes of hypoxaemia: severe ventilation/perfusion mismatch (intrapulmonary shunt) or anatomical shunting. These are not amenable to oxygen therapy, so that hypercapnia is less likely to go unsuspected.

Oxygenation can be measured to within 2% accuracy by pulse oximetry, provided the child is not in circulatory failure, that sufficient time is allowed for stabilization (a few minutes) and that the child is not hyperactive. Bright background lighting can reduce reliability. Sophisticated analysis provides a continuous check on quality.

Overnight oximetry, downloaded onto computer and printed out for inspection and analysis (Chapter 6) is commonly used to detect hypoxaemia during sleep, e.g. in upper airway, neuromuscular or sickle cell disease, or to monitor the adequacy of domiciliary oxygen therapy in chronic lung disease of prematurity for example. Where technically adequate recordings are possible these studies are informative. However they are less secure in screening children with adenotonsillar hypertrophy for obstructive sleep disruption, since some children awaken promptly (and often) when the upper airway becomes obstructed, before hypoxaemia develops. A normal trace cannot then exclude significant sleep disruption.

SPECIAL CONSIDERATIONS IN PRE-SCHOOL CHILDREN

Very few clinical problems in pre-school children are amenable to investigation by lung function tests, because few reliable techniques are available. *Plethysmographic* techniques are possible, with the toddler on his parent's knee.[23] *Forced expiratory manoeuvres* are possible: 30% of 5-year-olds[23] can perform a FEV_1 and rather more a PEF. The critical factor is maximal *in*spiration. *Impedance methods* such as forced oscillation technique hold promise but are not as well established as the R_{int} method, based on commercial equipment for which evidence of utility in toddlers is available.[19]

MEASURING LUNG FUNCTION IN INFANCY

Infant lung function tests are available in specialized centres throughout the industrialized world. It is easier to study children under 18 months (albeit sedated) than those between 18 months and 5 years.

The main clinical indications are: early detection of functional effects in CF, assessment of the effects of neuromuscular disease, investigation of isolated tachypnoea or measurement of the efficacy of treatments (bronchodilators, surgical procedures for example). Research applications are numerous (Further Reading 2).

Measurement conditions for infants clearly differ from those for older children (Table 7.2), but the principles of plethysmography, helium dilution lung volume measurement and oximetry are identical. Some tests are confined to infancy.

The rapid thoracic compression (RTC) method (Figure 7.10) mimics forced expiratory techniques in older children. The sudden inflation of a 'life jacket' surrounding the sleeping infant's chest and abdomen at end-tidal inspiration causes a passive, forced expiration through a facemask and flow-measuring device, to provide various indices of forced expiration. In a variant of the technique, the lungs are pre-inflated using PEEP, to 20 cm H_2O, which allows reproducible measurements of FEV_1 to be made, a theoretical advantage which has yet to be proven. Flow–volume curves generated by either technique provide useful qualitative information, as do curves in older children.

The test has clinical utility in the early detection of functional changes in CF, in bronchodilator evaluation and in assessing the functional effects of congenital airway disorders.

Plethysmography is feasible in infants. In combination with the single breath technique for measuring passive lung mechanics,[25] measurements of R_{aw}, FRC and C_{rs} can be made. Pressure–flow curves (Figure 7.8) allow airway dynamics to be studied, which can help in distinguishing tracheo- or bronchomalacia from other causes of airway obstruction. With all this information, children with congenital anomalies, unexplained tachypnoea (Case study 7.1) or persistent post-viral syndromes can usefully be studied.

Body surface measurements avoiding any contact with the face, are used to monitor breathing pattern, for example for sleep studies. Potentially they could replace many of the complex methods described above. Bands around the chest and abdomen which measure change of inductance with breathing, respiratory inductive plethysmography (RIP), are commercially available.

AIRWAY RESPONSES

Bronchoconstrictor responsiveness (BR)

CLINICAL PHYSIOLOGY
Intra-thoracic airways exhibit protective contractile responses to adverse stimuli. In diseases such as asthma, this type of response is exaggerated to a pathological degree: bronchial hyperresponsiveness (BHR). The concept is used daily in paediatric practice: 'When you run around, do you become wheezy and tight in the chest?' Increased bronchial responsiveness (BR) may have a genetic or developmental basis, or be acquired as a result of acute (neonatal or viral) or chronic (atopic or infective) inflammatory disease with structural airway consequences (remodelling). The degree of responsiveness in (untreated) asthma far exceeds that found in other lung diseases (Figure 7.11), but there is no clear cut-off. A continuum exists in the population, as a single, normal distribution.

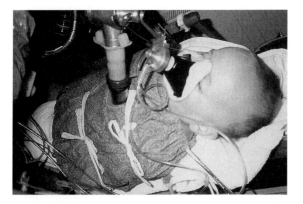

Figure 7.10: The rapid thoracic compression technique. The sleeping child is encased in an inflatable jacket. On inflation, the forced expiratory flow is detected by a flow meter attached to a sealed facemask.

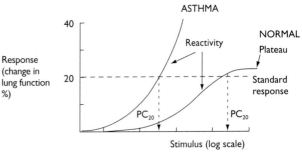

Figure 7.11: Bronchial responsiveness: the concept.

Tests of bronchial responsiveness are rarely used in the diagnosis of asthma: if there is clinical doubt, BR will fall in the 'grey area'. However it may be important in elucidating a child's airway problem, to measure the degree of BR, in order to provide appropriate treatment and monitoring. BR tests can be helpful in monitoring asthma therapy (although their advantage over simple physiological and clinical assessments has yet to be demonstrated in children).

BRONCHIAL CHALLENGE TESTING

The principle of measurement is that BR is a function of:

$$\frac{\text{degree of airway narrowing}}{\text{size of provocative stimulus}}$$

Bronchial challenge testing consists of:

1 applying a standardized stimulus (exercise or methacholine aerosol);
2 measuring a response (e.g. FEV_1 or PEF);
3 relating the two to give an index of BR (e.g. fall in $FEV_1\%$, after exercise, provocative concentration of methacholine giving a 20% fall in FEV_1, PC_{20}).

Exercise challenge provides a standardized, single shot stimulus (typically 6–8 minutes of jogging on a treadmill to produce a heart rate of >180/minute by the end) and the change in airway function (FEV_1 or PEF) from baseline gives an index of BR, the severity of exercise-induced asthma (EIA). EIA is more specific for asthma than methacholine PC_{20}.[26] It is classed as 'indirect challenge' since its effects are mediated by the airway epithelium (as a result of the osmotic and temperature effects of hyperventilation during exercise). Some pharmacological agents, such as adenosine also act indirectly.

Pharmacological challenge provides a sequentially increasing stimulus (usually doubling concentrations of the agent, normally methacholine or histamine, by nebulizer at intervals of about 5 minutes) until a significant target change in lung function has been exceeded (usually a 20% fall in FEV_1) or the maximum permitted concentration is reached. The index of BR is then the (virtual) concentration which caused the target change in lung function, determined by interpolation between the points on the log dose–response curve (Figure 7.11).

Pharmacological challenge tests can be performed in infants using the RTC (squeeze) technique to measure change in lung function[27] and in toddlers where transcutaneous Po_2[28] or an impedance technique requiring little co-operation[29] has been used. These procedures are in the research domain.

INTERPRETING RESULTS

False negative results may be due to technical factors (high humidity or air temperature during exercise challenge; nebulizer failure during pharmacological challenge), physiological factors ('big breath' tests such as FEV_1 can attenuate bronchoconstriction in mild- or non-asthmatics) or clinical factors (e.g. recent bronchodilator use). False positives are rarer, but seasonal variation in atopic subjects should be considered: BR is greater in non-asthmatic atopic rhinitis during the hayfever season, for example. Recent viral infection may transiently enhance BR.

A clearly negative test may be helpful in ruling out asthma as a cause of breathlessness (Case study 7.3). A positive test provides support for bronchodilator or anti-inflammatory therapy, even in the absence of a clear diagnosis of asthma.

Assessing bronchodilator responses

Although the procedure is one of the most widely used in clinical practice, there are few standards for measuring bronchodilator response. The principal points are as follows.

The subject should be capable of a response (i.e. no recent bronchodilator; some degree of airway obstruction).

The dose of bronchodilator should be adequate: for a therapeutic test, the 'normal' dose and device may be appropriate; for a diagnostic test, a big dose (2.5–5 mg of salbutamol or 5–10 mg of terbutaline) by nebulizer should be used. In acute severe asthma, repeated doses may be employed, or combinations (adding ipratropium bromide).

The airway response should be measured after an appropriate time interval (10–15 minutes for a β_2 agonist, or 30–40 minutes for ipratropium bromide), using an appropriate test. In most instances, the FEV_1 or PEF are appropriate, but the significance of the response is not easy to determine. A 15–20% improvement in FEV_1 is almost always significant, but lower values may fall within the 95% confidence interval for repeated measures. Whether the improvement should be expressed as '% baseline', '% best' or '% predicted' is not settled.

Electronic spirometers give additional 'free' information about indices of small airway function (MEF_{25} or FEF_{75}). These indices are poorly repeatable. It is wise only to accept a 40–50% improvement as significant.

RESEARCH ISSUES

TECHNIQUES

'Big breath' tests in schoolchildren have great simplicity and utility. Simple tests for toddlers (such as R_{int}) would be valuable, and techniques based on body surface measurements for infants, using advances in signal processing and mathematical modelling of the mechanical properties of the respiratory system, will enhance clinical practice. Body surface techniques will permit more reliable studies during sleep.

Bronchial challenge tests are time-consuming. Again, sensitive analysis of the changes in lung function brought about by single, low dose challenge would be valuable both for epidemiological research and clinical practice.

FUNCTION

For most clinical purposes, the single compartment 'tube and balloon' model of the respiratory system serves us well. Reliable ways of identifying the series properties of the airways (upper, large and small airways) would be valuable in diagnosis, and measurement of their parallel properties (inhomogeneity) will allow sensitive detection of early or mild dysfunction, in CF, for example. We will then be able to explore such factors as the neonatal (and therefore fetal) predictors of disease, the functional correlates of different wheezy infant phenotypes, and the physiological fate of aerosol therapy.

Functional imaging (MRI) and sophisticated computer modelling of lung function are likely to meet up soon.

CLINICAL NEEDS

Simple questions need answers. We have yet to establish:

- the diagnostic utility of some tests (direct or indirect challenge tests in asthma);
- the role of BHR as a surrogate for 'inflammation' and therefore a guide in the management of asthma;
- the role of domiciliary spirometry (or PEF) in the guided self-management of asthma;

CASE STUDIES

Case study 7.1: An infant with tachypnoea

Following a recent episode of RSV bronchiolitis, Poppy, a 4-month-old thriving infant was noted to breathe at about 60/minute when quiet. There were no other abnormal respiratory or cardiac signs, her SaO_2 was 97% in air and a CXR was clear. There were no dysmorphic features. Further questioning revealed that she had weighed only 2.9 kg at birth and that there had been 'very little water'.

Other investigations were also negative, including: congenital infection screen, sweat test and tests for gastro-oesophageal reflux. Lung function tests (plethysmography and RTC) were carried out to confirm the suspicion of hypoplastic lungs. The findings were as follows (SD score shown in brackets): FRC 113 mL(-2.5); C_{rs} 12.9 mL/cm H_2O (0.3); R_{aw} 2.0 kPa/L/s (+0.2); V_{maxFRC} 174 mL/s (+0.8). She had lungs of low volume, with appropriate compliance and normal airway function, compatible with lung hypoplasia, but not with interstitial lung disease or obliterative bronchiolitis.

Her tachypnoea gradually resolved over the subsequent 6 months, without further problem.

Case study 7.2: Difficult asthma

Heather, an ambitious 14-year-old elder daughter of professional parents, had spent long periods in hospital with troublesome asthma, apparently unresponsive to massive steroid doses. She had become obese and her growth had slowed. Peak flow charts and symptom diaries confirmed severe airway obstruction and breathlessness of a variable degree, disproportionate to her objective clinical state and relative freedom from sleep disturbance. On examination she had a strange pattern of breathing; inability to take a deep breath, active expiration against an upper airway obstruction, and manifest wheeze. Spirometry (repeated after a nebulized dose of salbutamol) showed the characteristic features of vocal cord dysfunction; inconsistency; a bizarre inspiratory pattern and no bronchodilator response (Figure 7.12). A subsequent microlaryngoscopy was normal.

She has improved with counselling and a phased, carefully structured reduction in steroid dose.

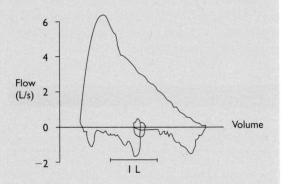

Figure 7.12: Flow–volume curves showing characteristic pattern of vocal cord dysfunction.

Case study 7.3: Breathless on exertion

Gareth was a successful teenage football player, but became breathless (with chest tightness and difficulty in breathing) during vigorous exercise. As a young boy he had moderate, atopic asthma and had been treated with inhaled corticosteroids and bronchodilators. His therapy was stepped up progressively to no avail. On examination, inspiration at rest seemed a little harsh. Spirometry was performed, both expiratory and inspiratory (Figure 7.13).

This revealed a truncated pattern during expiration and inspiration characteristic of fixed large airway obstruction. A barium swallow and echo-cardiograph were normal. Bronchoscopy revealed a symmetrical stricture of the mid-trachea with a 3 mm channel presumably of congenital origin. A treadmill exercise test was carried out. The change in FEV_1 was less than 5% after exercise. His anti-asthma therapy was completely withdrawn, with careful monitoring.

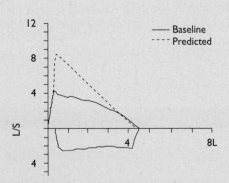

Figure 7.13: The truncated inspiratory and expiratory flow–volume curves characteristic of tracheal obstruction.

Case study 7.4: Scoliosis

Sunita had been monitored since the age of 8, because of progressive non-structural scoliosis. In her early teens, her lung function began to deviate increasingly from that predicted for her arm-span (arm-span = height under normal circumstances). In conjunction with radiological features, it was decided to intervene before completion of the pubertal growth spurt, to avoid progressive respiratory failure. Before surgery, overnight oximetry was performed (excluding significant hypoxaemia), and full plethysmographic measurements of lung volume and airway resistance were repeated as baseline for post-operative evaluations (Figure 7.14).

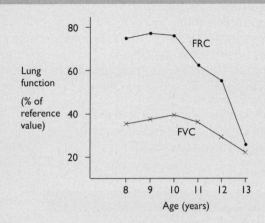

Figure 7.14: Deterioration of lung function in scoliosis. FRC: functional residual capacity; FVC: forced vital capacity.

Case study 7.5: A teenager with CF

Jane, a fourteen-year-old girl, was diagnosed as having cystic fibrosis after meconium ileus. She first grew *Pseudomonas aeruginosa* from a cough swab when aged 9. She developed marked nutritional problems two years ago. At this time her weight was 2 kg below the third centile, and her spirometry had deteriorated to FEV_1 of 54% predicted and FVC of 53% predicted. A percutaneous gastrostomy tube was inserted one month later. She required admission every two to three months for acute exacerbations. Despite aggressive nutritional measures, physiotherapy and anti-pseudomonal treatment her lung function continued to deteriorate (FEV_1 = 23% predicted, FVC = 33% predicted) with severe airway obstruction on the flow–volume curve (Figure 7.15a). She was hypoxic at rest (PaO_2 58 mmHg) and required supplemental oxygen therapy. Her $PaCO_2$ was 47 mmHg. She was listed for lung transplant.

Tests of lung function (Figure 7.15a) are used to determine timing of referral for assessment for lung transplant: (i) spirometry: FEV_1 <30% predicted; (ii) arterial oxygen tension (PaO_2) <60 mmHg (8 kPa) in air; (ii) arterial carbon dioxide tension ($PaCO_2$) >50 mmHg (6.66 kPa); (iii) exercise tests are sometimes used for quantitative assessment of 'functional impairment' (e.g. the 6 minute walk test).

After transplantation, her lung function was normal (Figure 7.15b).

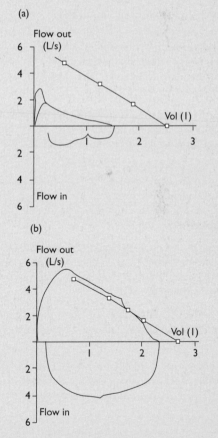

Figure 7.15: Spirometric traces (flow–volume curves): (a) before lung transplant at 13 years; and (b) after lung transplant at 15 years. Open squares indicate reference values.

- the limitations of nocturnal oximetry in assessing obstructive sleep disorders;
- the relative roles of lung function and imaging in the investigation of large airway disorders;
- the value of tidal breathing indices;
- lung function in the timing of lung transplantation (Case study 7.5).

When such questions are answered we will be able to learn more about the overall function of the respiratory system and its control.

REFERENCES

1. Polgar G, Promadhat V. *Pulmonary function testing in children*. London: WB Saunders, 1971.

2. Stocks J, Sly PD, Tepper RS, Morgan WJ. *Infant respiratory function testing*. New York: Wiley-Liss, 1996.

3. Gaultier C, Fletcher ME, Beardsmore C, England S, Motoyama E and the ATS/ERS Working Group on Standardisation of Infant Pulmonary Function Tests. Respiratory function measurements in infants; measurement conditions. *Eur Respir J* 1995; **8**: 1057–66.

4. Beardsmore CS, Thompson JR, Williams A, et al. Pulmonary function in infants with cystic fibrosis: the effect of antibiotic treatment. *Arch Dis Child* 1994; **71**: 133–7.

5. Busse WW, Banks-Schlegel SP, Larsen GL. Effects of growth and development on lung function. Models for study of childhood asthma. *Am J Respir Crit Care Med* 1997; **156**: 314–19.

6. Young S, Arnott J, Le Souef PN, Landau LI. Flow limitation during tidal expiration in symptom-free infants and the subsequent development of asthma. *J Pediat* 1994; **124**: 681–8.

7. Wensley DC, Silverman M. The quality of home spirometry in school children with asthma. *Thorax* 2001; **56**: 183–5.

8. Pelkonen AS, Nikander K, Turpeinen M. Reproducibility of home spirometry in children with newly diagnosed asthma. *Pediat Pulm* 2000; **29**: 34–8.

9. Miller MR, Pedersen OF. The Peak Flow Working Group: the characteristics and calibration of devices for recording peak expiratory flow. *Eur Respir J* 1997; **10** (Suppl. 24): 17s–22s.

10. Jones KP, Mullee MA. Measuring peak expiratory flow in general practice: comparison of mini-Wright peak flow meter and turbine spirometer. *BMJ* 1990; **300**: 1629–31.

11. Pedersen OF, Miller MR. The Peak Flow Working Group: the definition of peak expiratory flow. *Eur Respir J* 1997; **10** (Suppl. 24): 9s–10s.

12. American Thoracic Society. Standardisation of spirometry – 1994 update. *Am J Respir Crit Care Med* 1995; **152**: 1107–36.

13. Rebuck DA, Hanania NA, D'Urzo AD, Chapman KR. The accuracy of a handheld portable spirometer. *Chest* 1996; **109**: 152–7.

14. Enright PL, Johnson LR, Connett JE, Voelker H, Buist AS. Spirometry in the Lung Health Study. 1. Methods and quality control. *Am Rev Respir Dis* 1991; **143**: 1215–23.

15. Dubois AB, Botelho SY, Bedell GN, Marshall R, Comroe JH. A rapid plethysmographic method for measuring TGV. *J Clin Invest* 1956; **35**: 322–6.

16. Beardsmore CS, Stocks J, Silverman M. Problems in the measurement of thoracic gas volume in infancy. *J Appl Physiol* 1982; **52**: 995–9.

17. Helms P. Problems with plethysmographic estimation of lung volume in infants and young children. *J Appl Physiol* 1982; **53**: 698–702.

18. Rodenstein DO, Stanescu DC, Francis C. Demonstration of failure of body plethysmography in airway obstruction. *J Appl Physiol* 1982; **52**: 949–54.

19. Bridge PD, Ranganathan S, McKenzie SA. Measurement of airway resistance using the interrupter technique in preschool children in the ambulatory setting. *Eur Respir J* 1999; **13**: 792–6.

20. Tepper RS, Pagtakhan RD, Taussig LM. Non invasive determination of total respiratory system compliance in infants by the weighted spirometer method. *Am Rev Respir Dis* 1984; **130**: 461–6.

21. American Thoracic Society. Single-breath carbon monoxide diffusing capacity (transfer factor). Recommendations for a standard technique – 1995 Update. *Am J Respir Crit Care Med* 1995; **152**: 2185–98.

22. Koch G, Gaultier C, Boule M, Chaussain M. Transfer factor (diffusing capacity). Steady state method. *Eur Respir J* 1989; **2** (Suppl. 4): 164s–6s.

23. Klug B, Bisgaard H. Measurement of the specific airway resistance by plethysmography in young children accompanied by an adult. *Eur Respir J* 1997; **10**: 1599–1605.

24. Bisgaard H, Klug B. Lung function measurement in

awake young children. *Eur Respir J* 1995; **8**: 2067–75.

25. LeSouef PN, England SJ, Bryan AC. Passive respiratory mechanics in newborns and children. *Am Rev Respir Dis* 1984; **129**: 552–6.

26. Avital A, Springer C, Bar-Yishay E, Godfrey S. Adenosine, methacholine, and exercise challenges in children with asthma or paediatric chronic obstructive pulmonary disease. *Thorax* 1995; **50**: 511–16.

27. Clarke KR, Aston H, Silverman M. Delivery of salbutamol by metered dose inhaler and valved spacer to wheezy infants: effect on bronchial responsiveness. *Arch Dis Child* 1993; **69**: 125–9.

28. Phagoo SB, Wilson NM, Silverman M. Repeatability of methacholine challenge in asthmatic children measured by change in transcutaneous oxygen tension. *Thorax* 1992; **47**: 804–8.

29. Frey U, Jackson AC, Silverman M. Differences in airway wall compliance as a possible mechanism for wheezing disorders in children. *Eur Respir J* 1998; **12**: 136–42.

FURTHER READING

1. Stocks J, Sly PD, Tepper RS, Morgan WJ (eds). *Infant respiratory function testing.* Chichester: Wiley-Liss, 1996.

2. Hughes JMB, Pride NB, (eds). *Lung function tests: physiological principles and clinical applications.* London: WB Saunders, 1999.

3. Gibson GJ (ed). *Clinical tests of respiratory function*, 2nd edn. London: Chapman and Hall Medical, 1996.

4. Rosenthal M, Bain SH, Cramer D, *et al.* Lung function in white children aged 4–19 years: I–Spirometry. *Thorax* 1993; **48**: 794–802.

5. Rosenthal M, Cramer D, Bain SH, Denison D, Bush A, Warner JO. Lung function in white children aged 4–19 years: II–Single breath analysis and plethysmography. *Thorax* 1993; **48**: 803–8.

6. Quanjer Ph H, Stocks J, Polgar G, Wise M, Karlberg J, Borsboom G. Compilation of reference values for lung function measurements in children. *Eur Respir J* 1989; **2** (Suppl. 4): 184s–261s.

7. Quanjer Ph H, Tammeling GJ, Cotes JE, Pedersen OF, Peslin R, Yernault J-C. Lung volumes and forced ventilatory flows. *Eur Respir J* 1993; **6** (Suppl. 16): 5–40.

8. Hyatt RE, Scanlon PD, Nakamura M (eds). *Interpretation of pulmonary function tests: a practical guide.* Lippincott-Raven, 1997

CHAPTER EIGHT

IMMUNE FUNCTION, INFLAMMATION *AND* ALLERGY

M. Browning, J. Grigg and M. Silverman

- Immunodeficiency
- Inflammation
- Allergy

- References
- Further reading

IMMUNODEFICIENCY

BACKGROUND

The immune system has evolved to defend the host against infection. In a normal individual, the various components of the immune system act together to contain and eliminate invading organisms. Individuals with a defect in one or more components of the immune system suffer from an increased incidence of infections. Infections of the upper and lower respiratory tract are common in immunodeficient patients, and can lead to irreversible lung damage, or in severe cases to death. It is important, therefore, that *an underlying immune deficiency should be considered in any child that suffers from recurrent, persistent or unusual infections* (of any site), and that appropriate investigation of immune function should be undertaken. Other causes of recurrent infection, such as cystic fibrosis, ciliary dyskinesia or congenital pulmonary malformations, should also be excluded but are not considered further in this section.

The immune system can be divided into several functional components. The innate immune system consists of phagocytic cells and the complement system of serum proteins. The adaptive immune response is mediated by lymphocytes, and consists of the humoral (B-cell/antibody)

response, and the T-cell-mediated response. Defects of systemic immune function can involve any of these major components, leading to increased susceptibility to infections. Defects in immune function may be primary or secondary (Tables 8.1 and 8.2). (For a more detailed description of primary immunodeficiencies, readers are referred to the WHO Scientific Group Report on Primary Immunodeficiency Diseases.)[1] Secondary immunological deficiencies (Table 8.2) are much more common, and should be excluded first.

IMMUNODEFICIENCY AND RESPIRATORY DISEASE – PROBLEMS AND COMPLICATIONS

The major problem in patients with defective immunity is an increased susceptibility to infections (Table 8.3). The respiratory mucosa is under constant exposure to pathogenic and non-pathogenic microorganisms, and infections of the respiratory tract are a common presenting feature of a variety of primary and secondary immunodeficiencies. Each arm of the immune response plays its role in protecting against infection. Alveolar macrophages and neutrophils phagocytose and kill invading organisms. In this they are helped by antibodies and by complement components, which act as opsonins, increasing the efficiency of

Table 8.1: Main primary immunodeficiency diseases in children

Phagocytic cells chronic granulomatous disease leukocyte adhesion defect hyper IgE syndrome (Job's syndrome) Schwachman syndrome
Complement deficiencies can affect any component of the complement pathway
Predominantly antibody deficiencies transient hypogammaglobulinaemia of infancy X-linked agammaglobulinaemia (Bruton's disease) common variable immunodeficiency IgG subclass deficiency IgA deficiency specific antibody deficiency with normal immunoglobulins
Predominantly T-cell defects Di George syndrome chronic mucocutaneous candidiasis X-linked lymphoproliferative disease (Duncan's syndrome)
Combined T- and B-cell immunodeficiencies severe combined immunodeficiency (SCID) hyper IgM syndrome (CD40 ligand deficiency) Wiskott–Aldrich syndrome

Table 8.2: Causes of secondary immune dysfunction in children

Decreased synthesis	Loss/catabolism
Protein malnutrition	Nephrotic syndrome
Lymphoproliferative disease	Protein-losing enteropathy
Drugs	Burns
Infection	Infection

phagocytosis. T-lymphocytes co-ordinate the adaptive immune response, and play a central role in the clearance of viral infections. The different roles of the components of the immune response determine to a greater or lesser degree the types of infection that predominate in different types of immunodeficiencies.

In *antibody deficiencies*, infections of the upper and lower respiratory tracts, characteristically with encapsulated bacteria such as *Streptococcus pneumoniae* and *Haemophilus influenzae* type B, are the commonest presenting feature (Case study 8.1). Primary antibody deficiencies may present at any age. Granulomatous disease, with lymphadenopathy and hepatosplenomegaly, is a relatively common complication of common variable immunodeficiency (in up to 25%), and commonly affects the lung.

Deficiencies of cell-mediated immunity predispose predominantly to infections with viruses and fungi. Severe primary T-cell and combined immunodeficiencies tend to present early, often in the first weeks or months of life, and presenting features may include failure to thrive, chronic diarrhoea and/or severe respiratory infections, often with opportunistic, low virulence organisms such as *Pneumocystis carinii* or cytomegalovirus (Case study 8.2). The clinical profile may be similar to that seen in infants with AIDS.

Although relatively uncommon in Europe, the possibility of *paediatric AIDS* should be considered in children with a history suggestive of a cell-mediated immunodeficiency. Vertical transmission of HIV infection occurs in up to 10–30% of births to HIV-infected mothers (although maternal therapy and withholding breast feeding can reduce this very markedly). The range of opportunistic infections encountered in children with HIV infection is similar to that in adults, although bacterial infections are relatively more common in children. Infections of the respiratory tract are

Table 8.3: Types of infection in immunodeficient patients

Adaptive immunity		Innate immune defect	
Antibody	**T-cell**	**Phagocytes**	**Complement**
Bacteria	**Viruses**	**Bacteria**	**Bacteria**
(esp. encapsulated)		(esp catalase $+$)	
Strep. pneumoniae	CMV	Staphylococci	C3: pyogenic
Haemophilus (HIB)	herpes	Gram-negative	C5–9: *Neisseria* sp.
	RSV	(*Nocardia*)	
	rotavirus		
	measles		
	pox (vaccinia)		
Some viruses	**Fungi**	**Fungi**	
enteroviral (encephalitis)	*Candida*	*Aspergillus*	
polio	*Aspergillus*	*Candida*	
ECHO	*Pneumocystis*		
	carinii		
	Bacteria		
	(intracellular)		
	Mycobacteria		
	(incl. BCG)		
	Salmonella		
	Listeria		

Case study 8.1: Recurrent pneumonia

Jolene, a ten-year-old girl presented with pneumonia. She gave a history of recurrent respiratory tract infections since early childhood, and had been hospitalized on two previous occasions with pneumonia. Sputum culture grew *Strep. pneumoniae*.

Immunological investigations were as follows (normal range in brackets): IgG 8.6 g/L (5.4–16.1); IgA <0.1 g/L (0.5–2.4); IgM 1.6 g/L (0.5–1.8); IgG2 0.5 g/L (1.4–4.5); other IgG subclasses normal. Anti-tetanus and *Haemophilus influenzae* type B antibody levels were within normal limits (for an immunized child), but anti-pneumococcal antibody levels were undetectable.

A diagnosis of IgA and IgG$_2$ subclass deficiency was made. A thoracic CT scan revealed mild bronchiectatic changes. She was started on prophylactic amoxycillin. She made a modest IgG$_1$ antibody response but no IgG$_2$ antibodies to test immunization with Pneumovax. She remains well on a regime of prophylactic antibiotics and daily physiotherapy, with only occasional breakthrough infections.

---

common, and may be the presenting feature. The presence of *Pneumocystis carinii* pneumonitis is strongly suggestive of HIV infection or of a primary T-cell immunodeficiency. A more insidious form of respiratory involvement is lymphoid interstitial pneumonitis, a lymphoproliferative disorder which manifests with hypoxaemia, usually in children over 2 years of age without a preceding history of opportunistic infection.

Defects of innate immunity may also present with respiratory infections. Deficiencies of most of the components of the complement system have been described, but most are rare. Deficiency of the third complement component (C3) and the regulatory component factors H and I are associated with recurrent infections, especially with pyogenic bacteria. Patients with deficiencies of the late components of complement activation (C5–9) or

Case study 8.2: Unresponsive pneumonia

Zak, a five-month-old boy was admitted to the intensive care unit with bronchopneumonia, which had not responded to antibiotic therapy, and respiratory failure. He had been born at 38 weeks, of consanguinous parents. At 5 weeks old, he had been admitted to hospital with a slowly resolving bronchiolitis. At 8 weeks he developed diarrhoea, which lasted for over one month.

Chest X-ray showed extensive bilateral consolidation. A full blood count showed a raised total white cell count of 21.9×10^9 /L (6.0–17.5), but with a significant lymphopenia of 1.8×10^9 /L (4.0–10.5).

Immunological investigations: IgG 0.1 g/L (2.4–8.8); IgA undetectable (0.1–0.5); IgM 1.3 g/L (0.2–1.0). Lymphocyte phenotyping showed a reduced number and proportion of T-cells (both CD4+ and CD8+), with normal B-cell numbers. There was no HLA-DR (MHC class II) expression on B-cells or monocytes. A diagnosis of bare lymphocyte syndrome (a form of severe combined immune deficiency) was made.

Lung biopsy confirmed the presence of *Pneumocystis carinii*, which was treated with high dose co-trimoxazole and corticosteroids. Family members were HLA typed to identify a suitable related donor for bone marrow transplantation, but he died before an appropriate donor could be found.

properdin deficiency are particularly prone to infections with *Neisseria* sp., including meningococcal infections. Respiratory infections also occur in patients with phagocytic cell defects. In chronic granulomatous disease (CGD), infections with catalase-producing bacteria are typical, but pulmonary aspergillosis is a common complication, whilst in the hyper-IgE (Job's) syndrome, recurrent sinopulmonary infections with pyogenic bacteria are common, and may lead to pneumatocoeles.

There is a need to distinguish immunodeficiency from *other causes of respiratory infection*, such as cystic fibrosis, α-1 antitrypsin deficiency, primary ciliary dyskinesia and structural abnormalities of the respiratory tract. In addition, the causes

of secondary immunodeficiencies should be excluded (Table 8.2), although in most cases these are evident from the history, examination and basic investigation. The most significant respiratory complication of immunodeficiency diseases is the development of bronchiectasis in patients in whom infections are inadequately controlled.

INVESTIGATION OF IMMUNE FUNCTION

As with almost any branch of clinical medicine, a careful clinical history is the cornerstone. The nature, frequency, site and severity of the infections, the age of the patient at onset (Table 8.4),

Table 8.4: Typical age at presentation of primary immunodeficiency

Age (years)	Innate immunity	Antibody deficiency	Cell-mediated immunity
1–2	CGD Leukocyte adhesion defect Hyper IgE syndrome	Transient hypogammaglobinaemia X-linked agammaglobulinaemia	SCID Di George syndrome Chronic mucocutaneous candidiasis
		Hyper IgM syndrome Wiskott–Aldrich syndrome	
3–10	Leukocyte adhesion defect	Common variable immunodeficiency	Chronic mucocutaneous candidiasis
	Hyper IgE syndrome Complement deficiencies	IgG subclass deficiency	
>10	Complement deficiencies	Common variable immunodeficiency	

and other clinical features may give clues as to the underlying nature of the defect. The presence of associated symptoms or signs may indicate the presence of disease predisposing to secondary immunodeficiency. Wherever possible, documentation of current or past organisms causing infections should be obtained, and may give clues as to the nature of the immunological defect.

Each of the major arms of the immune response can be investigated for the presence of an abnormality which might predispose to infection (Table 8.5).

Full blood count

The simplest test of immune function is the full blood count, which gives important information on the numbers of the major immune cell populations such as neutrophils and lymphocytes. It should be noted, however, that the normal ranges

Table 8.5: Laboratory investigation of immunodeficiency

First line	Second line
General	
Full blood count	
Humoral immunity	
IgG, IgA, IgM	IgG subclasses
	Specific antibodies
	Responses to vaccines
Cell-mediated immunity	
Lymphocyte count (FBC)	Immunophenotyping
	Lymphocyte function tests
Phagocytic function	
Neutrophil count (FBC)	Neutrophil function tests
Complement	
C3, C4	Complement function (CH50, AP50)
	Indentification of individual components

First line investigations are widely available in most general hospitals; second line investigations may require specialist laboratories. It should be noted that normal results of first line investigations do not rule out underlying primary immunodeficiency disorders.

of these cell populations vary with age, and appropriate age-related normal ranges should be used.

Assessment of immunoglobulins and antibody formation

Serum immunoglobulin levels (IgG, IgA and IgM) should be measured in any child suspected of having an antibody deficiency. Serum immunoglobulin concentrations vary with age and environment, and local age related normal ranges should be reported with the individual's results. Low immunoglobulin results are not diagnostic of primary antibody deficiency, as reduced levels may be secondary to reduced synthesis of immunoglobulin for other reasons (e.g. protein malnutrition) or to increased loss (e.g. in nephrotic syndrome or through the gastrointestinal tract). Measurement of IgG subclasses or specific antibodies can also help to confirm a significant antibody deficiency. However, these are rarely of additional value in patients with total IgG levels <3 g/L, and it should be remembered that IgG2 antibody responses are usually deficient in children under two years of age. This subclass of antibody is particularly involved in the immune response to complex carbohydrate antigens, such as are found in the capsules of bacteria such as *Strep. pneumoniae* and *Haemophilus influenzae*, and patients with IgG2 subclass deficiency are prone to infections with encapsulated bacteria.

Specific antibody levels to common antigens, or to vaccines, can be used to assess the humoral immune response generally, or to specific antigens or types of antigen (e.g. bacterial capsular polysaccharides). Examples of common environmental antigens include testing for 'natural' antibodies to ABO blood group isohaemagglutinins or to common childhood viruses such as respiratory syncitial virus (RSV). If the child has been vaccinated, the specific responses to the vaccine can be assessed (e.g. antibody responses to diphtheria or tetanus toxoids). In addition, active immunization can be used to assess a specific immune response in a dynamic situation. This can be particularly useful in the assessment of IgG2 deficiency or specific antibody deficiency, where isotype and subclass specific antibody levels can be measured before and (4–6 weeks) after immunization with vaccines to pneumococcus,

Haemophilus influenzae type B or meningococcus. A three-fold increase or greater in specific antibody level is generally taken as indicating an adequate response to immunization.

Tests of cellular immunity

As indicated above, the full blood count gives valuable information on the integrity of neutrophil and lymphocyte cell numbers. More selective information can be gained from immunophenotyping of peripheral blood (or bone marrow) derived lymphocytes, using fluorescently labelled monoclonal antibodies to lineage-specific cell surface markers, which allows for both assessment of numbers of individual lymphocyte populations (B-cells, T-cells, NK-cells etc.) and for expression of certain relevant markers by these cells (e.g. CD18 deficiency in leukocyte adhesion defect; absence of MHC class II expression in the bare lymphocyte syndrome, a form of SCID). Monitoring of the CD4+ T-cell count is a useful marker of disease progression in HIV infection. However, a low CD4 count can have many causes, and the CD4 count should not be used as a diagnostic test for HIV infection. *In vivo* skin testing may be used to assess delayed cutaneous hypersensitivity (DCH) reactions as a measure of cell-mediated immunity to common recall antigens such as purified protein derivative (PPD), *Candida*, *Trichophyton* and tetanus toxoid. However, responses require prior sensitization of the individual to the antigens, and the results of the tests should be interpreted in the light of the age of the patient and the history of prior exposure. The use of delayed hypersensitivity skin testing in young children is therefore of questionable relevance.

In specialist centres, assessment of T-cell function can be carried out *in vitro* by stimulating the cells with mitogens such as phytohaemagglutinin (PHA) or concanavalin A (ConA), or using monoclonal antibodies against the CD3 component of the T-cell receptor complex. Absent responses to mitogens are indicative of severe T-cell deficiency. Antigen specific T-cell responses can also be determined by stimulation of lymphocytes *in vitro* with common T-cell antigens such as PPD, *Candida* or tetanus toxoid, although (as with DCH testing) such responses are lacking in individuals who have not been exposed to the relevant antigens, and so are of little value in neonates and young children. The execution and interpretation of these tests requires experience, and they should only be undertaken by specialist laboratories.

Tests of complement activity

Recurrent bacterial pneumonia may be a feature of complement deficiency, as well as of antibody deficiency. Most immunology laboratories test for serum levels of complement components C3 and C4, and for functional complement activity by the classical and alternative pathways of complement activation (the CH50 and AP50 tests). Interpretation of tests of complement function may be complicated by a number of factors. Firstly, a fresh serum sample is required, or reduced activity may be seen. Secondly, factors other than complement deficiency may be associated with reduced functional activity, e.g. intercurrent infection or immune complex disease. It is therefore advisable to test complement function in convalescence. If a defect of functional complement activity is detected, the individual component that is lacking should be identified. Both the clinical picture and the pathway(s) involved may give indications as to which components may be deficient. The definition of the specific absent component, however, is the responsibility of the specialist laboratory.

Tests of phagocytic function

A full blood count with differential should be carried out to determine the presence and numbers of phagocytic cells. A variety of tests are available for assessing phagocytic function, including tests of chemotaxis, phagocytosis and intracellular killing, and respiratory burst. The most widely used, and probably the most useful test is the measurement of nitroblue tetrazolium dye reduction (the NBT test), which measures super oxide production in stimulated neutrophils. The NBT test is used in the diagnosis of CGD (in which NBT reduction is virtually absent), and can also indicate carrier status for the disease.

Diagnosis of leukocyte adhesion defect is based on the absence or reduced expression of the common β chain, CD18, of the integrins CD11a, b and c, on immunostaining of cells with monoclonal antibodies specific for these markers.

Diagnosis and monitoring in HIV infection

The diagnosis of HIV infection may be complicated in young children (<18 months old), as the presence of HIV-specific antibody may reflect passively acquired maternal antibody in the absence of viral transmission. Additional tests, such as viral culture or polymerase chain reaction (PCR), may be required in order to make the diagnosis. Even these highly sensitive tests may be unreliable in the neonatal period, with the sensitivity of PCR being about 30% at birth, but rising to virtually 100% by 3 months. The estimation of viral loads and the CD4+ T-lymphocyte count are the main laboratory parameters for disease monitoring in the treatment and progression of HIV infection.

EVALUATING OUTCOME – INTERPRETATION OF THE RESULTS

In assessing a child's systemic immune function, it should be borne in mind that the development of the normal immune system, in particular adaptive immunity, continues after birth and, although functional, the neonatal immune system is immature. The age of the child and its immunological development need to be taken into account when considering the significance of immunological investigations (Table 8.4), and age related normal ranges should be used. Lymphopenia in a baby should not be ignored, as this is one of the cardinal signs of SCID, although other causes, including infection itself, should also be considered. If immunodeficiency is suspected, immunoglobulins and lymphocyte phenotyping should be carried out.

Interpretation of immunoglobulin levels in the first two years of life should take account of the development of the humoral (antibody) response. At birth, the term neonate is protected by maternally transferred immunoglobulin. Transplacental transfer of IgG takes place in the last weeks of pregnancy, and in premature infants this may be incomplete, resulting in hypogammaglobulinaemia. Endogenous antibody synthesis occurs mainly after birth, and is driven by exposure to antigens. Consequently, there is a physiological trough of serum antibody in the post-natal period

when maternal antibody has been catabolized, but endogenous antibody synthesis has not yet developed. This may result in transient hypogammaglobulinaemia of infancy, with increased susceptibility to infections, which may last for up to two to three years. Although by definition self-limiting, immunoglobulin replacement may be required if bacterial infections are a problem, until spontaneous recovery occurs. In addition, different antibody isotypes develop at different rates. In particular, IgG2 subclass antibodies tend to be amongst the last to develop, and in some children can take a number of years to develop fully. An apparent IgG2 subclass deficiency may therefore be due to maturational delay rather than to an underlying primary antibody deficiency in a child under 12 years. Selective IgA deficiency, although often asymptomatic, may also present with an increased incidence of respiratory infections. In these cases it is commonly associated with a deficiency of IgG2 or a specific antibody deficiency, and so patients should be screened for these associated humoral immune defects.

It should be remembered that infection itself may cause transient immunological abnormalities, including alterations to circulating cell numbers and subpopulations, and complement activation. If there is doubt, the test should be repeated in convalescence. Children with unexplained bacterial pneumonia or confirmed meningococcal disease should have their complement functional activity assessed in convalescence, to rule out an underlying complement component deficiency.

As indicated above, when an immunological abnormality is detected, it is important to rule out conditions predisposing to secondary immunodeficiency. In many cases these may be clinically apparent or diagnosed from routine investigations (e.g. nephrotic syndrome, acute leukaemia, malnutrition etc.). In other cases (for example, exclusion of cystic fibrosis, or congenital structural disorders) further investigation may be required.

INTEGRATING THE RESULTS INTO MANAGEMENT

The management of patients with immunodeficiencies depends on the underlying disease, and its clinical severity. In all cases, the aims should be to eliminate current infections, prevent further infections, and to treat complications and, where possible, the underlying disease.

The management of patients with antibody deficiency depends largely on the clinical severity. Patients with common variable immunodeficiency are at risk of infection, which is not usually adequately controlled with antibiotics, and therefore require immunoglobulin replacement therapy. As the half-life of IgG is in the order of 3 weeks, intravenous immunoglobulin replacement therapy is commonly given at three-weekly intervals, with the aim of maintaining a trough IgG level of >8 g/L (generally in a dose range of 200–400 mg/kg per infusion). More recently, the subcutaneous route as an alternative means of administering immunoglobulin has been introduced, but requires weekly administration to maintain adequate IgG levels. (It should be noted that there are separate preparations of immunoglobulin for intravenous and subcutaneous use.) In patients with selective antibody deficiencies (IgA deficiency, IgG subclass deficiencies, specific antibody deficiencies) there is a broad spectrum of clinical disease, and patients should be assessed on a case-by-case basis. In patients with mild antibody deficiencies, the prompt use of antibiotics at the first sign of bacterial infection may be sufficient. In more severely affected individuals, prophylactic antibiotics may be required to contain and prevent recurrent bacterial infections. If significant breakthrough infections continue, immunoglobulin replacement therapy may be required to control infections. Paradoxically, some patients with significant immunoglobulin subclass deficiencies have relatively few infections, whilst others with relatively mild deficiencies by serological investigation have a much greater susceptibility to infection. It is not possible, therefore, to base management guidelines on serological investigations alone. Immunization against common respiratory tract bacterial pathogens (such as pneumococcus, *Haemophilus influenzae* and meningococcus) may be useful, not only in boosting endogenous immunity, but also in determining the extent of the antibody deficiency by monitoring the antibody response to the vaccine. In addition to taking appropriate steps to minimize infections, patients with clinically significant antibody deficiencies

should have annual chest X-rays and lung function tests, to monitor for signs of disease progression. It is important to realize that in up to 50% of patients, bronchiectasis is not apparent on a standard chest X-ray. Children below 6 years of age cannot reliably perform lung function, and in this group, persistent or recurrent moist cough may be the only sign of developing suppurative lung disease. In all cases, the aim of treatment is to minimize infections and to prevent the development of permanent lung damage.

Whilst antibody deficiencies can be compensated for by replacement therapy with pooled normal human gammaglobulin, there is no equivalent form of therapy for severe T-cell or combined immunodeficiencies. Severe combined immunodeficiency is inevitably fatal unless treated. As in HIV infection, the cell-mediated immunodeficiency in SCID is associated with an increased risk of opportunistic infections, including *Pneumocystis carinii* pneumonia (PCP), and antimicrobial prophylaxis should be started. Many patients with SCID will also be immunoglobulin deficient (secondary to their T-cell immune dysfunction), in which case immunoglobulin replacement therapy is indicated. Live vaccines should be avoided, and only CMV-negative, irradiated blood products used, in patients suspected of having SCID (or any severe T-cell immunodeficiency), until cell-mediated immunity has been properly assessed, due to the risk of vaccine-related infection or donor leukocyte-versus-host disease. The only current curative treatment for SCID is bone marrow transplantation. With early diagnosis, good donor/recipient matching and an absence of pre-transplant infections the success rate of this treatment can be over 80%, but falls significantly with late diagnosis and infections.

For HIV infection in children, the use of combination anti-retroviral therapy has become standard practice. PCP prophylaxis (usually with septrin) can be added where there is a risk of infection, based largely on age of the child and the CD4 cell count. Antimicrobial prophylaxis is recommended in infants under one year of HIV-infected mothers until proven free of HIV infection, in patients between 1 and 5 years with CD4+ T-cell counts below 500 cells/μL, and in children over 5 years with CD4 counts below 200 cells/μL. As indicated above, bacterial infections are common in children with symptomatic HIV infection. In these cases, the use of intravenous immunoglobulin has been shown to reduce both frequency of infections and days in hospital.

Patients with CGD suffer from recurrent infections with catalase-producing bacteria or fungi (including pulmonary aspergillosis). The prophylactic use of antibiotics (usually septrin) is generally sufficient to control bacterial infections, supplemented with antifungal agents (itraconazole). The prophylactic use of gamma interferon remains controversial, although it may be a useful adjunct to the treatment of complications. Similarly, in patients with complement deficiencies the prompt or prophylactic use of antibiotics, combined with appropriate immunizations (e.g. against meningococcus for properdin or C5-9 deficiency), are the mainstays of management. Asplenic patients are susceptible to a range of infections, and the prophylactic use of antibiotics (penicillin, or erythromycin in penicillin-allergic patients), combined with immunizations against pneumococcus, *Haemophilus influenzae* and meningococcus is recommended.

CLINICAL RESEARCH ISSUES AND CONCLUSIONS

In the past few years, the genetic basis of many primary immunodeficiency diseases has been determined, and the defective genes and their functions identified. This has led to prospects of novel therapies, including the possibility of gene therapy for patients with single-gene defects. The cause(s) of common variable immunodeficiency, however, remains to be determined. Recent evidence suggests that there may be several subtypes of the disease, possibly with different aetiologies. The range of factors that are known at a research level to predispose to infection continues to grow faster than simple, reliable clinical and laboratory tests for these abnormalities. It is clear also that a number of the parameters currently used to measure immune function are relatively crude, and the results do not always translate readily to the clinical situation. The development of more sensitive and specific tests is therefore required. Vaccination remains an important tool in the management of patients with certain forms of immunodeficiency. Although an effective vaccine

against *Haemophilus influenzae* type B has been introduced, the vaccines for other encapsulated bacteria, such as pneumococcus and meningococcus, remain suboptimal. In addition, the levels of antibody that correlate with protection against these organisms remains to be evaluated (although this has been determined for antibody levels to *Haemophilus influenzae* type B).

Primary immunodeficiency diseases are uncommon but important causes of respiratory disease in children. There are registers of patients with primary immunodeficiencies in the UK and Europe. Assessment of immune function can be complex, and is best carried out by, or in consultation with specialist immunologists. Correct management of patients with disorders of immune function can reduce disease severity, improve quality of life, prevent irreversible lung damage and prolong life. Immunodeficiency should therefore be considered in any child presenting with recurrent, persistent or unusual infections.

INFLAMMATION

BACKGROUND

Leukocytes are inflammatory cells with the capacity to damage lung tissue and cause respiratory symptoms. Despite this, the pattern of leukocytes within the lung is rarely assessed in children with respiratory symptoms. There are two main reasons for this. First, there are ethical issues associated with the direct sampling of lung leukocytes from children with mild symptoms. Second, markers of lung inflammation both direct and indirect have, disappointingly, provided no more additional *clinical* information than history and examination. In contrast, sampling inflammatory cells from the lungs of children has significantly contributed to an understanding of the mechanisms of paediatric respiratory disease.

Lung leukocytes can be divided into two groups: those normally resident in the healthy lung, and those recruited from the systemic circulation during inflammation. Inflammation becomes a clinical problem when it leads to respiratory symptoms, but it is not necessarily associated with disease. For example, there is always a low-grade inflammatory reaction to inhaled particulates in the healthy airway. The most accessible populations of 'resident' leukocytes are in the bronchi and alveoli. The majority of cells in the lumen of the healthy airway are alveolar macrophages, and a representative sample can be removed by gentle washing (bronchoalveolar lavage) (Figure 8.1). In the healthy lung alveolar macrophages have an anti-inflammatory role: they remove potentially damaging particles, and release mediators that suppress other immuno-competent-cells. Alveolar macrophages can also initiate inflammation by releasing mediators that increase the stickiness of the lung endothelium for circulating leukocytes. The attachment of leukocytes to endothelial cells is critical to the development of lung inflammation, and depends on the expression of 'adhesion molecules' (e.g. intercellular adhesion molecule-1). Resistant leukocytes within the lung tissue can also initiate inflammation. For example, tissue lymphocytes from asthmatics are skewed towards a 'Th2' phenotype, and release mediators that are critical to eosinophil recruitment.

The *pattern* of adhesion molecules on the endothelium and counter-receptors on circulating leukocytes determines the type of cell that is recruited into the lung.[1] Thus asthma is associated with the preferential adhesion of eosinophils to lung endothelial cells, whereas neutrophil–endothelial adhesion occurs in bacterial pneumonia. During the resolution phase of acute inflammation, mechanisms are activated that limit tissue damage. If dying leukocytes disintegrated in the alveoli, mediators would be released that would cause additional tissue damage. To prevent additional damage, leukocytes undergo programmed cell death (apoptosis), in which the cell membrane remains intact. Alveolar macrophages rapidly phagocytose and destroy apoptotic leukocytes along with their damaging mediators[2] (Figure 8.2).

Since the pattern of lung inflammation determines the pattern of respiratory symptoms and signs, its measurement has the potential to provide a more objective assessment than clinical history and examination. Furthermore, measurement of inflammation could help to discriminate between conditions that share the same clinical symptom (e.g. cough), but have a different inflammatory aetiology. There are two approaches to measuring inflammation: leukocytes and their mediators can be sampled directly from the lung, or inflammation may be inferred from inflammatory markers at other sites (indirect assessment).

MEASURING PULMONARY INFLAMMATION

Lung biopsy

Lung biopsy is used to assess the inflammation associated with chronic interstitial lung disease

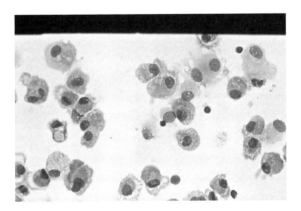

Figure 8.1: Bronchoalveolar lavage cells from a normal child stained with Diff-Quick. The majority of cells are alveolar macrophages; they are large and have an eccentric nucleus. The small cells with large nuclei are lymphocytes.

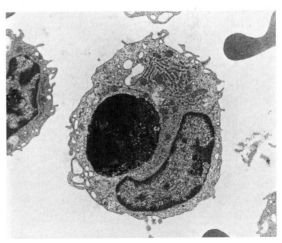

Figure 8.2: An apoptotic neutrophil within the phagosome of an alveolar macrophage. This specimen is from a premature infant during the resolution phase of hyaline membrane disease.

(ILD). Lung biopsy remains the gold standard for diagnosis of chronic ILD, primarily since this heterogeneous group is defined by specific leukocyte patterns.[3] Other reasons for lung biopsy are to exclude infection and structural abnormalities. The term 'interstitial' in ILD is misleading since abnormal inflammation involves most cellular components of the lung, including the endothelium and alveolar epithelium. In some acute forms of ILD, the underlying histology may be inferred from the clinical context: for example, lympho-cytic interstitial pneumonitis in children with HIV infection.[4]

WHAT TO DO

The classic presentation of chronic ILD is a child with long standing dry cough and/or shortness of breath on exercise and on examination, intercostal retractions, cyanosis, clubbing, and 'dry' crackles at the lung bases (Case study 8.3). Open lung biopsy has advantages over transbronchial biopsy performed through a flexible bronchoscope. First,

---

Case study 8.3: Interstitial lung disease

Hitesh, a six-year-old Asian boy, initially presented with jaundice, and the serum virology suggested cytomegalovirus (CMV) hepatitis. Three months later he presented in respiratory failure. He looked unwell, with mild recession, a non-productive cough, no wheeze or crepitations on auscultation, and a saturation in air of 88%. The chest X-ray showed widespread bilateral consolidation compatible with interstitial lung disease (ILD) (Figure 8.3). Pulmonary function tests showed a pure restrictive deficit with no bronchodilator response. The C-reactive protein, and blood film were normal. A Mantoux test was negative. There was no clinical response to parenteral broad spectrum antibiotics, and all microbial and virological cultures were negative. Whilst awaiting the results of the tests for specific aetiological factors for chronic ILD (autoantibodies, immune function tests, α-1 antitrypsin phenotype, cystic fibrosis genotype) all of which proved negative, a bronchoalveolar lavage (BAL) and open lung biopsy were performed. BAL cell findings were abnormal with an elevated percentage of lymphocytes and neutrophils. A silver stain of BAL cells for *Pneumocystis carinii* was negative, and no organisms, viruses, or fungi were isolated from the BAL fluid.

The lung biopsy revealed no granulomas or evidence of malignancy. Hyaline material was present in the alveoli, with hyperplasia of type II pneumocytes. The interstitium was hypercellular with mononuclear inflammatory cells. Inflammation extended from the air spaces into the terminal bronchioles. The final histopathological diagnosis was 'chronic pneumonitis'. Hitesh was treated with oral steroids and his clinical symptoms and lung function improved. Oral steroids were withdrawn after 7 months and he remains stable with no evidence of pulmonary hypertension, but with a mild restrictive lung deficit on lung function testing and moderate exercise intolerance.

The biopsy, by excluding infection and malignancy, gave the clinicians the confidence to treat Hitesh with high dose corticosteroids. In this case, the non-specific histopathological label for this child's interstitial lung disease did not affect therapy. CMV infection could have triggered the abnormal inflammatory process. As in this boy, complete recovery from ILD is unusual. Less than half of affected children recover normal lung function.

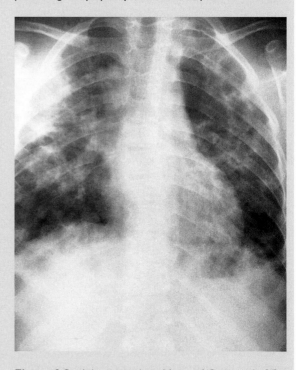

Figure 8.3: Admission chest X-ray of Case study 8.3 showing extensive bilateral consolidation compatible with an interstitial lung disease.

enough tissue is guaranteed . Second, there is less risk of missing significant pathology in conditions where relatively normal areas of lung alternate with areas of inflammation. Before the biopsy it is critical to liaise with all the relevant laboratories and the thoracic surgeon to ensure that the sample is handled correctly. Analysis should include direct culture for bacteria and viruses, immuno-fluorescence, electron microscopy, and light microscopy. Slides should also be saved to be sent, if necessary, to a pathologist with experience of paediatric ILD.

In 'usual interstitial pneumonitis' various stages of inflammation coexist with alveolar hyaline membranes (organized protein), invasion of the parenchyma with lymphocytes and macrophages, and fibrotic lesions. In 'desquama-tive interstitial pneumonitis' there is a more uniform picture with hyperplastic type II pneu-mocytes and large numbers of macrophages within the alveoli. Since both conditions are treated by systemic corticosteroids, there is a view that they should be grouped together as the 'chronic interstitial pneumonias'. Lymphocytic interstitial pneumonitis (LIP) is an inflammatory condition that is usually associated with HIV infection,[4] but occasionally with other triggers.[5] It is characterized by hyperplasia of bronchial lym-phoid tissue, and a diffuse interstitial infiltrate of mature lymphocytes, plasma cells and histiocytes. Systemic corticosteroids are the treatment of choice. Obliterative bronchiolitis is not usually classed as a chronic ILD, since it often has a better outcome. In this condition, the terminal bronchi-oles, respiratory bronchioles and alveolar ducts are invaded inflammatory cells. Abnormal repair processes lead to complete or partial obstruction by collagen. Recanalization can occur leading to histopathological and clinical improvement. The majority of cases of obliterative bronchiolitis are associated with therapeutic immunosuppression to prevent rejection. Repeated open lung biopsy to monitor for obliterative bronchiolitis or rejection is impractical in children with transplanted lungs, and transbronchial biopsy by fibreoptic broncho-scopy is the preferred sampling method.

INTEGRATING RESULTS INTO MANAGEMENT

The clinical reason for performing a lung biopsy in a child with radiological evidence of ILD is to rule out conditions where systemic corticosteroid treatment may be inappropriate (e.g. infection and malignancy). There is no evidence that in children the pattern of inflammation (and therefore the diagnostic category) in idiopathic ILD can be used to predict prognosis or response to corticos-teroids,[3] or to other immunomodulatory drugs such as hydrochloroquine.

Bronchoalveolar lavage

WHAT TO DO

Bronchoalveolar lavage (BAL) is particularly use-ful in the diagnosis of lung infection. In a group of seven children with severe respiratory disease (five of whom were ventilated) we detected a pathogenic organism in all lavage fluid specimens obtained by non-bronchoscopic BAL using a wedged suction catheter, and a pathogenic organ-ism was isolated from four out of eight immuno-suppressed children with respiratory disease using fibreoptic bronchoscopy and BAL.[6] Looking at the pattern of leukocytes *per se* in the BAL fluid is not helpful in diagnosing infection. A high pro-portion of BAL fluid neutrophils is found with bacterial infection, but this pattern also occurs with viral colds.[7] On the other hand, the presence of intracellular bacteria in BAL neutrophils is a useful marker of infection (Figure 8.4).[8]

BAL fluid can be obtained either by a fibreoptic bronchoscope inserted via a laryngeal mask for radiologically focal disease,[9] or by using a wedged suction catheter inserted blindly though an

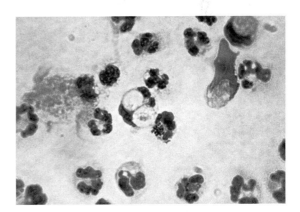

Figure 8.4: Bronchoalveolar lavage specimen from a child intubated for bacterial pneumonia. There is a significant increase in the proportion of neutrophils compared with the normal pattern. Intracellular bacteria are seen within a neutrophil.

endotracheal tube for diffuse disease.[10] The instilled volume of saline should be sufficient to reach the alveoli (approximately 1 mL/kg body weight). BAL by wedged suction catheter does not require specific training, and permits rapid diagnosis of infection in children who are ventilated for severe generalized lung disease. 500 μL of BAL fluid should be cytocentrifuged onto a microscope slide and stained by a rapid stain ('Diff-Quick™' or May–Grunwald–Giemsa). If the lavage fluid has sampled only the bronchi, there will be a high proportion of bronchial ciliated epithelial cells. In contrast, the presence of alveolar macrophages suggests alveolar sampling. Since staining for *Pneumocystis carinii* pneumonia (silver stain) or viral infection (immunofluorescence) is preferentially seen on alveolar macrophages,[11,12] it is possible to miss the diagnosis with a bronchial sample alone (Figure 8.5).

INTEGRATING RESULTS INTO MANAGEMENT

The leukocyte profile in the BAL fluid is always abnormal in chronic ILD, but the pattern is non-specific and cannot be used for diagnosis. One reason for this is that the pattern of leukocytes

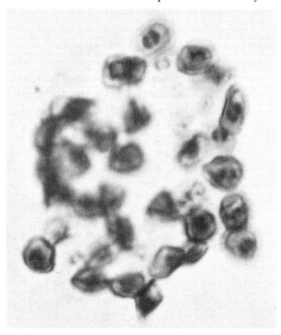

Figure 8.5: Silver stain of a bronchoalveolar lavage fluid preparation from an infant with *Pneumocystis carinii* pneumonia. The small circular structures are pneumocysts which are adherent to an alveolar macrophage (unstained).

within the small airways does not precisely match the leukocyte pattern within the lung interstitium (the key inflammatory site in ILD). Is there a role for BAL in asthma? Eosinophilia in the airway lumen *and* surrounding tissue is a hallmark of allergic lung inflammation. Analysis of eosinophils in BAL fluid or their products should in theory, provide useful information. Indeed, an eosinophil differential count of >5% in BAL fluid does appear to differentiate atopic children with asthma from those with isolated chronic cough.[13] In contrast, the absence of an airway eosinophilia does not exclude pulmonary allergic inflammation, especially in children treated with inhaled corticosteroids.

There is no doubt that BAL is a very useful research tool. For example, it has been shown that the group of children with isolated viral wheeze have lower levels of the eosinophil-derived mediator ECP (eosinophil cationic protein) in their BAL fluid than atopic asthmatics.[14] This finding suggests that isolated viral wheeze is a distinct inflammatory condition. However at an individual level, the distinction is less clear cut: some asthmatic children have low levels of ECP in their BAL fluid, and some viral wheezers have high ECP levels. Until a way is found of linking BAL findings to a clinically important effect in the individual child, its application in paediatric respiratory disease will continue to produce scientifically interesting, but clinically irrelevant results. Even if BAL could help to resolve some of the diagnostic dilemmas, the need for general anaesthesia or heavy sedation means that it would only be applied to the very small subgroup with severe symptoms.

Induced sputum

WHAT TO DO

Analysis of expectorated cells from the lower airway is a non-invasive method of directly assessing airway inflammation.[15] It is not suitable for children less than 7 years of age, since they are unable to expectorate vigorously on command.

The FEV_1 (forced expiratory volume in one second) should be measured prior to induction. If the FEV_1 is less than 80% of the predicted value, or there is a history of asthma, nebulized salbutamol should be given and the FEV_1 remeasured. Sputum induction can then be performed if the FEV_1 falls within the normal range. In mild asthma or normal adolescents, 4.5% saline should be given for 5 to 7 minutes by jet or ultrasonic nebulizer. The nebulized saline tastes 'like sea water', but it is not painful, and only very rarely causes nausea. The FEV_1 should then be checked, and if it has fallen by >10%, nebulized salbutamol given. The child should then blow its nose, and rinse its mouth with water.

Expectoration is hard work, and the technique should first be demonstrated by the clinician. To produce sputum in the absence of increased production is quite difficult and requires a lot of effort. Some adolescents are embarrassed by expectoration and appreciate being screened from view. The end result is a combination of saliva and small plugs of mucus. There is still debate whether the sputum should be processed as a whole, or the plugs processed separately. If only the plugs are to be examined, they should be picked out with sterile tweezers and the cells dispersed by mixing with a 0.1% dithiothreitol (DTT). The sputum should then be homogenized, the airway cells pelleted by centrifugation and resuspended in saline. Cytocentrifuge preparations (Cytospin, Shandon Ltd) can be stained with Diff-Quick or Romanovsky stain. The inflammatory cell differential can then be determined under oil microscopy ($\times 100$).

The cell population that is sampled by sputum induction is not the same as that sampled by BAL. During BAL, large numbers of macrophages are recovered from the alveoli, and these tend to overwhelm the relatively low number of cells removed from the bronchi (macrophages, neutrophils and ciliated bronchial epithelial cells). Induced sputum on the other hand preferentially samples the bronchi. This becomes an advantage when inflammation is predominant bronchial. The potential of induced sputum has been shown in several clinically important areas. Adults with non-asthmatic chronic cough (defined by absence of bronchial hyperreactivity, and no response to corticosteroids), have a higher number of neutrophils in their induced sputum when compared with healthy controls without asthma.[16] Induced sputum neutrophilia is also associated with 'difficult' asthmatics who are poorly controlled despite high dose corticosteroids,[17] but determining cause and effect is difficult. Analysis of induced sputum in adults has recently defined 'eosinophilic bronchitis'. This condition is not asthma and is characterized by a chronic cough and normal lung function.[18] The incidence of eosinophilic bronchitis in children is unknown.

INTEGRATING RESULTS INTO MANAGEMENT

There is currently no link between induced sputum studies and clinically important outcomes in children, but could it be used in the future? It is unlikely that induced sputum will be of any value in the *diagnosis* of children with clinical asthma. Testing the reversibility of small airways obstruction to bronchodilators, and clinical response to inhaled steroids, are usually adequate to identify the majority of affected children. If however, induced sputum can define an inflammatory phenotype associated with a poor response to steroids, it could be of clinical value. An additional explanation for a persistent induced sputum eosinophilia in a symptomatic adolescent on high dose inhaled corticosteroids would be non-compliance with therapy. Analysis of induced sputum could also help children whose respiratory symptoms are underperceived (they have symptoms but don't recognize them), or underreported (they have and perceive symptoms, but won't tell). Like non-compliant children, both of these groups are at risk of significant eosinophilic lung inflammation, and possibly permanent structural damage. If treating eosinophilic inflammation prevents irreversible lung damage, paediatricians will need to know the child's inflammatory status before reducing or stopping inhaled corticosteroids. To date, the debate on whether to treat 'asthmatic symptoms only' or 'symptoms *and* inflammation' has not been resolved (Case study 8.4)

Blood and urine markers

As the site of measurement moves away from the lung, there is the additional problem of specificity: i.e. how can the clinician tell that a particular serum marker reflects lung inflammation, or inflammation at another site? Serum markers of eosinophilic lung inflammation have been the most extensively studied and, of these, serum ECP and eosinophil protein X (EPX) have been clinically evaluated. ECP and EPX are granule proteins and are released by eosinophils on activation. EPX is excreted in the urine whereas ECP appears to be reabsorbed by the renal tubules. High serum levels of ECP and EPX

Case study 8.4: Difficult asthma

Every 2–4 weeks Gemma, a 14-year-old atopic girl, was admitted with an acute exacerbation of asthma, despite maximal inhaled and systemic therapy. There were concerns about non-compliance, but directly observed therapy by her mother did not lead to any improvement, and she missed most of her schooling. In addition to wheeze, she had a persistent cough, often productive of mucopurulent sputum. All tests for other chronic lung diseases and host defence defects were negative. Induced sputum showed neutrophilia of 45% (mean for normal adults is 38%[30]), and eosinophilia of 6.3% (normal mean 0.6%). Sputum culture was consistently negative. Regular admissions for intravenous steroids and antibiotics significantly improved her condition between episodes, reduced the number of admissions, and improved her school attendance.

This girl could represent an unusual phenotype of asthma, in which reversible airway obstruction is accompanied by neutrophilic bronchitis. The prognosis and treatment of this condition remains unclear, but the induced sputum analysis suggested that compliance may not be the only issue.

---

are associated with asthma, not because these proteins leak out of the lung into the blood, but because the assay reflects an increased sensitivity of systemic eosinophils (priming). Priming of systemic eosinophils to release ECP and EPX also occurs in eczema and hay fever.[19]

WHAT TO DO

At least one mL blood should be collected into a blood tube with clot activator (Vacutainer™). The sample has to stand for exactly 60 minutes at room temperature. This allows time for the serum to separate and for the eosinophils to release their granule proteins. Serum is then separated by centrifuging and stored at $-20°C$. It is critical to handle the sample in a standardized way, since deviation from the protocol by using a different blood container, changing the clot incubation time, or incubating at a higher temperature may significantly alter levels. There are two methods of assaying ECP (Pharmacia AB): radioimmunoassay, or the technically easier fluorometric method. The 'Uni-Cap™' (Pharmacial AB) assay machine is needed for the ECP fluorometric assay, whereas the radioimmunoassay may be performed using standard equipment. The EPX assay is only available as the radioimmunoassay kit. Urine samples for EPX can be frozen without processing and used directly in the radioimmunoassay. Urinary creatinine should be measured to correct for differences in urinary dilution.

INTEGRATING RESULTS INTO MANAGEMENT

There is a relationship between changes in ECP and EPX levels and changes in lung function in symptomatic asthmatic children.[20] However, as a recent review states 'even if ECP and EPX do reflect the disease process, this is of limited interest, because they are not really needed to establish disease activity: at this time medical history and physical examination seem superior'.[21] Are there any areas where serum markers could be used clinically? It would be interesting to know whether children with nocturnal cough, normal lung function, and no response to corticosteroids and bronchodilators,[22] could be identified by the *absence* of systemic eosinophil activation. Alternatively, serum ECP or EPX could be used as a screening tool for eosinophil activation before sputum induction. Another potential niche is in the differentiation of the two phenotypes of pre-school wheeze[23] for prognostic purposes (Case study 8.5). Clinical history and examination cannot distinguish those pre-school wheezy children who will continue as atopic asthmatics (persistent wheezers), from those whose wheezing illness resolves within the pre-school period (transient wheezers). However, pre-school wheezers with a high ECP (>20 μg/L) are more likely to develop more than three attacks a year and be wheezing 2 years later,[24,25] suggesting that 'transient' pre-school wheeze is not associated with eosinophilic lung inflammation.

Markers in the breath

Nitric oxide (NO) is present in the breath of healthy children.[26] Increased breath NO is associated with atopy (a positive skin prick test to allergens),[26] and asthma.[27] The source of the increased NO production from the lower respiratory tract in

Case study 8.5: Viral wheeze

Violet, a 2-year-old girl, was admitted with an acute attack of viral wheeze. There was a history of three previous severe attacks. Her serum ECP taken during the admission was 80 μg/L compared with the reference value of 7.1 μg/L for asymptomatic children (interquartile range 5.8–9.7 μg/L[25]). There was a good response to inhaled salbutamol, and she was discharged home on salbutamol via metered dose inhaler and spacer.

It may be possible in the future to say that she is at a significantly increased risk of developing asthma in later childhood, but currently there is not enough evidence to support the use of ECP as a predictive tool.

asthma is unknown in asthma. Corticosteroid therapy reduces NO excretion to normal levels,[28] possibly by a direct effect on inducible NO synthase (the enzyme responsible for NO production), rather than its specific effect on inflammation. However in chronic stable asthma there may be a direct link between the amount of eosinophil inflammation in the lung and breath NO.[29] Measurement of NO is still a research tool, and is likely to have the same problems of specificity as other indirect markers of lung inflammation. It may prove to be the least invasive test of lung inflammation.

CONCLUDING REMARKS AND RESEARCH ISSUES

There are clear indications for the direct assessment of lung inflammation in interstitial lung disease. For all the other sampling methods, the clinical usefulness of assessing lung inflammation is unproven. The key questions to ask for any marker of lung inflammation are: what is the sensitivity, specificity and accuracy of the measurement in diagnosing a clinically important condition, predicting a useful therapeutic response, and assessing prognosis. For markers of asthma, look at the graph of the individual data for the inflammatory marker. Is there a significant overlap between asthmatics and controls? Have the researchers included atopic controls without asthma? Has the 'cut off' value been derived retrospectively, or tested prospectively? Before accepting any test using direct sampling or indirect markers clinicians need to be convinced by the published evidence that it adds to rather than just confirms, the information gathered by traditional clinical techniques.

ALLERGY

BACKGROUND

Allergic disorders depend on an immunologically mediated hypersensitivity reaction to a foreign substance. In the major primarily atopic disorders, asthma, allergic rhino-conjunctivitis and eczema (atopic dermatitis), the mechanism is IgE-dependent, typically involving mast cells and eosinophils in inflammatory processes in the airways, nose, eyes and skin. IgE-dependent mechanisms may be partly responsible for allergy to *Aspergillus fumigatus* as a secondary phenomenon in children with chronic non-atopic airway inflammation (such as cystic fibrosis) but additional non-IgE-dependent mechanisms are also involved. The role of atopy in recurrent spasmodic croup is controversial. In some very rare situations in childhood (but more commonly in adults in the context of occupational asthma), entirely non-IgE mechanisms may lead, for instance, to acute allergic alveolitis in paediatric versions of 'pigeon fanciers' lung'. This section will deal mainly with the investigation of atopic disease.

The prevalence of atopic sensitization in children has risen progressively in industrialized countries for 30 years, together with atopic diseases. There is a definite causal link between these two events, although atopy is not usually a sufficient cause of any of the specific atopic diseases, merely a contributing factor. Adjuvant factors (infection, air pollution, tobacco smoke exposure and possibly dietary antioxidant imbalance) and other genetic factors in these polygenic conditions, may be important too. Atopy may be involved in airway disease in both initiating and sustaining chronic inflammation and in triggering acute episodes. In the first 2 years of life, a condition which falls within the asthma spectrum, episodic viral wheeze, appears to be almost completely independent of atopy.

It is important to recognize the contribution of allergic mechanisms to disease in individual patients because management can then be appropriately directed, for instance with anti-allergic drugs, general advice on avoiding exposures at home and advice on future career choices. The role of specific allergens should also be sought, to advise on environmental control to reduce specific exposures, for instance, in a house-dust mite-sensitive asthmatic, or to identify disorders of life-threatening importance, such as chronic allergic bronchopulmonary aspergillosis (ABPA) or acute food-induced anaphylaxis.

In a small proportion of asthmatic children, atopic sensitization cannot be detected. As in 'intrinsic' adult asthma, IgE-dependent mechanisms may still be operating locally, in the airways. But the importance of this unusual situation in children is that it should alert the health worker to the possibility of other important disorders, such as immune deficiency, another host-defence disorder, bronchomalacia or obliterative bronchiolitis. Failure to identify a specific allergen in a child with, say asthma and a raised total IgE level does not preclude an atopic mechanism.

A large proportion of children with severe rhinitis do not have any detectable allergies and are diagnosed as having perennial non-atopic rhinitis.

TECHNIQUES AND INTERPRETATION

Clinical evaluation

A good history is vital and provides important clues (Chapter 2). A personal or first-degree family history of atopic disease points to atopy as a probable factor. In asthma, the pattern of illness, especially the relationship between episodes and possible exposures to aeroallergens may occasionally pinpoint a specific allergic trigger (Case study 8.6) although this is rare in practice. The timing of exposure and onset of symptoms may be helpful. Amelioration of symptoms when on holiday away from home strongly suggests a local environmental factor. Intolerance to a specific food is usually more obvious from detailed questioning: it may begin in infancy (with weaning, for example); there may be associated eczema; occasionally the history is dramatic (in acute anaphylaxis, for instance). In IgE-mediated food hypersensitivity, most reactions begin within 30 minutes.

Symptom diaries are rarely helpful in specific antigen detection in chronic disease, except for food intolerance. For episodic illnesses such as anaphylaxis or episodic asthma, they can help to focus attention on potential exposures around the time of the attack. Often however, the choice of further investigations depends on probabilities and on the importance for clinical management of incriminating allergens that are amenable to avoidance measures.

Skin-prick tests (SPT) are performed to detect atopic sensitization to ingested or inhaled allergens. In the UK, over 40% of schoolchildren are

---

Case study 8.6: A highly atopic boy

Vivek, born in India, arrived in the UK 5 years ago, aged 2. He has had increasingly troublesome chronic perennial asthma, requiring high dose inhaled corticosteroids, long-acting bronchodilators and frequent short course prednisolone therapy for acute episodes. He also has eczema and perennial rhinitis, both treated with topical corticosteroids and antihistamines. Compliance was felt to be excellent. Daily records confirmed frequent nocturnal awakenings and variable PEF.

Spirometry confirmed airway obstruction, completely reversed by a nebulized ß$_2$ agonist. Two days after stopping antihistamines, skin prick tests were performed: the only reactions were to the positive (histamine) control (3 mm) and milk (8 mm).

A diet free of dairy products was supervised by a dietician. Vivek's rhinitis and eczema improved considerably within a week, while chest symptoms became more responsive to current therapy, allowing a step-down after 6 weeks. Non-dairy calcium supplements were provided. It is unusual but gratifying to find a single major allergen.

atopic (i.e. react on SPT to one or more allergens). The majority have no current atopic disease. The choice of test allergen solution is made as follows in the UK:

- Simply to identify atopy: house-dust mite (HDM), cat and mixed grass pollen.
- For perennial asthma: add mould mix, dog, eggs, milk, tree mix and cockroach.
- For seasonal asthma: spring – trees; summer – flowers and grasses; autumn – moulds.
- In intractable asthma or cystic fibrosis: *Aspergillus fumigatus* is included.
- Anaphylaxis: nuts, fish, shellfish, and other suspect foods (including soya, wheat, egg and milk).
- Other allergens as indicated by history.
- A negative control (diluent) and positive control (10% histamine solution) are always included, the former to detect a non-specific response to the trauma of SPT and the latter to ensure the potential for the skin to react (and to exclude inadvertent use of antihistamines).

The important aeroallergens vary with the climate and flora (Table 8.6).

The principle behind SPT is that by breaching the epidermis with a needle inserted through a drop of allergen extract, sufficient allergen (perhaps only a few hundred molecules) enters the dermis where it triggers the release of inflammatory agents including histamine, from specifically IgE-sensitized mast cells (Figure 8.6). A weal (capillary leakage with oedema) and flare (neural, axon-reflex-mediated vasodilatation) result. The mean diameter of the weal (but not the flare) is a measure of response. The size of the weal is partly dependent on the serum level of specific IgE, but the correlation is poor. Weals of 3 mm or more are positive (but not necessarily clinically relevant).

A number of technical variables may affect the results and their interpretation (Table 8.7). Allergen extracts vary in source and potency between

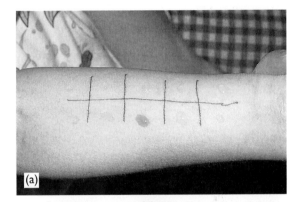

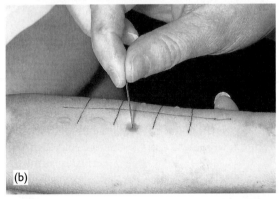

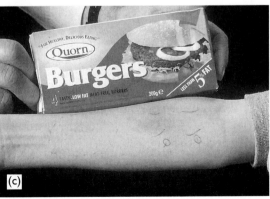

Figure 8.6: Skin-prick testing. (a) The extracts in a grid on the forearm; (b) pricking the skin; (c) the response in Case study 8.8.

Table 8.6: Important aeroallergens world-wide

Situation	Allergens
Temperate areas	House-dust mite (Derp1)* Cat (Fed d1) Grass pollen
Urban USA	Cockroach
Desert areas	Alternaria
Scandinavia	Birch pollen
Mediterranean	Olive pollen

* This agent is ubiquitous except in high altitude and low humidity environments.

Table 8.7: Interpretation of skin-prick tests in asthma and anaphylaxia

False positive	False negative
'Aggressive' SPT technique	Child too young
Sensitized but allergen unrelated to disease	Antihistamines taken within previous 48 hours
Dermographism or eczema causes exaggerated response	'Delicate' SPT technique
Pseudopodia (tend to exaggerate the size of response rather than cause true false positive)	Poor cutaneous expression of lung-selective immune process
	Very high levels of polyclonal IgE (nematode infection)
	Non-IgE-dependent mechanism for allergic disease
	Unreactive site chosen for tests
	Local corticosteroid creams

manufacturers. The technique for pricking the skin varies: in the traditional poorly standardizable Pepys method, a clean 23-gauge hypodermic needle is used for each allergen; modern pre-formed shouldered prick lancets (e.g. Morrow Brown needles) are inserted vertically until the shoulder engages the skin, to standardize the depth of penetration; multiple-prick devices allow several allergens to be tested at a single stroke, a boon for testing young or timid children; lancets pre-loaded with freeze-dried allergen (Pharmacia) which avoid the need for wet solutions have been available in the past and are convenient but expensive. The volar aspect of the arm or (in small infants) the area between the scapulae is used.

The size of the weal (but not the flare) is the mean of the greatest diameter and its perpendicular, avoiding the 'pseudopodia' which develop in extremely sensitive individuals. False results occur (Table 8.7). The correlation between the weal size and the clinical importance of any allergen is poor, but for aeroallergens in asthma the larger the weals the more likely they are to be clinically relevant.

Laboratory measurements

Total IgE is measured in serum. Because total IgE normally comprises less than 0.001% of total immunoglobulins, total IgE is measured by the very sensitive enzyme-linked immunosorbent assay (ELISA) technique. In industrialized countries, where parasitic infestations of the gastrointestinal tract are uncommon, the total serum IgE level is a useful clue to the presence of atopy, but is of little clinical value. An extremely high level (>10,000 IU/L) in a child with recurrent pulmonary and skin infections is diagnostic of Job's (hyper-IgE) syndrome. A normal level in a child with 'asthma' should alert one to alternative diagnoses. In the Third World, total IgE levels are dependent on parasite load as well as allergic factors.

IgE antibodies directed against specific allergens *(specific IgE)* are measured in serum using either a variation of the radio-allergosorbent test (RAST), or the enzyme-linked immunosorbant assay (ELISA). In the RAST, allergens are chemically bound to an insoluble matrix. When patients' serum is added allergen-specific IgE binds the immobilized allergen. Radioactively or fluorescently labelled anti-IgE is then added and this attaches to the specific IgE already bound to the allergen. The amount of specific IgE can then be determined by the amount of bound label. Antibody levels provide a crude indication of the likely importance of the allergen, but the correlation between levels and symptoms is poor.

Precipitins are usually IgG class antibodies against environmental proteins. It is important to seek them when acute allergic alveolitis or chronic extrinsic alveolitis are suspected – both rare in children. In ABPA multiple precipitins against *Aspergillus fumigatus* are pathognomonic.

Other measurements which may be useful include: C1-esterase levels in recurrent angio-oedema or anaphylaxis, and serum tryptase which has good diagnostic sensitivity and specificity in acute (<6 hours) anaphylaxis.[31]

Challenge tests

Allergen challenge tests are not appropriate for children with suspected aeroallergen-induced lung disease. They are too dangerous. Oral challenge with suspect foods in suspected anaphylaxis may be justified. They too are potentially dangerous. Guidelines have been published.[32] Our practice has been to do open food challenges in a number of specific circumstances (Box 8.1), using skilled staff and appropriate facilities for resuscitation in the event of an adverse reaction.

INTEGRATING RESULTS INTO PRACTICE

Asthma

Confirming the clinical relevance of an allergen is an iterative process. Directed history-taking may

---

Box 8.1: Some indications for oral challenge in anaphylaxis

- to determine tolerance, for instance to milk or egg;
- to identify an allergen when the cause of the reaction is not confirmed, e.g. nut challenge;
- to confirm or refute a diagnosis where history contradicts allergy tests; usually positive history – and negative test or very occasionally vice versa (e.g. a sibling);
- history not classical or typical, especially in nut allergy where diagnosis is so important as avoidance is absolute and diagnosis life-long;
- where allergy tests not available e.g. colourants or preservatives;
- in nut allergic patients who present with a history of an exposure to one nut, but SPT shows allergy to more than one nut.

---

help, aided by a symptom diary. It is rarely possible to prove symptomatic improvement by avoidance of aeroallergens, especially in highly sensitized children, since avoidance procedures in the home are not very effective, (for HDM, for example), and many allergens are ubiquitous (cat proteins, for example). Avoidance of ingested agents (foods) is easier although rarely the sole cause of asthma (Case study 8.6). In most children, allergy to one or two avoidable allergens is not the main factor in chronic asthma so that the options for environmental modification are, in any case, limited.

Advice to avoid new exposure to furry pets, for example, may be given. Career advice is also important, since exposure to animal proteins (laboratory or veterinary work) may be inadvisable.

The use of immunization ('hyposensitization') against specific allergens in asthmatic children is very contentious. It is dangerous in severe asthma, and not called for in mild disease.

Other disorders

Variable airway obstruction is common in other chronic lung diseases (cystic fibrosis, bronchiectasis, chronic lung disease of prematurity). Bearing in mind that 40% of all children are atopic, aeroallergen sensitivities in these groups should raise the possibility of IgE-dependent mechanisms complicating the picture, with consequences for management.

Asthma in a schoolchild with no evidence of atopy in SPT or blood tests, is unusual. Alternative causes should be sought (Case study 8.7).

Case study 8.7: Non-atopic asthma

At the age of 12, Melanie is referred for assessment. She has had episodes of wheeze and mucus production for many years and is now becoming breathless between episodes. She has no nocturnal symptoms, but is short of breath after exercise. 'Irritable bowel' had been a long-standing problem. Her symptoms have never clearly responded to inhaled corticosteroids and only responded partially to inhaled β_2 agonists. There was no family history of atopy.

On examination, she was slender for her (average) height and had minimal finger clubbing. There was chest overexpansion, with a few coarse upper lobe crackles. Her FEV_1 was reduced (65% predicted, with a 10% improvement after bronchodilator) and skin-prick tests were negative, and her serum IgE was at the upper normal limit. The absence of ENT symptoms made ciliary dyskinesia or immune deficiency unlikely. A sweat test was positive (sweat sodium 95 mmol/L; sweat weight 235 mg). Genotyping revealed Δ508/NI heterozygosity (NI: not identified).

Reconsider non-atopic children with chronic chest symptoms. CF variants are common!

Case study 8.8: Anaphylaxis

Algernon's family were strict vegans. On occasions he had suffered mild facial and tongue swelling, puffy eyes, generalized itching and some difficulty breathing. The symptoms settled on the first two occasions, but seemed to be more severe each time. He was brought to the Emergency Department on the third occasion, where anaphylaxis was diagnosed, responding quickly to intramuscular adrenaline (epinephrine) and oral antihistamine.

A careful history revealed that he had been eating Quorn (textured mycoprotein) burgers on each occasion. Skin-prick testing with an aqueous extract demonstrated hypersensitivity. There were no reactions to other commonly incriminated foods. Dietary avoidance measures were instituted. The family and school were provided with an emergency management plan, including antihistamines and adrenaline pens.

Anaphylaxis

The primary objective is to identify ingested allergens so that they can be avoided. The advice of a dietician will be needed where key nutrients or widespread allergens are involved. Avoidance should be backed up by a written, guided self-management plan including the provision of adrenaline for emergency use and antihistamines for mild reactions. (See Case study 8.8.)

FUTURE RESEARCH AND CONCLUSIONS

The poor correlation between atopic sensitivity and clinical disease is an area of intense research. Detecting organ-selective immune processes such as T-cell homing to the lung, which we cannot yet identify in human subjects, will allow us to increase the specificity of our measurements. Safe, subliminal inhalation challenge may be another means of identifying more specifically important allergic agents; such tests will depend on new methods of detecting pneumonary responses – perhaps by breath analysis.

Tied to identification, we need more effective and efficient measures to avoid environmental exposure to common agents such as HDM (Chapter 25) as well as safer more specific immunization procedures to reduce IgE-dependent allergic reactions.

At the moment, allergic disease is treated by crude pharmacological means, in the absence of population-based (public health) primary intervention measures or of allergen-specific, individual patient-based therapies.

ACKNOWLEDGEMENT

We thank Dr David Luyt for his advice on allergy.

REFERENCES

1. Carlos TM, Harlan JM. Leukocyte-endothelial adhesion molecules. *Blood* 1994; **84**: 2068–101.

2. Cox G, Crossley J, Xing Z. Macrophage engulfment of apoptotic neutrophils contributes to the resolution of acute pulmonary inflammation *in vivo*. *Am J Respir Cell Mol Biol* 1995; **12**: 232–7.

3. Fan LL, Langston C. Chronic interstitial lung disease in children. *Pediatr Pulmonol* 1993; **16**: 184–96.

4. Sharland M, Gibb DM, Holland F. Respiratory morbidity from lymphocytic interstitial pneumonitis (LIP) in vertically acquired HIV infection. *Arch Dis Child* 1997; **76**: 334–6.

5. Uziel Y, Hen B, Cordoba M, Wolach B. Lymphocytic interstitial pneumonitis preceding polyarticular juvenile rheumatoid arthritis. *Clin Exp Rheumatol* 1998; **16**: 617–19.

6. Riedler J, Grigg J, Robertson CF. Role of bronchoalveolar lavage in children with lung disease. *Eur Respir J* 1995; **8**: 1725–30.

7. Grigg J, Riedler J, Robertson CF. Bronchoalveolar lavage fluid cellularity and soluble intercellular adhesion molecule-1 in children with colds. *Pediatr Pulmonol* 1999; **28**: 109–16.

8. Meduri GU, Reddy RC, Stanley T, El-Zeky F. Pneumonia in acute respiratory distress syndrome. A prospective evaluation of bilateral bronchoscopic sampling. *Am J Respir Crit Care Med* 1998; **158**: 870–5.

9. Bandla HP, Smith DE, Kiernan MP. Laryngeal mask airway facilitated fibreoptic bronchoscopy in infants. *Can J Anaesth* 1997; **44**: 1242–7.

10. Koumbourlis AC, Kurland G. Nonbronchoscopic bronchoalveolar lavage in mechanically ventilated infants: technique, efficacy, and applications. *Pediatr Pulmonol* 1993; **15**: 257–62.

11. Wehle K, Blanke M, Koenig G, Pfitzer P. The cytological diagnosis of *Pneumocystis carinii* by fluorescence microscopy of Papanicolaou stained bronchoalveolar lavage specimens. *Cytopathology* 1991; **2**: 113–20.

12. Dakhama A, Hegele RG, Laflamme G, Israel-Assayag E, Cormier Y. Common respiratory viruses in lower airways of patients with acute hypersensitivity pneumonitis. *Am J Respir Crit Care Med* 1999; **159**: 1316–22.

13. Marguet C, Jouen-Boedes F, Dean TP, Warner JO. Bronchoalveolar cell profiles in children with asthma, infantile wheeze, chronic cough, or cystic fibrosis. *Am J Respir Crit Care Med* 1999; **159**: 1533–40.

14. Stevenson EC, Turner G, Heaney LG, *et al.* Bronchoalveolar lavage findings suggest two different forms of childhood asthma. *Clin Exp Allergy* 1997; **27**: 1027–35.

15. Magnussen H, Holz O. Monitoring airway inflammation in asthma by induced sputum. *Eur Respir J* 1999; **13**: 5–7.

16. Jatakanon A, Lalloo UG, Lim S, Chung KF, Barnes PJ. Increased neutrophils and cytokines, TNF-α and IL-8, in induced sputum of non-asthmatic patients with chronic dry cough. *Thorax* 1999; **54**: 234–7.

17. Hargreave FE. Induced sputum and response to glucocorticoids. *J Allergy Clin Immunol* 1998; **102**: S102–5.

18. Brightling CE, Ward R, Goh KL, Wardlaw AJ, Pavord ID. Eosinophilic bronchitis is an important cause of chronic cough. *Am J Respir Crit Care Med* 1999; **160**: 406–10.

19. Grigg J, Venge P. Inflammatory markers of outcome. *Eur Respir J* (Suppl.) 1996; **21**: 16s–21s.

20. Koller DY, Halmerbauer G, Frischer T, Roithner B. Assessment of eosinophil granule proteins in various body fluids: is there a relation to clinical variables in childhood asthma? *Clin Exp Allergy* 1999; **29**: 786–93.

21. Hoekstra MO. Can eosinophil-derived proteins be used to diagnose or to monitor childhood asthma? *Clin Exp Allergy* 1999; **29**: 873–4.

22. Chang AB, Phelan PD, Carlin JB, Sawyer SM, Robertson CF. A randomised, placebo controlled trial of inhaled salbutamol and beclomethasone for recurrent cough. *Arch Dis Child* 1998; **79**: 6–11.

23. Martinez FD, Wright AL, Taussig LM, Holberg CJ, Halonen M, Morgan WJ. Asthma and wheezing in the first six years of life. The Group Health Medical Associates. *N Engl J Med* 1995; **332**: 133–8.

24. Villa JR, Garcia G, Rueda S, Nogales A. Serum eosinophilic cationic protein may predict clinical course of wheezing in young children. *Arch Dis Child* 1998; **78**: 448–52.

25. Koller DY, Wojnarowski C, Herkner KR, *et al.* High levels of eosinophil cationic protein in wheezing infants predict the development of asthma. *J Allergy Clin Immunol* 1997; **99**: 752–6.

26. Franklin PJ, Taplin R, Stick SM. A community study of exhaled nitric oxide in healthy children. *Am J Respir Crit Care Med* 1999; **159**: 69–73.

27. Artlich A, Busch T, Lewandowski K, Jonas S, Gortner L, Falke KJ. Childhood asthma: exhaled nitric oxide in relation to clinical symptoms. *Eur Respir J* 1999; **13**: 1396–401.

28. Lanz MJ, Leung DY, White CW. Comparison of exhaled nitric oxide to spirometry during emergency treatment of asthma exacerbations with glucocorticoids in children. *Ann Allergy Asthma Immunol* 1999; **82**: 161–4.

29. Mattes J, Storm van's Gravesande K, Reining U, *et al.* NO in exhaled air is correlated with markers of eosinophilic airway inflammation in corticosteroid-dependent childhood asthma. *Eur Respir J* 1999; **13**: 1391–5.

30. Spanevello A, Beghe B, Bianchi A, *et al.* Comparison of two methods of processing induced sputum: selected versus entire sputum. *Am J Respir Crit Care Med* 1998; **157**: 665–8.

31. Enrique E, Garcia-Ortega P, Sotorra O, Gaig P, Richart C. Usefulness of UniCAP-Tryptase fluoroimmunoassay in the diagnosis of anaphylaxis. *Allergy* 1999; **54**: 602–6.

32. Luyt D, Dunbar H, Baker H. Nut allergy in children: investigation and management. *J R Soc Med* 2000; **93**: 283–7.

FURTHER READING

IMMUNODEFICIENCY

1. WHO Scientific Group Report on Primary Immuno-deficiency Diseases. *Clin Exp Immunol* 1997; **109**. (Suppl. 1): 1–28.

2. *Consensus document for the diagnosis and management of patients with primary antibody deficiency.* Royal College of Pathologists, Royal College of Physicians, and Primary Immunodeficiency Association, 1995.

3. Stiehm ER (ed). *Immunologic disorders in infants and children*, 4th ed. Philadelphia: WB Saunders, 1996.

4. Ziegler JB, Blanche S and Loh R. Children with HIV. *Med J Austral* 1996; **164**: 672–9.

5. Spickett G. *Oxford handbook of clinical immunology.* Oxford: Oxford University Press, 1999.

INFLAMMATION

6. European Respiratory Society Taskforce. Methods for assessment of airway inflammation. *Eur Respir J* 1998; **11**: (Suppl. 26).

7. Silverman M, Pedersen S, Grigg J. Measurement of airway inflammation in children. *Am J Respir Crit Care Med* 2000; **162**: (Suppl.): S1–S55.

ALLERGY

8. Warner JA, Warner JO. Allergy. In: Silverman M (ed). *Childhood asthma and other wheezing disorders.* 2nd edn. London: Arnold, in preparation.

CHAPTER NINE

CILIARY STRUCTURE *AND* FUNCTION

M.A. Chilvers and C. O'Callaghan

- Background
- Techniques
- Interpretation of results

- Research issues
- References

BACKGROUND

Respiratory cilia beat in a regular co-ordinated manner, propelling overlying mucus from the airways to the oropharynx where it is either swallowed or expectorated. Approximately 200 cilia project from each epithelial cell surface and beat at a frequency between 12–15 Hz.[1] They have recently been shown to beat in a forward and backwards motion without a sideways motion in their recovery stroke.[2] Each cilium has a uniform ultrastructure that repeats precisely every 96 nm. This is constructed from microtubule doublets, dynein arms and radial spokes surrounding a central microtubular pair and forms the classical '9+2' arrangement. (Figure 9.1).[1]

Primary ciliary dyskinesia may be caused by one of a number of different ciliary ultrastructural defects involving the dynein arms, radial spokes, microtubules or complete absence of cilia.[3,4] Such ultrastructural abnormalities result in cilia which are either stationary or beat in a slow or dyskinetic fashion. Ineffective movement impairs mucociliary clearance resulting in mucus retention. This leads to recurrent chest infections, which may progress to bronchiectasis, and chronic sinusitis.[5]

Primary ciliary dyskinesia is inherited in an autosomal recessive fashion.[6] The incidence is approximately 1 in 16,000 of whom 50% will have situs inversus.[1,3,4] Given this incidence, there should be approximately 3000 patients in the United Kingdom with 70 new cases occurring each year. It is suspected that primary ciliary dyskinesia is significantly under diagnosed.[4,7]

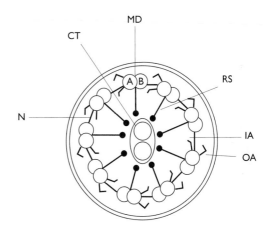

Figure 9.1: Diagram of the classical '9+2' cross section. Two central microtubules (CT) are enclosed within a central sheath to form the central axis of the axoneme. This is surrounded by nine microtubule doublets (MD). The doublets consist of an A and B doublet. Each doublet is connected by nexin links (N) to the next. From the A doublet, inner (IA) and outer (OA) dynein arms project to the adjacent doublet. Radial spokes (RS) connect the central sheath to the outer microtubule doublets.

Table 9.1: Features of primary ciliary dyskinesia

Neonatal	Unexplained respiratory distress or neonatal chest infection
	Situs inversus
	Congenital anomalies: cardiac defects, hydrocephalus, oesophageal atresia, biliary atresia
Childhood	Chronic 'wet' cough
	Bronchiectasis
	Atypical asthma failing to respond to treatment
	Hearing impairment due to chronic otitis media
	Situs inversus
	Learning difficulties
Adulthood	Bronchiectasis
	Male infertility due to impaired sperm motility
	Female ectopic pregnancy

Primary ciliary dyskinesia can present in infancy or late adulthood due to the varying patterns of symptoms[4,6] (Table 9.1). Symptoms frequently start in the neonatal period and include a chronic nasal discharge and a moist cough. Hearing problems may occur in approximately 50%, with glue ear being common. It is assumed that 50% of patients will have situs inversus. All siblings of index cases require assessment.[8]

WHY MAKE A DIAGNOSIS OF PRIMARY CILIARY DYSKINESIA?

The diagnosis of primary ciliary dyskinesia (PCD) should be considered in patients under investiga-tion for suspected bronchiectasis or in patients with a persistent 'wet' cough. At which point one should consider investigating for primary ciliary dyskinesia dependent on the pattern of symptoms (Case studies 9.1 and 9.2).

Diagnosis of primary ciliary dyskinesia is diffi-cult. While false positive diagnoses occur the greatest problem is late diagnosis.[4] Late diagnosis is of concern as lung function progressively declines in undiagnosed patients[7] and hearing related problems are often poorly managed. Antibiotic therapy and aggressive physiotherapy halts this decline and causes the fall in lung func-tion to plateau.[7] Early diagnosis is essential to achieve a good prognosis and to minimize the high morbidity from progressive bronchiectasis and rhinosinusitis.[4,7]

Case study 9.1

Celia, a 10-year-old girl, was referred with a history of a chronic cough productive of yellow sputum. Her exercise tolerance was reduced. On examination she had a 'wet' sounding cough. Her weight which had been on the 50th centile 2 years ago, had fallen to the 10th centile. Harrison's sulci were noted and chest auscultation revealed coarse crackles at both lung bases. A chest radiograph showed areas of lobar and segmental collapse and a CT scan revealed disseminated bronchiectasis.

The following investigations were negative; sweat test; CF genotype; oesophageal pH monitoring; barium swallow; bronchoscopy with bronchiolar lavage; immunoglobulins and subclasses; functional antibody levels; serum comple-ment; nitroblue tetrazolium (NBT) test.

This patient had bronchiectasis of unknown cause. At this point primary ciliary dyskinesia should be considered. Ciliary biopsy revealed cilia with a normal beat frequency that were beating dyskinetically on slow motion replay of high-speed video footage. The diagnosis of PCD secondary to a ciliary transposition was confirmed on electron microscopy.

Case study 9.2

Hassan, a 9-year-old Asian boy, was referred for assessment of chronic cough. He was born at term to parents who are first cousins. At 8 hours of age he was transferred to the neonatal unit with respiratory distress and required 30% headbox oxygen. He was discharged home after three days with a diagnosis of delayed clearance of lung fluid.

Since then he had persisting problems with nasal discharge and a moist sounding cough. He recently failed a hearing test due to glue ear and is due to have grommets inserted. He was being treated with inhaled steroids and β_2-agonists with little improvement. His FEV_1 had fallen to 50% of its predicted value.

On examination he had a wet sounding cough and was mouth breathing. His weight was on the third centile. Harrison's sulci were noted and chest auscultation was normal. A chest radiograph showed situs solitus with slight perihilar changes.

The most likely diagnosis was primary ciliary dyskinesia and in this case investigation for PCD was one of the initial investigations. Neonatal respiratory distress in a term infant is not an uncommon presenting feature of primary ciliary dyskinesia. The fact the parents are related also increases the likelihood of an inherited disease such as primary ciliary dyskinesia. A combination of a moist cough with nasal discharge starting in the neonatal period, with glue ear, is also strongly suggestive. The diagnosis was confirmed on functional and structural studies of a nasal ciliary biopsy.

The diagnosis of primary ciliary dyskinesia in a child may be delayed for a number of reasons:

- young children are usually unable to expectorate sputum even when they have a very moist sounding cough;
- children usually remain apyrexial despite ongoing chronic lung inflammation and infection;
- chest auscultation is usually normal despite bronchiectasis;
- the chest radiograph may be normal despite extensive bronchiectasis; only 50% of patients with PCD have situs inversus;
- young children are unable to perform objective lung function testing such as spirometry.

Thus a persistent moist sounding cough with nasal blockage or discharge, starting in infancy, may be the only features of PCD in this age group.

TECHNIQUES

SCREENING TESTS

Various screening methods have been developed to identify patients with primary ciliary dyskinesia. These cannot be recommended to screen for children suspected of having PCD at present.

1 The *saccharin test* is inappropriate for children; it involves the application of a small particle of saccharin to the inferior nasal turbinate. The time for a sweet sensation to be tasted is noted. A time greater than 30 minutes is abnormal and requires further investigation. The test is difficult to perform and may only identify cases with immotile cilia.[9] Cases in which cilia are beating dyskinetically may be missed.[9]
2 *Exhaled nitric oxide* is low in primary ciliary dyskinesia. Although research is continuing in this area it is considered premature to use nitric oxide as a screening test.[4]

DIAGNOSTIC PROCEDURES

The gold standard tests for the diagnosis of PCD are:

- measurement of ciliary beat frequency;
- assessment of ciliary beat pattern;
- electron microscopic evaluation of ciliary ultrastructure.

Ciliated epithelium is obtained by nasal brush biopsy of the inferior turbinate without local anaesthetic (Figure 9.2). It is important that the patient is free of an upper respiratory tract infection for at least 4 weeks prior to the biopsy as this may confusingly cause secondary ciliary dyskinesia. The sample is processed at 37°C to look at the ciliary beat frequency and beat pattern.

Two popular methods, the photomultiplier and photodiode techniques are used to determine beat frequency indirectly by detecting changes in the intensity of a light beam passing through beating cilia. More recently the development of digital high speed video-imaging not only allows ciliary beat frequency to be rapidly measured, but allows the exact movement of a cilium throughout the beat cycle to be visualized.[2]

Measurement of ciliary beat frequency alone may be unreliable. Beat frequency is influenced by temperature, pH and a variety of different drugs.[10] Certain ultrastructural defects such as ciliary transposition that cause primary ciliary dyskinesia, may result in a beat frequency within the normal range. However, an abnormal ciliary beat pattern is seen on slow motion analysis.[2,11]

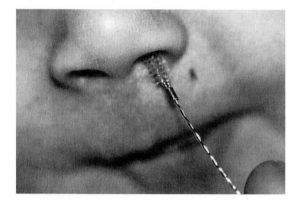

Figure 9.2: Patient undergoing nasal brush biopsy of their inferior nasal turbinate.

Assessment of beat pattern by slow motion analysis in conjunction with beat frequency may have a greater chance of identifying these defects.[2] Investigations should be performed at centres with extensive expertise in the evaluation of ciliary structure and function who have their own normal reference ranges, because of the importance of measurement conditions.

Part of the sample is stored in gluteraldehyde to allow assessment of ciliary ultrastructure by transmission electron microscopy. The absence of inner or outer dynein arms, microtubules and ciliary disorientation are all features of PCD.

INTERPRETATION OF RESULTS

An abnormal ciliary beat frequency of less than 12 Hz accompanied by immotile or dyskinetically beating cilia, together with specific abnormalities of the ciliary axoneme on electron microscopy are found in patients with primary ciliary dyskinesia.[4] This combined with a supportive clinical history allows the diagnosis of PCD to be confirmed. If primary ciliary dyskinesia is strongly suspected or any doubt exists about the diagnosis then the patient should have a repeat nasal brush biopsy. It is important to remember that PCD due to ciliary transposition may give a normal beat frequency. However, a dyskinetic beat pattern is seen on slow motion analysis.

Treatment is aimed at preventing lung damage and halting the evolution of bronchiectasis and decline in lung function (Table 9.2).[4]

With optimal treatment the prognosis is thought to be good with a near normal life expectancy.[4]

RESEARCH ISSUES

The genetic loci responsible for primary ciliary dyskinesia are unknown and currently under investigation.[8] This is an extremely complex area as several hundred genes are involved in the construction of a cilium.[12] It is therefore thought unlikely that a diagnostic genetic test will become

Table 9.2: Main aspects of management of primary ciliary dyskinesia

Respiratory	Aggressive use of antibiotics in respiratory exacerbations Twice daily physiotherapy and exercise Inhaled bronchodilators +/− corticosteroids Regular review with formal lung spirometry Yearly review by specialist centre Yearly flu vaccination
Hearing	Regular audiometry Temporary hearing aids may be required for severe hearing loss
Fertility	May require assessment at assisted conception unit
Psychosocial	Genetic counselling Entitlement to economic benefits Primary ciliary dyskinesia patient support group Educational provision appropriate to learning difficulties (if any)

available in the foreseeable future. Research is underway to determine if the combined analysis of ciliary beat frequency, beat pattern and ultra-structure may reduce the risk of misdiagnosis.[2]

REFERENCES

1. Chilvers MA, O'Callaghan C. Local mucociliary defence mechanisms. *Paed Respir Rev* 2000; **1**: 27–34.

2. Chilvers MA, O'Callaghan C. Analysis of ciliary beat pattern and beat frequency using digital high speed imaging: comparison with the photomultiplier and photodiode methods. *Thorax* 2000; **55**: 314–17.

3. Schidlow DV. Primary ciliary dyskinesia (the immotile cilia syndrome). *Ann Allergy* 1994; **73**: 457–68.

4. Bush A, Cole P, Hariri M, *et al.* Primary ciliary dyskinesia: diagnosis and standards of care. *Eur Respir J* 1998; **12**: 982–8.

5. Rossman CM, Newhouse MT. Primary ciliary dyskinesia: evaluation and management. *Pediatr Pulmonol* 1988; **5**: 36–50

6. Sturgess JM, Thompson MW, Czegledy-Nagy E, Turner JA. Genetic aspects of immotile cilia syndrome. *Am J Med Genet* 1986; **25**: 149–60.

7. Ellerman A, Bisgaard H. Longitudinal study of lung function in a cohort of primary ciliary dyskinesia. *Eur Resp J* 1997; **10**: 2376–9.

8. Meeks M, Bush A. Primary ciliary dyskinesia. *Curr Paediatr* 1998; **8**: 231–6.

9. Canciani M, Barlocco EG, Mastella G, *et al.* The saccharin method for testing mucociliary function in patients suspected of having primary ciliary dyskinesia. *Paed Pulmonol* 1988; **5**: 210–14.

10. Rusznak C, Devalia JL, Lozewicz S, Davies RJ. The assessment of nasal mucociliary clearance and the effect of drugs. *Respir Med* 1994; **88**: 89–101.

11. Rossman CM, Forrest JB, Lee RM, Newhouse MT. The dyskinetic cilia syndrome. Ciliary motility in immotile cilia syndrome. *Chest* 1980; **78**: 580–2.

12. Afzelius BA. Genetics and pulmonary medicine. Immotile cilia syndrome; past, present, and prospects for the future. *Thorax* 1998; **53**: 894–7.

CHAPTER TEN

RADIOLOGICAL PROCEDURES

C. Wallis and I. Gordon

- Introduction
- Imaging techniques
- Further reading

INTRODUCTION

Radiology is an invaluable tool for the paediatrician who cares for children with respiratory conditions. Imaging can assist in establishing a diagnosis and provide an assessment of the extent of disease. For children with chronic respiratory disorders, judicious use of radiological procedures can monitor the progression of the disease process and help tailor medical and surgical intervention.

Radiological investigations need careful planning to ensure that the most appropriate test is chosen to provide the information that is sought. In paediatrics, especially in children with chronic respiratory conditions, the number of tests and exposure to radiation should be minimized. Consultation with a radiologist, following a detailed history and examination, will assist in planning the best radiological approach and the appropriate sequence of tests for an individual patient.

The case studies illustrate only some of the respiratory cases that paediatricians may encounter. The images presented are illustrative only. For more comprehensive reviews and studies of radiological imaging, a number of atlases are available and are listed at the end of this chapter.

IMAGING TECHNIQUES

PLAIN RADIOGRAPHY

Upper airways – post-nasal space and lateral neck

The lateral neck/post-nasal space (PNS) and sinuses are frequently included on the same X-ray. Frontal and lateral views are required. The frontal projection visualizes the facial sinuses but in children under 1–2 years of age the relatively small size of the facial bones makes it exceedingly difficult to interpret. The antra are usually aerated sufficiently by the age of 18–24 months to be seen on the X-ray. In this young age group, CT may be invaluable (see Upper Airway section p.122). In older children the ethmoid and frontal sinuses, the nasal septum and turbinate bones should be seen. The lateral view assists in visualizing the frontal sinus or in assessing its lack of development but there is a wide range of ages in the normal development of these sinuses. Aeration of the ethmoid/sphenoid air cells is also further aided by this view. The palatine tonsils as well as the adenoidal area must be studied. The relationship of the trachea to the cervical spine as well as the general tracheal calibre is well visualized. The lateral view has certain technical limitations and it is important to be sure that the projection is adequate, i.e. the floors of the anterior, middle and posterior fossae of the skull are overlapping and that the cervical spine is truly lateral. The normal space between the trachea and the cervical spine is one vertebral body; an apparent increase in this space may be pathological, but may also be due to the radiograph being taken in expiration – in this situation the trachea shows an acute angle.

Chest

For a frontal posteroanterior (PA) chest radiograph (anteroposterior, AP, in younger children), the patient must be straight, best evaluated on the film by the relationship of the medial ends of the clavicles to the pedicle of the vertebral body. Even slight rotation can cause unusual appearances in a normal chest X-ray. The medial ends of the clavicles should lie at the level of the fourth vertebral body. X-rays in inspiration are generally preferred, the degree of inspiration judged by counting either the anterior rib ends in the right mid-clavicular line down to the level of the diaphragm – there should be 5–6 ribs present – or counting the posterior aspect of the ribs where one should see down to the 10th rib on inspiration. An expiration film is often regarded as being of little value but such a film demonstrates good compliance of the lungs suggesting that no overinflation or air trapping is present. The expiration film should not be disregarded but rather carefully reviewed to consider whether it needs to be repeated. Pathological conditions which result in a loss of compliance, e.g. opportunistic

---

Case study 10.1: Recurrent chest infections

Karl, a 2-year-old boy had been admitted to his local hospital with three episodes of pneumonia that required in-patient treatment. On each occasion, the left lower lobe had been affected. The frontal chest radiograph showed patchy consolidation behind the heart on the left with loss of the medial aspect of the left hemi-diaphragm. He had recovered well from each infection although on the last admission, his recovery was more prolonged and further assessment was sought. There was no history of feeding difficulties, Karl had not been troubled by infections involving other systems and no other abnormalities were present on clinical examination.

Radiological comment: There are a number of underlying factors to be considered in a child with recurrent chest infections (Table 10.1). In this boy, a number of causes can be excluded on history and examination, but the repeated involvement of the left lower lobe required exclusion of a local pulmonary abnormality at this site. A chest radiograph taken when the child was well shows subtle abnormalities in the left lower zone but no obvious congenital abnormality (Figure 10.1A). To define the anatomy more precisely, a CT was performed. The transaxial slice through the lower zones showed a multi-loculated cystic structure in keeping with a cystic adenomatoid malformation in the left lower lobe (Figure10.1B). No further radiological studies were considered necessary.

Outcome: Surgical excision successfully removed the area that was vulnerable to repeated infection and a congenital adenomatoid malformation was confirmed on histological examination.

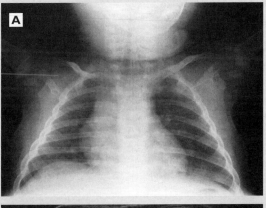

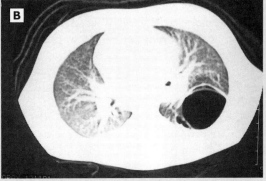

Case study 10.1: Recurrent chest infections (continued)

Table 10.1: Causes of recurrent chest infections

Generalized abnormalities of defence	Immunodeficiency
	Immunosuppression
	Primary ciliary dyskinesia
	Cystic fibrosis
Upper respiratory tract abnormalities	Sinusitis, tonsillitis
	Cleft larynx
	Inco-ordinate swallowing
	Tracheo-oesophageal fistula
Congenital structural abnormalities	Sequestration
	Cystic adenomatoid malformation
Acquired pulmonary abnormalities	Foreign body
	Bronchiectasis
	Aspiration / gastro-oesophageal reflux
	Obliterative bronchiolitis
	Airway compression e.g. nodes, mass
Cardiac pathology	Left heart failure
	Enlarged left atrium
	Left to right shunt
	Primary pulmonary hypertension
Musculo-skeletal abnormalities	
Unusual or resistant organism	

infection in the immune-suppressed child, cause repeated 'expiration films' to be obtained.

In the infant or sick child, supine AP chest X-rays are commonly carried out. The classical signs of well-known pathological conditions can alter, e.g. pleural effusion may only be seen as an 'apical cap'; pneumothorax may not appear peripherally and a pneumomediastinum may appear only as a vague transradiancy in the mediastinum. A lateral chest radiograph with a horizontal beam is useful when doubt persists following the AP view.

The normal visualization of the cardiac outline as well as the diaphragm is due to an aerated lung being adjacent to a 'solid non-aerated organ'. Loss of the normal outlines means that the adjacent lung tissue is no longer aerated; this can occur with consolidation (i.e. fluid in the alveolar spaces due to infection, inflammation or pulmonary oedema). If the airway remains patent throughout then consolidation without major collapse may occur. If there is collapse in a lobe of lung, i.e. loss of volume, bronchial pathology, e.g.

foreign body, mucus or extrinsic compression, must be borne in mind. When consolidation occurs first it is not possible for this solid pulmonary parenchyma to lose volume to any major extent. The diagnosis of a collapsed lobe is made by either identifying a displaced fissure, failing to identify the normal hilum or observing a displaced hilum with fewer vessels in the remaining lung parenchyma.

The lateral chest radiograph requires a greater exposure than the frontal film and because the two lungs are superimposed, it makes interpretation of this film difficult. This film should not be part of a 'routine' chest radiograph in paediatrics, but rather reserved for certain clinical situations. The presence or absence of overinflation may be best assessed on this view. Metastases in children with known solid tumours are less likely to be overlooked when the frontal and lateral films are taken together routinely. In a child with recurrent chest pathology undergoing investigation, a lateral film at the time of the first chest radiograph is strongly recommended. In the long-term follow-up of

Case study 10.2: Acute chest infection

Judy, a 10-year-old girl who had been previously well presented to casualty following a 10-day history of chest pain and fever. She had responded initially to oral antibiotics, but had returned with ongoing fever, lethargy and anorexia. Examination revealed a toxic child with stony dullness throughout the right hemithorax. Her white cell count was significantly raised.

Radiological comment: The frontal chest radiograph shows an almost complete opaque right hemi-thorax with a slight shift of the mediastinum to the opposite side. There is crowding of the ribs on the right but little in the way of a scoliosis (Figure 10.2A). A review of the causes of an opaque hemi-thorax (Table 10.2) favoured a purulent effusion in this clinical scenario. An ultrasound of the chest confirmed the presence of fluid with loculations in the chest (Figure 10.2B). The ultrasonographer was able to mark the site of maximum fluid.

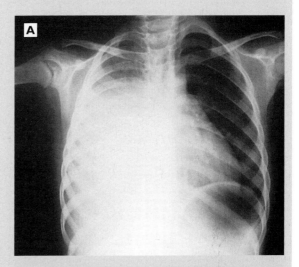

Outcome: An intercostal drain was inserted at the designated site that initially drained 300mL of purulent fluid, but was unsuccessful at complete drainage. Because of ongoing fever and an elevated white cell count after 5 days, a CT of the chest was ordered. The transaxial cut through the mid chest after IV contrast shows the consolidated compressed right lung which enhances with contrast. The pleura is also noted to enhance. The large collection with the drain *in situ* is also noted (Figure 10.2C). The empyema was drained with re-inflation of the lung over the next 5 days. A follow-up frontal chest radiograph after removal of the drain shows slight residual pleural thickening in the lower axiallary aspect on the right, this is likely to resolve completely with time and requires no further treatment (Figure 10.2D).

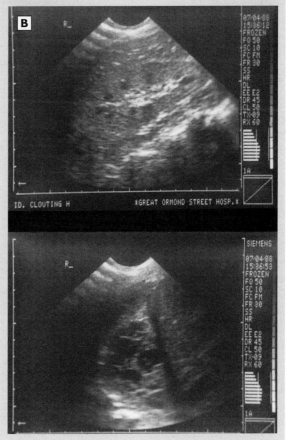

Integrated imaging: In the ill child who has a pleural effusion, which goes on to empyema, it can be valuable to undertake both CT and US. The CT will ensure that a lung abscess is not mistaken for an empyema and will also provide a base line for follow-up especially as one cannot guarantee resolution of the empyema with no sequelae. The US will show loculations that may not be seen on CT.

Comment: Some centres would proceed to a minithoracotomy when loculations are detected, but there is no consensus on management.

Case study 10.2: Acute chest infection (continued)

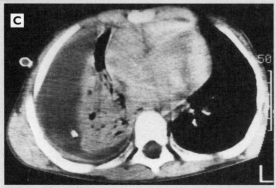

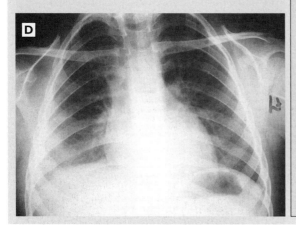

Table 10.2: Causes of an opaque hemithorax

1   Ipsilateral pathology
With mediastinum central or same side:
■ lung aplasia
■ lung hypoplasia
■ collapse/consolidation of lung/lobe
■ empyema with collapse/consolidation
 	
With mediastinum pushed to opposite side:
■ pleural fluid
  – chylothorax
  – haemothorax
  – empyema
■ diaphragmatic hernia (fluid-filled)
■ cystic hygroma
■ thoracic meningocoele
■ tumours

2   Contralateral pathology – with mediastinal shift +/− compression ■ emphysema–congenital lobar   – obstructive secondary to tumour, foreign body ■ cystic adenomatoid malformation ■ tension pneumothorax ■ diaphragmatic hernia (air-filled)

chronic chest disease, e.g. cystic fibrosis, many would recommend that a lateral view be carried out whenever the PA film is obtained.

The normal lateral chest radiograph should show progressive transradiancy over the dorsal spine, i.e. the lower vertebral bodies are blacker than the upper ones. The lateral film may detect smaller volumes of pleural fluid than are seen on the frontal view by revealing obliteration of the posterior costophrenic angle. The trachea is well seen; displacement and narrowing are readily detected on this projection. Compression is rarely detected on the frontal view.

Filter view

A filter view is a frontal (AP) coned view of the mediastinum using a high voltage (130–140 kV) technique and a copper/tin/aluminium filter very close to the X-ray tube. Magnification is routinely employed. This gives good visualization of the trachea, carina and main bronchi on a single film. When the intra-thoracic pathology results in shift of the mediastinum then the child must be positioned obliquely to allow the mediastinum to be seen more adequately. Narrowing of the airway due to either intrinsic pathology such as bronchomalacia or extrinsic pathology such as glands or vessels may be detected. Thoracic situs can also be assessed, important in the neonate with congenital heart disease.

Tomography allows radiographic sections of the lung fields and mediastinum to be obtained. Tomography requires a co-operative child and is unsuitable for those under 2 years of age. Where computerized tomography (CT) scanning and an appropriate high kV filter X-ray are available, tomography has no role.

Case study 10.3: Wheezing

Hugh, a three-year-old boy presented to casualty at midnight. He had been completely well that day and had joined a cocktail party in celebration of his father's 40th birthday. During the night he had had difficulty sleeping, was coughing intermittently and was breathing fast. Examination of the chest revealed tachypnoea with soft unilateral wheezing on the left and decreased breath sounds.

Radiological comment: A plain chest radiograph shows a radiolucent left hemi-thorax with decreased vascular markings (Figure 10.3A). The high KV filter view fails to identify the left main bronchus shortly after its origin (Figure 10.3B). A foreign body was suspected and no further imaging advised.

Outcome: A peanut, partially obstructing the left main bronchus was removed via a rigid bronchoscope.

Additional radiological comment: A foreign body is not always static. This can lead to changing signs both clinically and radiologically. Also, a foreign body can have two pathophysiological effects: it can cause a complete blockage and collapse or it can result in an incomplete blockage to the bronchus. This results in a ball valve effect with air trapping distal to the blockage. In the case presented, the air-trapping is immediately obvious. In other situations, however,

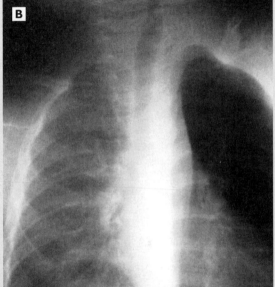

where the bronchus is partially obstructed, the inspiratory frontal chest radiograph may appear normal and an expiratory frontal chest radiograph is required to reveal the localized air trapping. Figure 10.3C is a frontal chest radiograph showing air trapping in the right lower zone with reduced vessels in this area and a flat right hemi-diaphragm. The inspiratory frontal chest radiograph (not shown) was normal.

The role of imaging in suspected foreign body is well established: a rigid bronchoscopy is required whenever there is a strong suspicion of a foreign body. Other imaging techniques become important when you wish to exclude a suspected foreign body that was not detected via bronchoscopy. In such circumstances a normal V/Q scan virtually excludes the diagnosis. The same is probably true for a normal CT.

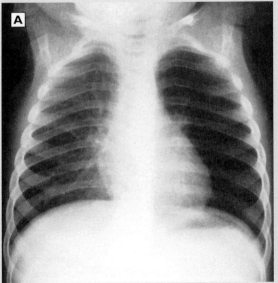

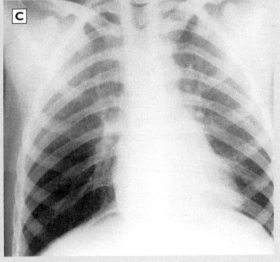

FLUOROSCOPY

Airways and diaphragms

Fluoroscopy of the thorax includes the lungs, diaphragm, pleura, mediastinum and the trachea. Whenever there is a complicated unexplained chest problem, valuable information can be obtained when an experienced radiologist fluoroscopes the thorax. Prior to beginning any fluoroscopic examination, the clinical questions to be answered should be well formulated and the previous and current chest radiographs reviewed.

Fluoroscopy should occur prior to any barium examination. The information available includes details of the movement of both hemidiaphragms with spontaneous and forced ventilation and the position of the mediastinum and the effect of respiration on both the mediastinum and trachea. If consolidation is present, its exact position, mobility and the presence of

---

Case study 10.4: Chronic productive cough

A 3-year-old boy had been seen repeatedly by the general practitioner for coughing. Chest examination was normal but because of suspicions of early clubbing and an evolving history of a 'wet' cough, the patient was referred for further investigation. Additional history revealed additional problems of otitis media and rhinitis and a maternal brother had died in childhood from pneumonia. On examination he was growing on the third centile, had mild clubbing and produced purulent sputum when encouraged to expectorate. His heart was normally situated. A co-ordinated clinico-radiological approach of investigation into the child with chronic coughing included evaluation of his immunoglobulin levels that showed severely reduced levels of IgG, IgA and IgM in keeping with X-linked agammaglobulinaemia.

Radiological comment: The frontal chest radiograph showed minor changes to the lower lobe bronchi. Although there was insufficient evidence on this frontal chest radiograph to diagnose bronchiectasis, the depression of the right lower lobe bronchus is very suspicious of loss of volume in the right lower lobe. Further evidence of collapse of the right lower lobe is the inability to see the right decending pulmonary artery (Figure 10.4A). A high resolution CT scan was more successful in demonstrating the collapse with bronchiectasis in the right lower lobe and also dilatation of the left lower lobe bronchi (Figure 10.4B). The CT is a more sensitive tool to establish the presence and extent of bronchiectasis. This should be coupled with a V/Q scan to assess the function of the lobes as well. In this case the left lower lobe, although affected by bronchiectasis, was functioning normally on V/Q scan (not shown).

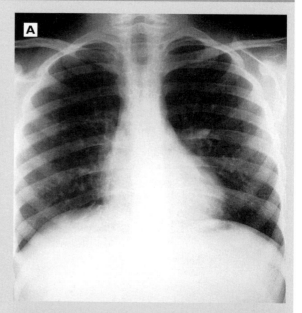

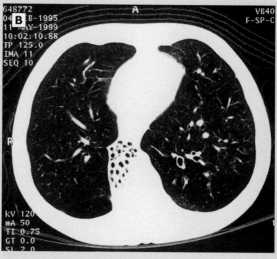

calcification can be ascertained. Fluid may be localized on fluoroscopy. If a diagnostic tap is thought necessary with small amounts of fluid, then both ultrasound and fluoroscopy may aid in a successful tap.

It is possible to look at all these features every time one fluoroscopes the chest, but since fluoroscopy does have a radiation burden, it is preferable to attempt to answer specific clinical problems in each case rather than to attempt to look at all aspects in every child.

ULTRASOUND (US)

Aerated lung prevents the US waves from reaching the pathological area and for this reason, the pathology must lie adjacent to the pleura or heart.

Effusions and masses

In the opaque hemi-thorax on chest X-ray, i.e. lung white-out, the US may distinguish between the presence of fluid, a mass or lung collapse. When a peripheral lung mass is present then ultrasound can determine if this is cystic, e.g. hydatid or solid, e.g. tumour. Occasionally in a child with pneumonia it is difficult both clinically and radiologically to assess how much fluid is present in addition to the consolidation; US is useful if the consolidation is basal, especially on the right. Effusion and empyema may require tapping or draining and US has proven useful in defining the appropriate site. The diaphragm is well visualized by US especially on the right and therefore may be useful when defects are suspected. Antenatal diagnosis of thoracic pathology is no longer a rarity; diaphragmatic hernia, adenomatoid malformations as well as fluid collections in the lungs may alert the paediatrician to the birth of an infant who may require the facilities of a neonatal intensive care team.

In cases of suspected sequestrated segment, US has been able to show the feeding vessel arising from the abdominal aorta.

Children with stridor, in whom the diagnosis of extrinsic compression is being considered should undergo a US examination. The US is sensitive in the detection of the aortic arch and may thus pick up the right-sided aortic arch and ligamentum

teres or the double aortic arch. The detection of an aberrant left pulmonary artery arising from the right pulmonary artery and swinging back to the left between the oesophagus and trachea may be missed on US.

Diaphragms

When diaphragmatic palsy or paralysis is suspected on chest radiograph, an ultrasound should be the first investigation. There may be difficulty in visualization of both hemi-diaphragms simultaneously and in such cases fluoroscopy may still be required. Occasionally, when there is partial hemi-diaphragmatic palsy, this may only be seen on the oblique views during fluoroscopy.

Larynx

The use of a high frequency probe with a good near focus allows clear visualization of the true and false vocal cords. This examination can be undertaken quickly and causes little discomfort. Vocal cord paralysis is readily recognized, however a paresis may be difficult to detect. With modern bronchoscopic equipment, this should be undertaken if either there is doubt about the US findings or there is no appropriately trained person to undertake the US examination.

Thymus

An opacity in the upper zone which cannot be separated from the mediastinum may be due to a normal thymus. This situation is encountered most often in the child who has undergone a CXR for a mild chest infection and the child is soon asymptomatic. The thymus has a characteristic echo pattern on US and is easily identified so that the shadowing on the CXR may be safely ignored.

RADIOISOTOPE INVESTIGATION

Isotope scans provide a functional image which may be quantified; this contrasts with the anatomical information available from radiology and makes the two examinations complementary.

Case study 10.5: Persistent wheezing

A 4-month-old child called Tara presented with a history of regular recurrent episodes of wheezing since birth. Initially the child had thrived, an infective cause was not suspected and a presumptive diagnosis of laryngomalacia had been made. Direct visualization of the cords at bronchoscopy showed a normal larynx with no evidence of malacia. A pH probe for gastro-oesophageal reflux was normal. At the time of referral, there was intermittent but increasing inspiratory and expiratory effort with wheezing and clinical evidence of decreased air entry and hyper-resonance to percussion on the left.

Radiological comment: A structured radiological approach was arranged. Firstly, the plain chest radiograph shows the trachea displaced to the right with few vessels present in the hypertranslucent left lung and the suspicion of a sub-carinal mass. The left hemidiaphragm is low and flat with the right affected to a lesser degree. In a 4-month-old such overinflation is pathological (Figure 10.5A). The barium swallow was normal (not shown). The transaxial cut of the CT during the dynamic phase with contrast shows a non

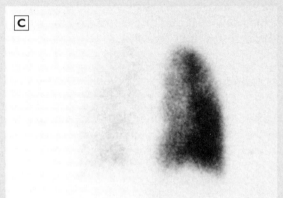

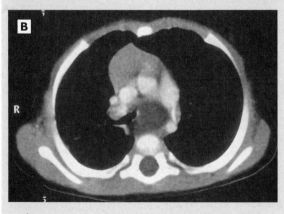

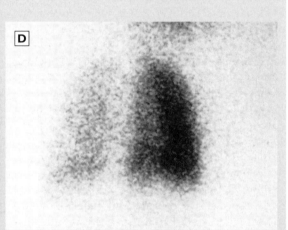

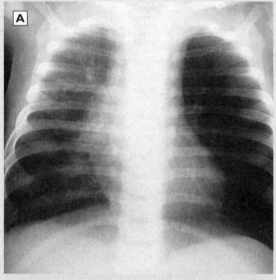

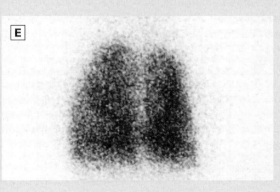

Case study 10.5: Persistent wheezing (continued)

enhancing 'cyst' behind the great vessels in the posterior mediastinum. The right main bronchus is seen (Figure 10.5B), The VQ scan shows virtual absence of perfusion on the left lung (Figure 10.5C) and slightly better ventilation (Figure 10.5D). With a change of the child's position to the left posterior oblique, the left lung is noted to have improved ventilation, the phenomena of ventilation that switches 'on-off' depending on position (Figure 10.5E). Surgical removal of the lesion was recommended.

Outcome: Histological examination of the surgical specimen confirmed the mediastinal mass to be a bronchogenic cyst (Table 10.3). A follow-up ventilation-perfusion study demonstrated complete return to normal function of the left lung (not shown).

Comment: With the radiological features on the plain chest radiograph, there is no need to proceed to bronchoscopy, rather a CT is required to show the mass.

Table 10.3: An approach to the mediastinal mass

Anterior mediastinum	Thymus
	Thyroid
	Glands
	Cystic hygroma
	Germinal cell
	tumours
Middle mediastinum	Glands
	Bronchogenic cyst
	Oesophageal
	dilatation
	Pulmonary artery
	dilatation
Posterior mediastinum	Duplication cyst
	Lateral thoracic
	meningocoele
	Neural tumour
	Ganglioneuroma
	Neuroblastoma
	Ewing's tumour
	Abscess –
	paravertebral
	Haematoma –
	especially with
	fractured ribs
	Kidney

81m Krypton (Kr) ventilation (V)/99m technetium (Tc) macroaggregate (MAA) perfusion (Q) lung scan (81m Kr V/99m Tc MAA Q)

Sequential images of both ventilation and perfusion can be obtained in children of any age including the newborn. Multiple views are obtained so that a three-dimensional image of the lungs is built up. 81m Kr is an inert radioisotope gas with a half-life of 13 seconds. The inspired air/81m Kr mixture never reaches equilibrium in the alveoli air spaces. The image is therefore of alveolar ventilation and not lung volume. This holds true for all children over 1–2 years but in the neonate/infant the high respiratory rate may invalidate this situation so that the 81m KeV scan may reflect a complex lung volume/specific ventilation situation.

Xenon (133 Xe) is used in many institutions where Kr is unavailable. The advantages of this gas are its free availability and relatively long half-life of 5.3 days; the disadvantages are the relatively high radiation dose. It is absorbed when given via IV infusion resulting in a high background activity and most importantly it requires very good patient co-operation so that it is used with difficulty in the child under 6 years old. Only a single posterior view can be obtained and therefore it is difficult to compare the 99m Tc MAA Q scan images to the 133 Xe image. In the older co-operative child the ability to carry out a wash in, equilibrium image and wash out allows assessment of gas trapping.

The use of labelled particles to monitor muco-ciliary clearance requires a co-operative child breathing 99m Tc-labelled microspheres. Relatively large particles are required and imaging must take place over some hours. In this circumstance a 99m Tc MAA perfusion scan should be done at 48 hours preceding the muco-ciliary study.

Case study 10.6: Feeding difficulty

A 3-week-old term neonate had remained in the neonatal intensive care unit following intermittent episodes of cyanosis and considerable difficulty in establishing feeding. Breast feeding was associated with bouts of coughing and cyanosis and the child was receiving all feeds via nasogastric tube. There was no further relevant history and the only additional feature on examination was a weak cry.

Radiological comment: The history is suggestive of aspiration and a plain chest radiograph showed patchy areas of consolidation and hyper-inflation consistent with significant aspiration (Figure 10.6A). The first line of investigation required exclusion of any connection between the oesophagus and trachea. A tube oesophagram study failed to demonstrate the presence of a fistula (not illustrated) but a videofluoroscopy of the infant swallowing showed the first bolus penetrating the vocal cords, outlining the trachea and entering the lungs (Figure 10.6B). An ultrasound study of the larynx revealed bilateral paralysis

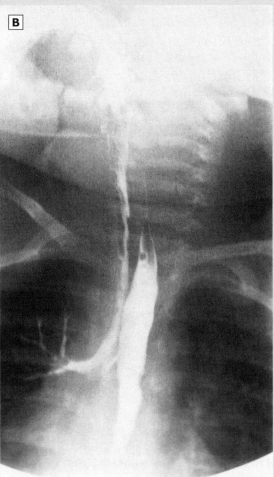

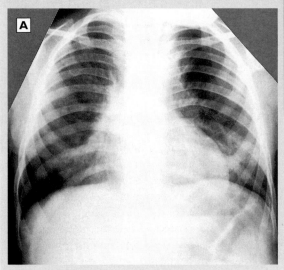

of the vocal cords which was subsequently confirmed by bronchoscopy.

Outcome: No specific cause for the vocal cord palsy could be found. The child continued to have significant problems with aspiration and required a gastrostomy and tracheostomy to allow safe feeding and effective tracheal toilet.

99m Tc MAA are injected intravenously and are stopped by the first capillary bed, normally the lungs. This gives images of pulmonary perfusion. In pulmonary hypertension, caution should be exercised, but a perfusion scan may be undertaken if clinically indicated. In the presence of right to left shunts perfusion lung scans have been used without ill effect; the 99m Tc MAA are then seen in the systemic circulation (kidneys and brain).

The V/Q images reflect regional lung function. There is no other non-invasive method available to assess regional V/Q. Indications for V/Q scanning include establishing the diagnosis, assessing the effectiveness of treatment or, in cases of known pathology, assessing the extent of the disease for follow-up (Table 10.4). Following surgery on the pulmonary artery, a Q scan is the only non-invasive means for follow-up.

Table 10.4: Indications for V/Q scans

I   Establish a diagnosis
   ■ The small lung/hypertranslucent lung on CXR
     – hypoplasia
     – hypoplasia with sequestrated segment
     – hypoplasia with interrupted pulmonary artery
     – McLeod syndrome
     – lobar emphysema
     – cystic adenomatoid malformation
   ■ Pulmonary embolus
 	
2   Follow-up
   ■ Extent of known disease
     – following foreign body removal
     – post-infection such as bronchiolitis obliterans
     – chronic lung disease of infancy
     – cystic fibrosis
   ■ Effect of treatment in
     – cystic fibrosis
     – aspiration
     – bronchiectasis
   ■ nocturnal hypoxia
   ■ after pulmonary artery/bronchial surgery

The 81m Kr V lung scan gives a very small radiation dose so that when estimating the dose to a patient from a V/Q scan the majority of the dose is from the 99m Tc MAA. The dose varies with age and is equivalent to 1.5 minute screening by fluoroscopy.

Milk scan

This is used for evaluation of gastro-oesophageal reflux and pulmonary aspiration. 99m Tc sulphur colloid (10 MBq) is added to a normal feed. Following the feed a small volume of non-radioisotope fluid is given to clear any activity from the oesophagus. Infants are cuddled for 5 minutes; all children are placed supine over the gamma camera. Continuous imaging for 1 hour then takes place with delayed images of the lungs 3–5 hours after completion of the feed. The Tc sulphur colloid is a small particle which adsorbs onto the milk and is not absorbed by the gut mucosa. When aspiration occurs the activity may be seen in the lung. Ciliary movement and bronchial clearance seem to be relatively

ineffective in removing the aspirated isotope. It is imperative to have the gamma camera linked to a computer system in order to analyse the results since one must be able to look at the oesophageal area and lung fields independently of the high activity in the stomach.

This test is more sensitive than a barium swallow in detecting gastro-oesophageal reflux since the oesophagus is studied for up to 60 minutes continuously and also has a very much lower radiation burden than barium swallow. Quantification of the reflux permits assessment of therapy. Early reports suggested that this technique might be useful in detecting lung aspiration but this has not been substantiated.

Computerized axial tomography scanning (CT)

Upper airway

The nasal sinuses and upper airway are readily identified on CT. The diagnosis of choanal atresia can be established on CT while on radiography this diagnosis is made with difficulty. Rarely, CT may be used in the older child for inflammatory processes of the sinuses but in most cases the radiograph is sufficient.

Mediastinum / pleura / trachea

Masses in either the mediastinum, chest or pleura require a CT. Examples include children with known solid tumours, primary thoracic cage masses e.g. Ewing's tumour, or tumour involving the pleura. Mediastinal pathology is well visualized and tissue characterization allows differentiation of solid from cystic lesions. The use of contrast is essential when the mediastinum or pleura is being evaluated. When there is suspicion of major airway pathology including the diagnosis of congenital tracheal pathology, then a CT should be studied after the CXR and filter view. With an aberrant left pulmonary artery origin, the association of tracheal stenosis and an eparterial bronchus arising from the trachea and going to the right upper lobe are so important that a CT should be undertaken in these children. 'Virtual bronchoscopy' is under evaluation. Here, fine section images are acquired with overlap so that computographic reconstruction can recreate a bronchoscopic view of the inner wall of the trachea and main bronchi.

Lungs

Indications for CT include lung parenchymal pathology such as bronchiolitis obliterans, unusual infections (especially occurring in the immunodeficient child) certain cases of bronchiectasis, as well as in shadowing of undetermined cause (e.g. allergic alveolitis). In other diffuse lung disease, e.g. cystic fibrosis, the role of CT is not well established. In cases of suspected sequestrated segment, CT has been able to show the feeding vessel arising from the

---

Case study 10.7: Acute intermittent dyspnoea

A premature neonate born at 30 weeks' gestation required 4 weeks of ventilation in the neonatal intensive care. She had respiratory distress syndrome but responded well to treatment including surfactant. She weaned off all ventilatory support and was well oxygenated in room air by 8 weeks of age. She remained in a high dependency unit because of intermittent episodes of cyanosis. These were most often associated with crying and feeding. Positive pressure bagging was required to maintain saturations until the episodes subsided although, on two occasions, she required reintubation and positive airway support. There was no evidence of a cardiac lesion or vascular ring on echocardiographic studies. Further investigation was required when, having been reintubated for the third time, respiratory support could not be withdrawn without life-threatening symptoms.

Radiological comment: A review of her neonatal X-rays showed the early changes of hyaline membrane disease. Subsequent frontal chest radiographs demonstrate good recovery and her recent imaging showed normal lung fields. A barium swallow was normal and there was no evidence for aspiration. The history supported the possibility of malacia of the large airways.

A contrast study of the large airways was performed whilst ventilated. The image on the right shows marked narrowing of the left main bronchus over the proximal and middle third, while there is almost complete occlusion of the origin of the right main bronchus. The left hand image shows the airway with a PEEP of 20 cm H_2O where the left main bronchus appears of good calibre and the origin of the right is now patent but narrow and irregular (Figure 10.7). Images were obtained at various levels of PEEP and the bronchomalacia could only be overcome by a PEEP of > 15 cm H_2O.

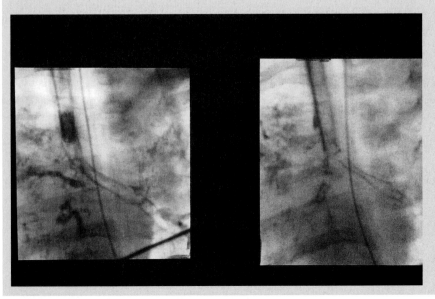

Outcome: Continued use of nasal prong PEEP allowed for growth of the infant and a gradual improvement in the malacic segment such that non-invasive respiratory support could be withdrawn by 6 months of age. Isolated areas of malacia in premature infants without any evidence of external compression may be secondary to insults on the developing airways such as intubation and repeated suctioning.

abdominal aorta but not always the venous drainage.

Interpretation of the CT requires high quality images acquired with a short exposure time to ensure little or no movement artefact. The images should be displayed so that images with both 'lung' and 'mediastinal' content can be identified. The anatomy of the airway, arteries and veins must be known and followed down slice by slice.

The relatively high radiation burden of CT means that this examination should be carried out only after CXR and re-evaluation of the child.

CONTRAST STUDIES

Oesophageal and stomach examination

In the vast majority of cases this is simply a barium swallow looking for normal swallowing, extrinsic masses in the mediastinum compressing the oesophagus (vascular rings or bronchogenic cyst), the gastro-oesophageal junction (its position and function for reflux) as well as the stomach's emptying capacity and the position of the duodenal jejunal flexure to exclude mal-rotation of the small bowel. A fully distended oesophagus is essential for an adequate barium swallow result. This examination is aimed at showing extrinsic lesions pressing or displacing the oesophagus. The aberrant left pulmonary artery may only be visible on the true lateral projection. Intrinsic diseases, e.g. hiatus hernia, gastro-oesophageal reflux or in-coordinate swallowing with aspiration may be diagnosed.

When an H-type tracheo-oesophageal fistula (TOF) is suspected, a normal swallow does not exclude the diagnosis. The tube oesophagogram is confined to those patients with a normal barium swallow, in whom an H-type TOF is still suspected. It requires an injection of water-soluble, non-ionic contrast down an oesophageal tube with the child in the prone position. A video recording of the fully distended oesophagus in the lateral projection is essential since static films are too slow to detect the small TOF.

Bronchography

This examination is infrequently performed since surgical treatment for bronchiectasis is uncommon now, CT scanning successfully shows bronchiectatic change and regional lung function can be assessed accurately by radioisotopes. It has found a role when one is looking for tracheal or bronchomalacia with intermittent closure of the major airways. This has proven useful in a neonate with suspected localized pathology of the major airways and 'stuck' on the ventilator in intensive care. In this setting, since this examination is almost always undertaken on the intubated child, the PEEP at which the airway remains open is a crucial part of the examination once the anatomical limits of the malacia have been shown. A small catheter (3.8 French) is placed in the distal trachea and 1–1.5 mL Omnipaque 280 mg/iodine per mL is instilled as a bolus. Following this instillation, fluoroscopy is undertaken at different positive end expiratory pressure (PEEP) settings to determine the PEEP required to keep the airway open if any area of tracheal and or bronchial narrowing has been detected.

Angiography

This is the investigation of choice for severe haemoptysis. Therapeutic intervention may be possible at the same time. Embolization of the artery feeding a sequestrated segment is sometimes a definitive treatment.

MAGNETIC RESONANCE IMAGING

Magnetic resonance imaging (MRI) creates images by rapidly changing the strong magnetic field applied to the body; no radiation is involved. The images are very sensitive to motion artefact and so normal cardiac pulsation as well as respiratory movements create artefacts. With cardiac gating, the cardiac motion can be removed, but this is not yet true for respiration. This equipment is expensive and therefore not widely available. Its role in chest pathology is still being established. The technique is proving of great value in looking at the anatomy of the pulmonary veins, and for certain pathology related to the pulmonary artery, e.g. aberrant left pulmonary artery. The advances in this area are rapid and the full potential of MRI in respiratory imaging may still be unrealized.

Case study 10.8: Miliary shadowing

Jan, a 6-year-old boy presented to his paediatrician with cough and shortness of breath. There was no additional history of relevance although the parents were first cousins. Examination revealed some restriction to chest wall movement but clear lung fields. His oxygen saturations were 90% in room air and lung function testing showed a restrictive pattern. The chest radiograph was remarkable in that it demonstrated a diffuse miliary pattern (Figure 10.8A). A tuberculin test was negative and all baseline blood investigations were within normal limits.

Radiological comment: The radiological term 'miliary' is used to describe the presence of fine discrete nodules less than 5 mm in size and extending uniformly throughout the lung fields. This pattern of densities is commonly associated with tuberculosis in areas where the disease has a high prevalence. There is, however, a wide range of conditions that can provide this picture and some to consider are listed in Table 10.5. The unremarkable history and examination ruled out many of these conditions. A CT of the chest was arranged to evaluate the lung parenchyma in more detail and to image the mediastinum looking carefully for lymphadenopathy (Figure 10.8B). The CT images provided no further useful information and a bronchoscopy was the next investigation of choice with a view to performing a bronchoalveolar lavage (BAL) and transbronchial biopsy.

Outcome: The BAL showed alveolar macrophages and scattered lumps of calcium and the transbronchial biopsy had the histological features of pulmonary microlithiasis: intra-alveolar calcospherites in virtually all alveolar spaces and staining periodic acid–Schiff positive. No specific therapy could be offered for this unusual condition.

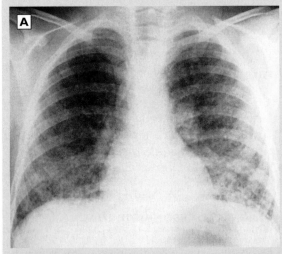

Table 10.5: Miliary pattern on chest radiograph: causes of diffuse, fine (1–4 mm), sharply defined nodules

Infectious diseases Fungal	Disseminated histoplasmosis, coccidioidomycosis, blastomycosis, aspergillosis, and cryptococcosis
Bacterial	Nocardiosis Tuberculosis
Viral	Varicella zoster
Metastases	Thyroid carcinoma, melanoma and lymphangitic carcinomatosis
Granulomatous	Eosinophilic granulomata, sarcoidosis
Inhalation disorders	Berylliosis, silicosis, pneumoconiosis, siderosis, and extrinsic allergic alveolitis
Inherited disorders	Niemann–Pick disease, Gaucher disease, and pulmonary alveolar microlithiasis
Other disorders	Haemosiderosis

Case study 10.9: A child with CF and haemoptysis

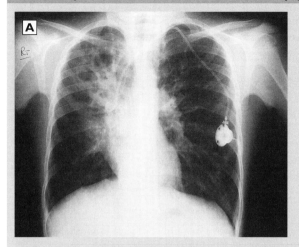

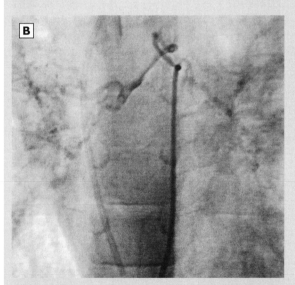

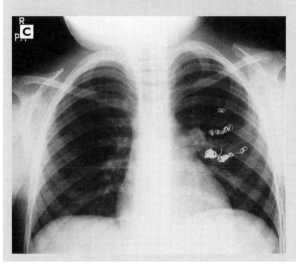

Simon, a ten-year-old boy with cystic fibrosis and fairly advanced lung disease had been troubled by small amounts of haemoptysis and increasing sputum production. He was admitted to hospital and started on a course of appropriate intravenous antibiotics. His clotting profile was normal. Three days after initiating therapy Simon had two large fresh blood haemoptyses of 500 mL each. He was resuscitated and a chest radiograph showed marked overinflation of both lungs, flattened diaphragm, a narrow heart, as well as added shadowing in the right upper and mid zones. In the right upper lobe there are also cystic spaces. These are the changes of cystic fibrosis affecting both lungs but especially severe in the right upper lobe (Figure 10.9A). Whilst in the radiology department he had a further large haemoptysis.

Radiological comment: Bronchoscopy is rarely useful in isolating or managing a large haemoptysis in this clinical situation. The investigation of choice is angiography looking for an unusually large and often tortuous bronchial feeder artery and may also show a characteristic blush if there is active bleeding from the vessel. A large vessel leading to the severely affected right upper lobe with an associated blush was identified at emergency angiography and successfully embolized (Figure 10.8B). No further intervention was necessary.

In a child with haemoptysis due to an arterio-venous malformation (AVM), angiography is only indicated if the bleeding is life-threatening since they are usually multiple and as one AVM is embolized so another becomes dominant. This is seen in a different child who had no underlying condition apart from the AVMs. Here the frontal chest radiograph shows the multiple coils which were introduced when he had a life-threatening haemoptysis (Figure 10.9C).

Case study 10.10: Acute stridor

Larry, a 10-month-old child presented with a one day history of fever, poor feeding and stridor. The chest was clear to auscultation and viral croup was diagnosed. No radiological investigations were indicated and after a 24-hour period of observation, the child had improved considerably and was discharged home.

Radiological comment: Stridor can be acute or persistent and an approach to the causes of stridor are listed in Table 10.6. The lateral radiograph neck is not generally helpful in acute stridor and the clinical history and examination usually allow the diagnosis to be made. The illustrative radiograph for this case demonstrates a caution in interpretation: the lateral neck view shows displacement of the trachea forwards and also the trachea has an acute angle. These features cause an increase in the retropharyngeal space (Figure 10.10A). The film repeated minutes later when the infant was more settled, shows a normal retropharyngeal space (Figure 10.10B). The abnormal retropharyngeal space may be 'physiological' when the child is crying and the buckling of the trachea is an important clue to this expiratory phase with a venous plexus which is full.

An ill child with suspected croup should not be sent to an X-ray department (especially after hours) to have an X-ray plate applied to the neck for a lateral film. The casualty radiology department is often cold and the X-ray plate is also cold. The airway may be significantly compromised and such manipulation may precipitate a respiratory arrest in a poorly staffed department. If an X-ray is really required, the child should be admitted to a high dependency area and the radiograph undertaken in a well equipped environment.

Table 10.6: Causes of stridor – acute and persistent

In the lumen:
- congenital cyst
- laryngeal web/cleft/papilloma
- vocal cord palsy
- foreign body
- infective or inflammatory membrane

In the wall:
- laryngotracheobronchitis
- laryngomalacia
- tracheomalacia
- complete tracheal rings
- subglottic stenosis

Outside the wall:
- vascular ring
- mediastinal mass e.g. lymph nodes

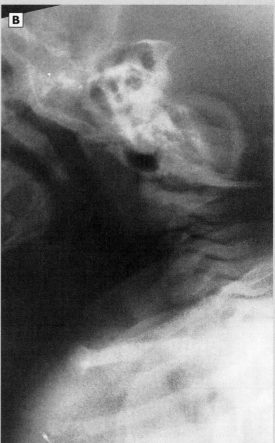

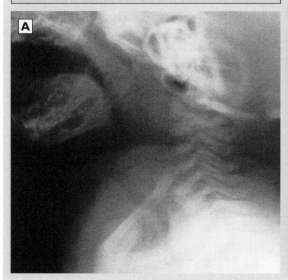

Case study 10.11: An infant with tachypnoea due to a hypoplastic lung with a sequestrated segment

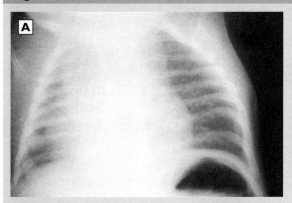

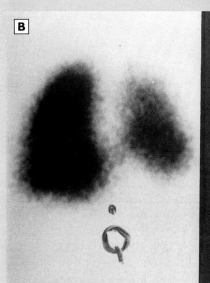

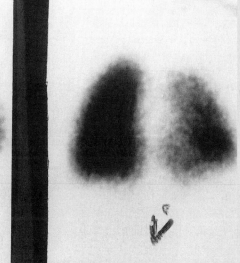

This one-month-old infant called Poppy presented with tachypnoea. The frontal chest radiograph shows the mediastinum displaced to the right with obliteration of the right heart border and poor visualization of the vessels in the right lung. The right hemi-diaphragm is clearly seen (Figure 10.11A). The posterior projection of the 99m Tc MAA perfusion/krypton ventilation lung scan shows normal perfusion and ventilation of the left lung. The right lung reveals good ventilation of both upper and lower lobes, but the ventilation is reduced compared with the left lung (marked V) (Figure 10.11B). A similar appearance is noted on the perfusion scan. In addition, there is total absence of perfusion in the right postero-medial basal segment (marked Q). At surgery, a sequestrated segment in the hypoplastic right lung was resected.

Radiological comment: Sequestrated segments of the lung receive their blood supply from the systemic circulation and are therefore seen as segmental areas of reduced perfusion. The intra-lobar sequestrations are in communication with the bronchial tree and therefore are usually ventilated. When a sequestration is suspected, an ultrasound examination specifically searching for the feeding artery which comes off the abdominal aorta can not only provide the final clue but can also alert the surgeon to the exact origin of the artery. Angiography is indicated when consideration is given to embolization of the vessel as one form of final treatment.

INTEGRATED IMAGING TECHNIQUES

The radiologist and clinician must both be well versed in paediatric chest pathology. There are studies where one imaging technique is compared with a second, but the quality of the first may be substantially reduced compared to the second and so the second technique is considered 'more sensitive'. This is particularly obvious with the aberrant left pulmonary artery where the barium swallow is considered 'less' sensitive than CT or US yet when a fully distended oesophagus is seen in the true lateral projection, this examination has a high pick-up rate.

When pleural pathology is suspected, inevitably both US and CT are required if resolution is not rapid (e.g. empyema) since the placing of a chest drain with or without a thoracotomy requires exact anatomical knowledge of the extent as well as the internal nature of the pleural collection. CT may not pick up septa or loculations as well as US.

The paediatrician and radiologist should view the different imaging techniques as each having

Case study 10.12: Hypoplastic lung with an interupted pulmonary artery

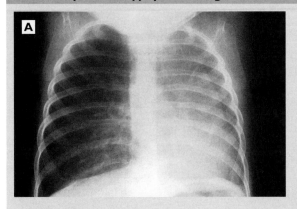

This 11-month-old infant called Henry presented with cough and wheeze for a few days. There was no other relevant history. The frontal chest radiograph shows the mediastinum deviated to the left with loss of the inferior aspect of the left heart border. There are reduced vessels in the left lung. The left main bronchus as well as the left lower lobe bronchus are clearly seen and occupy a normal position, suggesting that there is no loss of volume in the left lung. The hemi-diaphragm is in a normal position. There is overinflation of the right lung, but the vascular pattern in the right lung is normal (Figure 10.12A). The child underwent a CT scan which shows the over expanded right lung with normal vessels. The heart is displaced to the left. The left main bronchus is clearly seen as are vessels in the small left lung (Figure 10.12B). The 99mTc-MAA perfusion/krypton ventilation lung scan shows that the ventilation to the left lung is good, however reduced compared with the right lung. Note on the left posterior oblique projection the right lung still has higher activity compared with the left lung. These are typical ventilation scan findings of a hypoplastic lung. The perfusion scan reveals perfusion only to the right lung (Figure 10.12C).

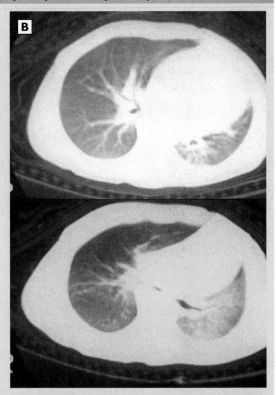

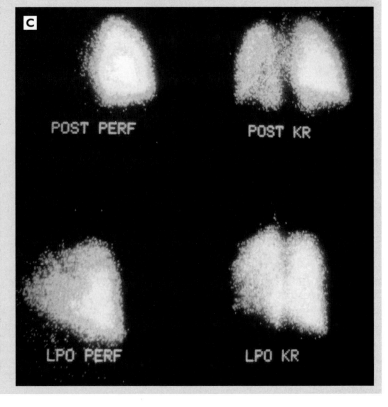

Radiological comment: In hypoplastic lungs, there is an increased incidence of sequestrated segments, interruption of the pulmonary artery as well as abnormal venous drainage from the hypoplastic lung.

pros and cons and ask what is required for the imaging to influence management.

FURTHER READING

1. Felman AH. *The paediatric chest*. Illinois: Charles C Thomas, 1983. ISBN 0-398-04730-8.
2. Singleton EB, Wagner ML, Dutton RV. *Radiologic atlas of pulmonary abnormalities in children*. Philadelphia: WB Saunders, 1988. ISBN 0-7216-2062-0.
3. Carty H, Brunelle F, Shaw D, Kendell B. *Imaging children*. Chapters 1 and 2. London: Churchill Livingstone, 1994. ISBN 0-443-04260-8.

CHAPTER ELEVEN

AIRWAY ENDOSCOPY, LUNG BIOPSY *AND* BRONCHOALVEOLAR LAVAGE

A. Moir, S. Kotecha and G. Jones

INTRODUCTION

With the advent of flexible paediatric and neonatal bronchoscopes, bronchoscopy and bronchoalveolar lavage (BAL) have become more widespread in clinical practice. In a well organized and equipped unit, bronchoscopy can provide useful information on both the upper and lower airways with safety. The most common indications for bronchoscopy are shown in Table 11.1.

Both flexible and rigid bronchoscopy can be useful in aiding the diagnosis of upper or lower airway abnormalities and pathological conditions, for assessing the severity of disease (for instance in broncho- or tracheo-malacia), and for therapeutic interventions (removal of mucous plugs or foreign body). When other investigations fail to provide an answer, bronchoscopy may provide an unsuspected diagnosis (Case study 11.1). In addition, bronchoalveolar lavage fluid may be obtained to diagnose infection in both the immunocompetent and immunocompromised child. Bronchial and transbronchial biopsies may also be obtained to aid or confirm diagnosis.

BRONCHOSCOPY

INSTRUMENTS USED FOR BRONCHOSCOPY (TABLE 11.2)

The rigid bronchoscope

This is used in an anaesthetized patient and permits artificial ventilation through the instrument. Anaesthetic gases can be delivered through the rigid tube and visualization is obtained via a Stortz–Hopkins rigid telescope. The picture quality is considerably better than the flexible scope. The sizes used in practice have an outer diameter of 4.0 mm for neonates and up to 12 mm for adolescents.

The flexible bronchoscope

This is more easily portable and can be used in a sedated patient. It can also visualize more peripheral airways and more awkward segments, particularly the right upper lobe. Thinner bronchoscopes can be used to visualize the tracheobronchial tree in ventilated patients on the paediatric and neonatal intensive care units. Flexible bronchoscopes range from 2.2 mm to 4.5 mm

Table 11.1: Indications for bronchoscopy and related procedures

Upper airway disorders (may be able to use awake microlaryngoscopy)

Obstruction:
  nasopharyngeal obstruction
  stridor (including biphasic stridor)
  sleep apnoea

Laryngeal:
  vocal cord dysfunction
  dysphonia

Lower respiratory disorders Congenital abnormalities Persistent lobar disease (segmented collapse or   hyperinflation) Suspected foreign body aspiration Unexplained cough

Infection:
  unresponsive to antibiotics (BAL)
  suspected TB (BAL)
  in an immunocompromised child (BAL)
  repeated infections (e.g. bronchial biopsy to
  assess ciliary function)

Unexplained haemoptysis
Failure to extubate in NNU or PICU
Difficult asthma or unresponsive airway
  obstruction
Suspected interstitial disease (consider open lung
  biopsy and BAL)

Other disorders Recurrent aspiration of unknown cause Post-lung transplant assessment

BAL = bronchoalveolar lavage

for older children. The most commonly used instrument which is satisfactory for children older than 18 months has an external diameter of 3.5 mm with a 1.2 mm suction channel.

THE PROCEDURE

Patient preparation

The decision to use local anaesthetic (with or without sedation) or a general anaesthetic[1] depends on the age of the child, the nature of the procedure (elective or emergency), the underlying condition and the experience of the operators.

In our practice we have chosen to use a general anaesthetic to ensure optimum conditions for the bronchoscopists with maintenance of normal oxygenation. This practice requires a skilled and experienced anaesthetist and access to appropriate anaesthetic facilities. General anaesthesia is more labour intensive, but the advantage is that the children recover from anaesthesia and regain their laryngeal reflexes more rapidly than with sedative techniques. Full anaesthetic monitoring is required for these patients. This includes blood pressure, heart rate, oxygen saturation and end tidal CO_2. Patients should be breathing spontaneously on emerging from anaesthesia, to allow proper assessment of a floppy larynx and also vocal cord dysfunction. Again bronchomalacia should be evaluated when the patient is breathing spontaneously. It is important to remember that the positive end expiratory pressure induced by the bronchoscopy may interfere with assessment. Many bronchoscopists nevertheless use sedative techniques especially for children over two years of age. The most commonly used combination of drugs would be intravenous midazolam (a benzodiazepine) supplemented with small increments of fentanyl (an opioid) to help to suppress laryngeal reflexes. This technique is often perceived as requiring less personnel but it is essential that appropriate equipment and skilled personnel for resuscitation are available.[2] Ready access to paediatric intensive care unit (PICU) facilities must be available as the child may require endotracheal intubation. In adults, local anaesthetic without sedation is frequently used but in paediatric practice this is only practicable for the co-operative teenager. The child should not suffer any distress or discomfort.

It is difficult to assess the larynx and to exclude tracheo- or bronchomalacia if the patient is paralysed and ventilated. Therefore, in our practice spontaneous ventilation is maintained throughout the procedure. Short acting muscle relaxants (e.g. suxamethonium) are not routinely used to aid intubation because they increase the frequency of post-operative apnoea. Bronchoscopy is therefore carried out with deep halothane anaesthesia plus local anaesthetic spray to the vocal cords. To prevent reflex and halothane-induced bradycardia, all patients receive intravenous atropine in a dose

Case study 11.1: An ex-preterm child with stridor

Ed was born at 27 weeks' gestation, with birth weight 900 g, and required mechanical ventilation for respiratory distress syndrome for 7 days. He was completely weaned off oxygen by 3 weeks of age. The remainder of his neonatal course was uneventful. His progress was excellent thereafter: his development was normal, he was thriving and had no respiratory symptoms. However, during his second year of life, Ed had three admissions in four months where a diagnosis of croup was made. On two occasions Ed required mechanical ventilation for his airway obstruction. Due to the severity and frequency of the episodes, a bronchoscopy was performed. Ed was noted to have a circumferential subglottic stenosis (Figure 11.1), a consequence of neonatal intubation. The stenosis was not severe enough to consider surgical correction. It was anticipated that Ed would grow and the severity of the croup would become less with time. Ed did not have any further episodes of airway obstruction and is now asymptomatic at the age of five.

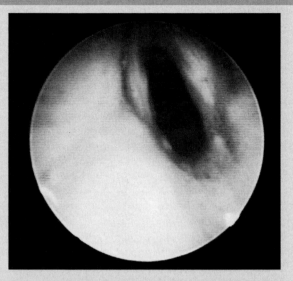

Figure 11.1: Circumferential subglottic stenosis immediately below the vocal cords.

Table 11.2: Comparison of the characteristic features of the rigid and flexible bronchoscopes

	Rigid	Flexible
Picture quality	Excellent	Good
GA needed?	Always	Sometimes
Biopsy possible?	Yes	Yes
BAL possible?	Limited	Yes
Therapeutic manoeuvres possible?	Yes	Limited
Ventilation possible?	Yes	No*
Visualization of segmental bronchi?	Difficult	Yes

GA: general anaesthetic; BAL: bronchoalveolar lavage.
* Oxygen can be delivered through the suction port of the bronchoscope.

of 10–20 µg/kg. This has the added benefit of reducing airway secretions. We often use a laryngeal mask as this maintains the child's airway and prevents contamination of the instrument from the nasal passages should samples be required for microbial studies.[3]

Prior to the examination, in particular a detailed history and examination of the respiratory system is essential, the assessment must include routine questioning about previous anaesthetic experiences, general health and current medication. The respiratory status of the child should be optimized prior to the procedure. Antibiotics should be used to eradicate infection (unless the procedure is being performed to identify an infective process), physiotherapy to improve sputum clearance and bronchodilators or corticosteroids, as appropriate, to reduce the likelihood of bronchospasm. Lung function tests (and blood gases) should be noted, if relevant, to indicate whether or not the child might require high dependency care after the procedure (for instance, due to critical airway obstruction or a neuromuscular disorder). The investigation of a coryzal child should be postponed since airway reflexes are heightened and may therefore compromise respiratory function. In infants, it is important to establish any history of apnoeic episodes. An apnoea monitor should be used post-operatively in all such patients as well as routinely in all those under 60 weeks post-conceptional age. On occasions, severe upper airway obstruction may occur after instrumentation, particularly in children with subglottic stenosis. We routinely give such patients dexamethazone in theatre, and they are observed in a place of safety such as a paediatric intensive care unit.

Some bronchoscopists routinely use nebulized salbutamol with or without lignocaine in the preoperative period. In our practice, the vocal cords are routine sprayed with lignocaine under general anaesthetic prior to bronchoscopy.

For a child in the paediatric intensive care unit the risks of the procedure need to be balanced with the benefits that may be obtained by performing the procedure. In immunosuppressed children and in those who may have lobar collapse thus preventing extubation from mechanical ventilation, bronchoscopy may provide essential information about the microbial flora in the lung and facilitates therapeutic removal of a mucous plug respectively. When a child undergoes bronchoscopy on the paediatric intensive care unit, skilled personnel especially in resuscitation must be involved with one such individual maintaining a close eye on the child's clinical condition whilst the bronchoscopist performs the procedure. Wherever possible the child's ventilation should continue e.g. through the end-porthole of the mechanical ventilator circuit. It may be necessary in the unstable child to perform the bronchoscopy with repeated insertions and removal of the instrument with each attempt assessing the essential areas of the lung. Heart rate and oxygen saturation must be closely monitored in these children. The procedure may need to be curtailed should the child's condition deteriorate.

Personnel

In addition to an experienced nurse who will assist the operator, it is essential that the anaesthetist has an assistant who is experienced in endoscopy. During the procedure the child must undergo continuous ECG, oxygen saturation and non-invasive blood pressure monitoring.[2]

Upper respiratory tract

Both the upper and lower respiratory tracts are examined during the procedure. Good visualization of the upper respiratory tract can only be achieved with a general anaesthetic and is better with a rigid bronchoscope. Abnormalities including bifid uvula, vallecular cysts, laryngeal cleft and more commonly vocal cord palsies may be seen. The latter will often present with a cough that does not appear to improve with medical treatment including bronchodilators for asthma. The view of the upper respiratory tract with the rigid Hopkin's rod is excellent but any procedures

on the upper respiratory tract would then be undertaken using a microscope in combination with microlaryngeal instruments (Case study 11.2). The airway is then maintained either by naso-endotracheal intubation or a cricothyroid needle puncture and high frequency jet ventilation, for example when an infant is diagnosed as having a life-threatening laryngomalacia at bronchoscopy. The tension in the ary-epiglottic folds can then be released by incising with micro-scissors, allowing the epiglottis to come forward off the laryngeal inlet to relieve the upper airway obstruction. It is important to realise that surgical procedures for straightforward laryngomalacia are very rarely needed. In the Leicestershire paediatric population of 200,000 children, such a procedure is required once or twice a year only.

Lower respiratory tract

Once through the vocal cords, the subglottis is viewed and any stenosis measured. Due to the wide-angle lens of the flexible bronchoscope, subglottic stenosis especially of minor degree may be difficult to assess (Case study 11.1). Below the cricoid ring, the lower respiratory tract can be examined with either the flexible or rigid bronchoscope.

Particular attention needs to be paid to the dynamic movements of the airways especially the trachea and bronchi (which could indicate tracheo-bronchomalacia) and whether there is excessive extrinsic pulsation from an abnormal vessel or an enlarged pulmonary artery. Equal attention should be paid to all the components of the respiratory tree including the trachea, bronchi and smaller airways to ensure that major obvious abnormalities are not missed. A knowledge of the normal anatomy is important (Figure 11.3). Tracheal abnormalities such as complete tracheal rings (Case study 11.3) are rare but can mimic obstructive respiratory diseases such as asthma. The carina is flattened in young children but sharpens with age. The right main bronchus is more vertical than the left and is easier to visualize. Because of this, foreign body inhaled into the lower respiratory tract will tend to go into the right main bronchus. Normal variations such as tracheal origin of right upper lobe bronchus (so called 'pig bronchus') may occasionally be seen. Narrowing of the airways from extrinsic

Case study 11.2: Delayed speech and dyspnoea

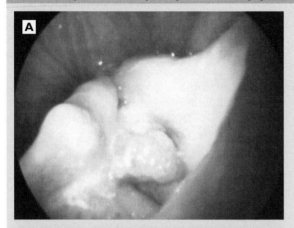

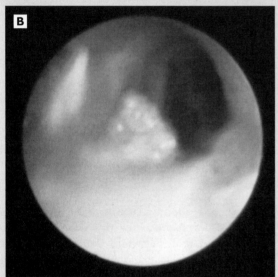

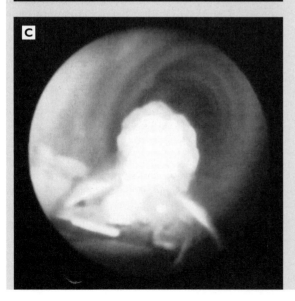

Steve presented at the age of four years with aphonia and dyspnoea. The aphonia had been present since birth, but it was the dyspnoea that precipitated the admission. He had severe upper respiratory tract obstruction with mild inspiratory stridor, suprasternal tug, intercostal and subcostal recession. His respiratory rate was 40/minute, heart rate 140/minute, Pao_2 was within normal limits but his $Paco_2$ was raised at 8.5 kPa. He was apyrexial and there was no evidence of an infective process. His chest radiograph was normal but the admitting doctor arranged for a lateral soft tissue X-ray of the neck which demonstrated an abnormal laryngeal airway. Steve had an urgent laryngoscopy under general anaesthetic and was noted to have extensive laryngeal papillomatosis (Figure 11.2A). The extent of the airway obstruction was so severe that a tracheostomy was necessary. Monthly laser therapy was unsuccessful as was 12 month treatment with interferon. The tracheostomy was removed at the age of eight and a bronchoscopy at that time showed that the papillomata were regressing spontaneously. A papilloma was also seen on the posterior tracheal wall which may have seeded during one of the procedures (Figure 11.2B). It was removed endoscopically with optical forceps (Figure 11.2C) and has not recurred. Steve is now eleven years old and is free of disease.

The outcome may not be as good as in this case. Papillomas can often carry on life-long, causing an intermittent hoarse voice and airway obstruction, requiring therapy.

Figure 11.2: (A) Papillomata seen on vocal cord (Case study 11.2). They did not respond to laser therapy or to beta-interferon but regressed spontaneously from the age of eight years. (B) Papillomata on posterior tracheal wall probably seeded during a previous procedure. (C) Removal by microforceps.

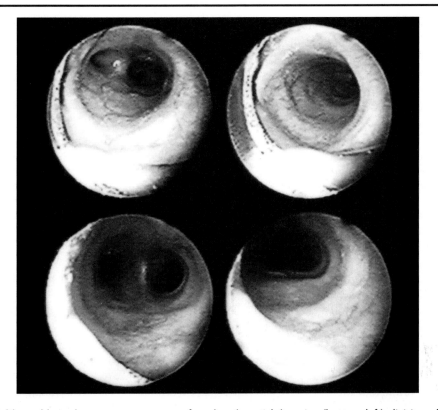

Figure 11.3: Normal bronchoscopy appearances of trachea (top right), carina (bottom left), division of right upper lobe and right lower divisions (top left) and left main bronchus (bottom left).

Case study 11.3: Infant wheeze

Rob presented as an infant with recurrent cough and wheeze. He was treated with bronchodilators with no improvement in his condition. When he was three months old lung function tests using the squeeze technique showed irreversible, fixed pattern, obstruction of the larger airways (see Chapter 7). At bronchoscopy, complete tracheal rings were diagnosed extending from just below the cricoid ring into the right main bronchus. Rob's exercise tolerance has been excellent until recently. Bronchoscopy at the age of 14 years showed that the trachea was still narrowed extending into the right main bronchus (Figure 11.4). Tracheal reconstructive surgery had been discussed in the past, but the risks were deemed to be high and the benefits small as Rob's exercise tolerance was good. Rob who is now 15 years old has recently found exercise more difficult – he can no longer play sports, he is short of breath on walking and is now a strong candidate for reconstructive surgery, despite its risks.

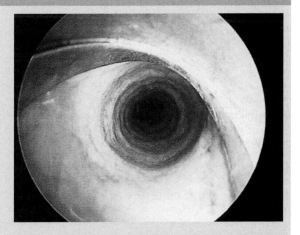

Figure 11.4: Complete tracheal rings (stenosis). Note any lack of trachealis muscle posteriorly.

Note: Infant lung function testing is not routinely advocated as a clinical tool in infancy. Symptoms alone would have led to a bronchoscopy being performed in this case.

compression is usually due to aberrant blood vessels within the chest or mediastinal masses. Marked pulsation would normally suggest an abnormal vessel (such as an enlarged pulmonary artery), but in the absence of pulsation, mediastinal masses such as enlarged lymph nodes should be suspected.

RELATED PROCEDURES

Bronchoalveolar lavage

Bronchoalveolar lavage has been useful for research purposes but has applications in the diagnosis of unusual infection in children.[4] Samples can be obtained from the lower airways for microbiological investigations to identify opportunist infections, such as *Pneumocystis carinii*. Care must be taken not to contaminate the instrument or the specimen in the upper respiratory tract. Our practice to use 10 mL N-saline at room temperature for lavage whilst others base fluid volumes on either weight (e.g. two aliquots of 1 mL/kg) or lung function parameters such as FRC. The proportion recovered is usually about 50% of the volume instilled depending on the underlying disease, dwell time, suction pressure and airway size. The sample should be taken to the laboratory with specific instructions within 20–30 minutes to look for the organisms of interest in fresh samples. Procedures include: cytological preps (for *Pneumocystis* for example), viral bacterial and fungal cultures and special diagnostic techniques (e.g. PCR-based diagnosis). Cell differential counts and measurements of soluble constituents of the supernatant are largely research activities but may occasionally give a clue to the underlying diagnosis. Bronchoalveolar lavage is also a useful method for removing mucous plugs. Mucolytic drugs may be instilled through the suction channel but their efficacy is unproven.

Biopsy

Bronchoscopy readily permits the collection of ciliated epithelium from the lower airways using a brush inserted through the suction channel. The function and structure of the cilia can be investigated with high-speed video (to assess beat frequency) and by electron microscopy respectively (See Chapter 9). Tissue biopsies can be obtained by cup forceps but are rarely required in children in contrast to adults where they are used frequently to diagnose carcinomas. Transbronchial biopsies should only be performed in experienced hands using fluoroscopy since complications including pneumothorax or intra-thoracic bleeding can occur. In children open lung biopsy is preferred to transbronchial biopsy since more reliable tissue samples are obtained. The role of biopsy, even in confirmed 'interstitial' lung disease is controversial. Transbronchial biopsy is not without risk especially of bleeding and air leaks and may not sample accurately due to the diffuse nature of lesions within the lung.

POST-OPERATIVE MANAGEMENT

Particular attention must be applied to care of the upper airway as any airway narrowing may be exacerbated by instrumentation. Airway complications can be reduced by the use of intravenous corticosteroids given at the time of the bronchoscopy or nebulized adrenaline (epinephrine) in the early recovery period. These drugs are required when there is clinical suspicion of a compromised airway. Children should be monitored appropriately during recovery, but after an hour are allowed to drink freely, as in our experience the lignocaine spray used during the procedure does not compromise swallowing for longer than an hour.

Most complications occur soon after the procedure but infection may not be obvious for several days (Table 11.3). Early complications are more likely to be manifestations of upper airway obstruction and in severe cases may require endotracheal intubation and additional intensive care. Airway obstruction can occur after the immediate recovery period and is usually related to the underlying lung pathology, such as exacerbation of an unsuspected infective process.

CARE OF THE BRONCHOSCOPE

Thorough cleaning and sterilization of the instruments between cases is extremely important to prevent cross-infection and also contamination of specimens collected. Rigid bronchoscopes can be autoclaved but flexible ones are destroyed

Table 11.3: Complications of bronchoscopy

Exacerbation of pre-existing pathology:
    oedema in airway narrowing e.g. subglottic
      stenosis
    infection

Complications of sedation and general anaesthetic:
    apnoea
    oxygen desaturation
    bradycardia
    laryngospasm

Bleeding

Pneumothorax

Infection

Aspiration

Perforation of major airways (main risk with
bronchial biopsy)

Pyrexia following bronchoalveolar lavage usually
within 6 hours of the procedure

with this procedure. Glutaraldehyde is still the commonest agent used for sterilizing flexible bronchoscopes but peracetic acid is used in some centres although there are concerns about damage to flexible bronchoscopes. Nevertheless a minimum of 20 minutes for routine cases is essential and this time is increased to at least 60 minutes for high risk infections such mycobacteria. Stringent Health and Safety Executive regulations (in the UK) require a closed system when glutaraldehyde is used to reduce exposure. After cleaning with glutaraldehyde the instrument should be thoroughly cleansed with sterile water and most modern systems will do this automatically but great care needs to be applied to the biopsy channels. The cleaning time determines the interval between cases, when the number of instruments are limited.

RESEARCH ISSUES

Bronchoscopy has become established in the management of children with respiratory disorders. As the instruments become widely available, they are increasingly used to study respiratory diseases in children. Where once it would have been impossible to obtain samples from children, these instruments have permitted the study of the airway milieu. Bronchoalveolar lavage has been firmly established to study diseases such as asthma and wheezing disorders in pre-school children. Bronchial biopsies are often obtained to study epithelial cells including ciliary function. With increasing usage, increasingly questions are being raised about the ethics of the use of bronchoscopes in obtaining lung biopsies from children. Although accepted in many adult studies, acquisition of bronchial biopsies for research in children with underlying respiratory disease or in normal controls is associated with many ethical questions.

Bronchoalveolar lavage samples are easier to obtain but may not reflect the whole pulmonary environment. Sampling sites, non-homogenous disease, sampling error (e.g. with transbronchial biopsies), estimation of epithelial lining fluid all generate controversies. The lack of universally accepted criteria to represent both cellular and non-cellular measurements have further complicated the area especially when comparing results between studies. The European Respiratory Society has recently attempted to provide guidelines for bronchoalveolar lavage in children of all ages including neonates (Further Reading, de Blic 2000).

CONCLUSIONS

A bronchoscopy service is an essential part of a clinical paediatric respiratory service. The majority of procedures are undertaken as part of an elective service, but facilities for emergency bronchoscopy should be available. In order to obtain and maintain the necessary skills, we would recommend that at least 50 bronchoscopies are performed each year in any centre. This would also allow the endoscopists to see a wide range of clinical conditions and normal variations. For teaching and record keeping, a camera and monitor, a video recording system and a hard copy printer should be routinely used. Digital capture and recording of the images in the future will enhance teaching and allow the transfer of material between departments and hospitals. Accurate records should be kept of each bronchoscopic procedure and a regular audit performed, to ensure that any adverse effects are accurately assessed and any shortfalls quickly addressed.

REFERENCES

1. Tobias JD. Sedation and anesthesia for pediatric bronchoscopy. *Curr Opin Pediatr* 1997; **9**: 198–206.

2. Kociela VL. Pediatric flexible bronchoscope under conscious sedation: nursing considerations for preparation and monitoring. *J Pediat Nursing* 1998; **13**: 343–8.

3. Boehringer LA, Bennie RE. Laryngeal mask airway and pediatric patient. *Inter Anesthesiol Clin* 1998; **36**: 45–60.

4. Scheinmann P, Pedersen S, Warner JO, de Blic J. Methods for assessment of airways inflammation: paediatrics. *Eur J Respir* 1998; **26**: 53S–58S.

FURTHER READING

1. Barbato A, Landau LI, Scheinmann P, Warner JO, Zach M. *The bronchoscope – flexible and rigid – in children.* Treriso, Italy: Arcari-Editore, 1995.

2. Bolliger CT, Mathur PN. Interventional bronchoscopy. Basel, Switzerland: S Karger AG, 2000.

3. Brownlee KG, Crabbe DC. Paediatric bronchoscopy. *Arch Dis Child* 1997; **77**: 272–5.

4. de Blic J, Midulla F, Barbato A, *et al.* Bronchoalveolar lavage in children. ERS Task Force. European Respiratory Society. *Eur Respir J* 2000; **15**: 217–31.

5. Wood RE. Pediatric bronchoscopy. *Chest Surg Clin N Am* 1996; **6**: 237–51.

6. Forte V, Gaffney R. Bronchoscopy in the pediatric age group: An ear-nose-throat surgeon's experience. In: Kerem E, Canny GJ, Branski D, Levison H (eds). *Advances in pediatric pulmonology.* Switzerland: Karger, 1997. 105–11.

CHAPTER TWELVE

SPECIAL PROCEDURES *TO* IDENTIFY INFECTION

M . W i s e l k a a n d C . O ' C a l l a g h a n

- Background
- Pneumonia in children
- Diagnostic techniques

- Conclusions and future prospects
- Acknowledgement
- References

BACKGROUND

The epidemiology of paediatric respiratory infection has changed over recent years due to a variety of factors (Table 12.1). These factors have contributed to the emergence of opportunistic pathogens as major causes of morbidity and mortality. New antibiotics and antiviral drugs are being developed but require prompt diagnosis of the cause of infection and determination of antimicrobial sensitivities to be of maximal benefit.

Clinicians treating children with serious respiratory infection therefore require rapid and accurate diagnostic facilities in order to identify the pathogens present and to deliver appropriate therapy. It is also essential to be able to distinguish infections from other pathogenic processes affecting the lungs including chronic aspiration, malignancy, graft versus host disease, lymphoid interstitial pneumonitis and drug or radiation induced effects.

Conventional diagnostic techniques have included the use of chest X-rays and microscopy and culture of nasopharyngeal or sputum specimens. These methods are helpful, particularly in uncomplicated bacterial infections but are less useful for viral or atypical infections due to lack of sensitivity. Serological tests can be useful to make a retrospective diagnosis of infection but are seldom positive in the acutely ill patient. There has been a resurgence of tuberculosis and atypical mycobac-

Table 12.1: The changing epidemiology of paediatric respiratory infection

Increasing numbers of susceptible and immunocompromised patients
- survival of low-birthweight babies / bronchopulmonary dysplasia
- recognition and treatment of congenital immunodeficiencies
- increased survival of patients with cystic fibrosis
- human immunodeficiency virus (HIV) infection
- chemotherapy for malignant disease
- organ transplantation
- expansion of paediatric intensive care facilities

Wider range of microbial pathogens
- opportunistic and atypical infections
- spread of resistant organisms
- nosocomially acquired infection
- resurgence of tuberculosis and other mycobacterial infections
- imported infections due to increased travel / migration

Novel treatments
- newly introduced antibiotics
- increasing use of antifungal and antiviral agents
- out-patient antimicrobial therapy

terial infections over recent years, however diagnostic techniques for mycobacteria remain inadequate and standard culture can take several weeks.

Well established diagnostic tests have now been augmented by increasingly sophisticated imaging and sampling techniques and molecular diagnosis of microbial disease. This chapter will review these recent advances and potential future developments.

PNEUMONIA IN CHILDREN

Outside the neonatal period patients with acute pneumonia have respiratory symptoms and signs. If these are absent, pneumonia is unlikely. Occasionally a child with very high temperatures may have radiographic evidence of pneumonia in the absence of obvious respiratory illness.

In the developing world the WHO has suggested that tachypnoea (respiratory rate higher than 50 breaths per minute in children under 12 months: higher than 40 per minute from 13 months to 5 years) and chest indrawing should

lead to a presumptive diagnosis of pneumonia. In developed countries the vast majority of children with pneumonia are seen in a general practice setting and are given antibiotics with no investigation. It is likely that a high percentage of these patients have non-bacterial infection.

Whether to investigate and which investigations to perform will depend on the clinical situation. Those requiring admission to hospital and those with infection not responding to empirical treatment in a primary care setting should be subject to at least basic investigation. In children who are immunocompromised or seriously ill there is an urgent need to make a rapid and accurate microbiological diagnosis (Case studies 12.1, 12.2 and 12.3), particularly since the introduction of newer antiviral agents which may be life-saving in these circumstances. In such patients more invasive procedures are justified including bronchoscopy and bronchoalveolar lavage (BAL) and occasionally transbronchial, percutaneous, thoracoscopic or open lung biopsy.[2] The basic

---

Case study 12.1: Pneumonia and leukaemia

May, a 9-year-old girl receiving combination chemotherapy for acute lymphoblastic leukaemia developed a high fever and right upper lobe shadowing on the chest X-ray which persisted despite treatment with broad spectrum antibiotics. The differential diagnosis included viral pneumonia (e.g. CMV pneumonitis), *Pneumocystis carinii* infection, fungal infection, tuberculosis and other opportunistic infections. In view of her immunosuppression and failure to respond more invasive diagnostic procedures were considered.

A bronchoscopy and lavage was performed and the fluid grew *Nocardia asteroides*, an opportunistic bacterium that eventually responded to prolonged antimicrobial therapy.

Comment: This case demonstrates the value of early BAL in the immuno-compromised patient. The result of culture influenced the management and antibiotic choice leading to a favourable outcome.

Figure 12.1 shows a flow diagram for the diagnosis of pneumonia in immuno-compromised hosts.[28]

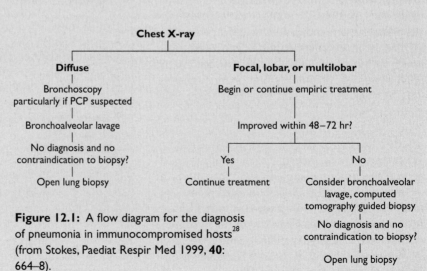

Figure 12.1: A flow diagram for the diagnosis of pneumonia in immunocompromised hosts[28] (from Stokes, Paediat Respir Med 1999, **40**: 664–8).

Case study 12.2: Pneumonia and immunosuppression

June, a six-year-old girl developed severe pneumonitis three weeks after a bone marrow replacement for acute myeloid leukaemia. All cultures were negative. She deteriorated and required extra-corporeal membrane oxygenation (ECMO) as she was unable to maintain her arterial blood gases despite maximal ventilatory support. June clearly had a severe and life-threatening opportunistic infection in view of her recent bone marrow transplant and a blind bronchoalveolar lavage was performed.

The BAL revealed influenza A virus that was detected by immunofluorescence and subsequently isolated in tissue culture. In addition to broad spectrum antibiotics Amantadine was administered, an antiviral agent with activity against influenza A. Despite initial improvement the patient subsequently died.

Comment: This case demonstrates that the use of invasive tests such as BAL may allow accurate virological diagnosis of infection. This has become increasingly important with the advent introduction of specific and effective antiviral agents including neuraminidase inhibitors for influenza infection.

investigations and the more invasive procedures for obtaining diagnostic samples are discussed below. Their use in patients with immunosuppression or cancer are also mentioned briefly.

The results of *non-specific investigations*, such as increase in neutrophils, C-reactive protein (CRP) plasma viscosity or ESR, have poor sensitivity and a poor predictive value.

DIAGNOSTIC TECHNIQUES

BACTERIAL AND FUNGAL DIAGNOSTIC PROCEDURES

Traditional culture techniques and serology have recently been augmented by an array of molecular diagnostic methods. However, even the most sensitive diagnostic tests are limited by the quality of the clinical material received.

Obtaining diagnostic specimens (Table 12.2)

In addition to obtaining good quality specimens it is important to arrange transport to the laboratory as soon as possible as many pathogens are very fragile outside the body and in addition, delay may permit the growth of contaminating organisms. Clear communication with the microbiology laboratory is crucially important to ensure that the appropriate investigations are performed.

Table 12.2: Techniques for diagnosing microbial infection

Bacterial microscopy and culture
Viral isolation in tissue culture
Serological techniques:
complement fixation test
haemagglutination inhibition test for influenza antibodies
immunofluorescence
enzyme-linked immunosorbent assay (ELISA)
Molecular techniques:
gene probes
polymerase chain reaction (PCR) and other gene amplification techniques
gene sequencing
restriction fragment length polymorphism (RFLP) analysis (Case study 12.4)

Sputum examination is difficult in young children. An excess of squamous cells rather than epithelial cells in the sputum suggests oral origin (i.e. saliva). Features suggestive of lower respiratory tract secretions include presence of polymorphonuclear leukocytes and a relatively monotonous bacterial morphology. Diagnosis made from sputum correlates poorly with organisms recovered from blood or pleural fluid, due to upper airway contamination. Mycobacteria and certain fungi are unusual contaminants of the upper airway and their presence may provide diagnostic information.

Nosocomial transmission of tuberculosis has been associated with sputum induction on the

Case study 12.3: Severe pneumonia in early infancy

Tobias, a three-month-old boy was admitted in respiratory failure with a severe pneumonia which did not respond to broad spectrum antibiotics. He had an uncomplicated birth, had been breast fed and showed normal development. He had received no immunizations at the time of admission. His mother had emigrated from Africa several years previously. There was a family history of tuberculosis.

The immediate need was for mechanical ventilation followed by further diagnostic investigation. Blind broncho-alveolar lavage revealed the presence of *Pneumocystis carinii*. Treatment was changed to high dose co-trimoxazole.

Pneumocystis carinii pneumonia is associated with immunosuppression and HIV infection. Following appropriate counselling the child and his mother were screened for HIV infection and both were found to have antibodies to HIV. Active HIV infection in the child was confirmed by performing an HIV polymerase chain reaction that showed HIV viraemia.

Comment: The diagnosis of PCP in this child led to testing for HIV infection. Unfortunately the risk factors for HIV infection in this case had not been identified in the antenatal clinic. Prophylactic co-trimoxazole would normally be given to all children born to HIV-positive mothers and continued until the HIV status of the child became apparent.

Figure 12.2 shows a flow diagram for the diagnosis of pulmonary disease in patients with AIDS.[29]

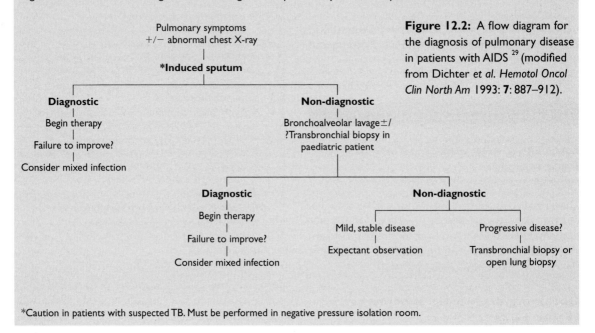

Figure 12.2: A flow diagram for the diagnosis of pulmonary disease in patients with AIDS [29] (modified from Dichter *et al. Hemotol Oncol Clin North Am* 1993: **7**: 887–912).

*Caution in patients with suspected TB. Must be performed in negative pressure isolation room.

---

open ward and if TB is suspected sputum should be induced in an isolation room, with negative-pressure ventilation. There may be practical difficulties achieving this on many paediatric units.

Nasopharyngeal aspirates are relatively easy to obtain from infants using a trap device. The yield for viral culture is greater than for simple nasal and throat swabs.[3] Virological specimens should not be neglected and these should be placed in virus transport medium and transported to the laboratory as soon as possible.

Blood cultures are positive in only 3 to 12% of presumed cases of pneumonia.[4] Results take over 24 hours, and contamination of cultures can occur.

Bronchoscopy with bronchoalveolar lavage (BAL) can be performed safely in children.[5] For children intubated for intensive care a non-bronchoscopic technique may be used. Flexible bronchoscopy provides excellent culture material (Box 12.1).

Although yield from gastric aspirate is probably superior to bronchoscopy for the diagnosis of tuberculosis, bronchoscopy gives additional information about the state of the lower respiratory tract (Chapter 11).

Bronchoalveolar lavage is the most useful technique for identifying the cause of infection in the immunocompromised host. It is generally safe even when the platelet count is low. BAL is particularly helpful in the diagnosis of *Pneumocystis carinii* infection, mycobacterial infection, cytomegalovirus and other opportunistic infections. Brushings at bronchoscopy can be used for cytological examination and viral culture, but the yield is low.

There are limitations. In patients on empirical broad spectrum antibiotics, the bacterial yield is low. In patients without AIDS, the density of infection with *P. carinii* is often low which may give a false negative result. Although CMV can be rapidly diagnosed, other complicating infections may be missed. *Aspergillus* and other fungi are often difficult to diagnose by bronchoscopy.

Transbronchial biopsies are relatively safe in older patients but are rarely performed in young children. They are most useful when *P. carinii* or granulomatous lesions are likely.

Gastric aspirates are useful when the pathogen sought does not usually colonize the upper airways, for example tuberculosis.

The diagnostic yield from *endotracheal aspirates* is improved by using protected microbiological brushes or non-bronchoscopic BAL.

Aspiration of pleural fluid for culture is usually performed when pleural fluid is present (see Case study 12.5).

Transthoracic needle aspiration and lung puncture are normally done under radiological guidance. The pleural space should be aspirated to detect an effusion that was too small to detect clinically prior to entering the lung. Results of transthoracic needle aspiration biopsy using an ultra-thin needle in the diagnosis of nosocomial pneumonia in non-ventilated adults showed it to be specific (100%) and have a high positive predictive value (100%). However, the sensitivity of 60% was relatively low as was its negative predictive value (34.1%).[6] Lung aspiration, which is an attempt to aspirate from an area of consolidation using a needle and syringe, is rarely done in children. Although the rate of complications following lung aspiration are relatively small it should only be done by an experienced operator and only when thought to be of clinical help.

Transthoracic needle aspiration biopsy may be useful for the diagnosis of PCP in paediatric patients with cancer and for localized infections in other immunosuppressed patients.[7,8] Pneumothorax has been reported as a complication in approximately one third of needle aspirations done for PCP. Haemorrhage may be serious but is less common. CT or fluoroscopic guidance greatly

Case study 12.5: Empyema

Paul, a 15-year-old boy presented with a severe pneumonia which responded poorly to broad spectrum antibiotics. He developed swinging pyrexia and continued to lose weight. The possible reasons for his failure to respond included antibiotic resistance, secondary nosocomial infection, localized abscess or empyema or underlying immunosuppression.

A repeat chest X-ray and subsequent CT scan of the chest revealed a loculated empyema. The biochemical blood profile showed a normal albumin and low total protein level. On questioning he admitted to recurrent attacks of sinusitis and otitis media. A 'mini' thoracotomy was performed to break down loculations and to remove infected fluid and debris. This was followed by a rapid clinical improvement.

Immunological investigation revealed the presence of hypogammaglobulinaemia and a diagnosis of common variable immunodeficiency was made. There have been no further problems following treatment with regular immunoglobulin infusions.

Comment: The presence of an empyema is strongly supported by presence of pus, bacteria in pleural fluid following Gram stain, pH less than 7.3 and a glucose concentration less than 60 mg/dL. In exudative pleural effusions, protein content is rarely less than 3 g/dL and lactate dehydrogenase concentration is high. The average white blood cell count in empyema fluid is 19,000 cells\m.[3] Pleural fluid should be obtained and cultured appropriately for aerobic and anaerobic bacteria, fungi and mycobacteria. Detection of bacterial antigens in pleural fluid may be useful.

improves the yield and safety. It still remains an accepted procedure for children with suspected peripheral fungal lesions.

Open lung biopsy is sometimes considered for patients with cancer or immunosuppression to provide tissue for diagnostic investigation. Open lung biopsy generally has a low morbidity. How frequently results of open lung biopsy have led to a change in therapy of patients when non-specific histological findings and organisms treated by empirical therapy are excluded, has been questioned. In immunocompromised paediatric patients, diagnostic yields have ranged from 36–94%.[9]

It has been suggested that any patient with a condition not clearly responding to the therapy chosen on the basis of other diagnostic tests including bronchoscopy or therapy chosen empirically would usually benefit from a biopsy to obtain specific diagnosis. The risk increases when biopsy is delayed until the patient has become critically ill. With diffuse disease, only a limited thoracotomy with a superficial subsegmental dissection is necessary.

Bacteriological diagnosis

Microscopy and staining: The Gram stain gives information on the number and morphology of the organisms present. Although certain bacteria give characteristic staining patterns it is often not possible to make a precise bacteriological diagnosis and the method is relatively insensitive requiring over 10^5 organisms/mL for reliable detection.

Ziehl–Neelsen staining must be performed if tuberculosis is suspected. The increasing numbers of children with human immunodeficiency virus (HIV) infection and other causes of severe immunosuppression has led to the use of additional staining techniques to identify opportunistic organisms including silver staining for *Pneumocystis carinii* and Indian ink staining for cryptococcus and other fungi.

Bacteriological culture is performed on a variety of media, selected according to the source of the clinical material and the predicted pathogens present. Aerobic or anaerobic cultures allow growth of different organisms. A positive isolate can then be characterized and antibiotic sensitivities determined.

A positive culture helps to guide treatment decisions for individual patients and also provides important epidemiological information on the prevalence of different strains and antibiotic resistance patterns in the community. This has allowed the spread of organisms such as *Burkholderia cepacae* in cystic fibrosis patients, methicillin-resistant *Staphylococcus aureus* and penicillin-resistant *Streptococcus pneumoniae* to be documented. Information collected on national and local antibiotic resistance patterns is used to guide antibiotic prescribing policies.

In addition to the standard culture media, specific media may be helpful to isolate certain fungi or fastidious organisms. Improved culture systems are now available for tuberculosis including the BACTEC system of liquid broth media which allows *Mycobacterium tuberculosis* culture in under two weeks.[10]

Immunodetection of bacterial antigen (*S. pneumoniae*, *H. influenzae* type B, *Neisseria meningitidis*, Group B streptococci) may be performed with commercially available methods. False positive and false negative results are not infrequent. Results can be difficult to interpret, as patients may be asymptomatic carriers of organisms such as pneumococcus. These tests are routinely used to diagnose suspected bacterial meningitis and are also used in some centres to enhance the diagnosis of pneumococcal pneumonia.

Serological diagnosis is rarely done due to the delay in gathering results. An immature immune response may often be present at the time of infection especially in young children. For example with *H. influenzae* type B antibody response to infection may be absent.

Success has been claimed in diagnosing pneumonia by performing immunoassays on convalescent sera to detect antibodies against *S. pneumonia* (pneumolysin), *H. influenzae* Type B, *Moraxella catarrhalis* and *Mycoplasma pneumoniae*.

Identification and characterization of positive cultures

Further techniques that are used to define and characterize cultured bacteria include biochemical analysis (biotyping), antimicrobial susceptibility testing, serotyping and phage typing. These methods are expensive and labour intensive but are of particular importance in epidemiological studies that investigate the source and spread of infections in the community. More recently molecular methods have been used to characterize microbial isolates including restriction fragment length polymorphism analysis (RFLP) and comparison of nucleic acid sequences.

RFLP analysis shows whether strains of bacteria are genetically similar and can be used to investigate the transmission of bacterial infection in the community. RFLP has been particularly useful in the investigation of tuberculosis infection and most studies have used the conserved insertion sequence known as IS6110 that is present in multiple copies in strains of *Mycobacterium tuberculosis*. Comparison of the RFLP profiles from *Mycobacterium tuberculosis* isolates from different patients has helped to show how TB is acquired and spread through a population.[11] The value of this technique is illustrated by Case study 12.4.

DIAGNOSIS OF VIRAL INFECTION

Virus isolation

Virus isolation in tissue culture is a useful technique, however sensitivity depends on the quality of the clinical material received and the pathogens present. Most laboratories use a variety of tissue culture cell lines to isolate respiratory viruses including human embryonic lung cells (e.g. MRC5 cells), monkey kidney cells, and human epithelial cells (e.g. hEP2 cells). Cell cultures are regularly checked for the presence of the characteristic cytopathic effects associated with virus infection. Immunofluorescence may help to detect the growth of viruses at an early stage, before the cytopathic effect appears. An example is the detection of early antigen in cells infected with cytomegalovirus. Many respiratory viruses grow relatively slowly or poorly in tissue culture and viral isolation remains a very skilled and labour-intensive process that does not provide rapid diagnosis.

Serological tests

Serological tests seek antibody to the pathogen responsible for causing the disease. Tests in common use include the haemagglutination-inhibition test for influenza and the complement fixation test which exploits the ability of antigen–antibody complexes to fix complement and is used to detect antibodies to a variety of respiratory pathogens including *Mycoplasma pneumoniae*, *Chlamydia psittaci*, *Coxiella burnetti*, respiratory syncytial virus and adenoviruses. Serological tests are particularly helpful in viral or atypical chest infections where organisms are difficult to isolate using conventional culture techniques. However, the complement fixation test has a relatively poor sensitivity and is best for detecting IgG antibodies that only appear in the convalescent stages of infection.

Accurate serological diagnosis of infection is usually made by comparing the antibody titres in acute and convalescent samples. A fourfold rise in titre is conventionally taken as evidence of recent infection. Serological tests are therefore largely unhelpful in the acute stages of infection, although it is sometimes possible to diagnose infection at an earlier stage by looking for the appearance of specific IgM. Serological tests are generally more helpful in providing epidemiological information on the incidence of pathogens in the community rather than as a guide to the management of the seriously ill patient.

Enzyme-linked immunosorbent assay (ELISA)

The ELISA test can be adapted to identify the presence of antigen or specific antibody. To detect antibodies microtitre well-plates are coated with microbial antigen and incubated with the patient's serum. Any antibody present will bind to the antigen on the plate and can be detected using an enzyme-labelled anti-human immunoglobulin. The test measures the colour change after the addition of the enzyme substrate.

The ELISA technique is rapid, fairly sensitive, gives a semi-quantitative result depending on the degree of colour change, and is relatively cheap. It can be automated for testing multiple specimens and screening for a number of respiratory viruses simultaneously.[12] ELISA tests are now routinely used to diagnose viral, bacterial and parasitic infections. However, in the field of respiratory virus infections ELISA has not yet replaced conventional serology.

Immunofluorescence

The direct immunofluorescence technique is used to identify the presence of microbial antigen in clinical material using fluorescein-labelled specific antibodies. Infected clinical material is dried on a slide or microtitre well-plate and is incubated with the labelled specific antibody. If antibody binds to the specimen intense fluorescence is seen by UV microscopy.

The technique is rapid and specific, but is not particularly sensitive and gives best results on nasopharyngeal aspirates or bronchial lavage specimens.[13,14] Commercially available fluorescein-labelled monoclonal antibodies are now available to detect *Legionella pneumophila*, *Pneumocystis carinii*, *Chlamydia pneumoniae*, *Mycoplasma pneumoniae* and a number of respiratory viruses including RSV, influenza A and B, adenovirus, parainfluenza, cytomegalovirus and herpes simplex. Cellular samples such as bronchial lavage specimens are particularly suitable for immunofluorescence.

The indirect immunofluorescence technique detects the presence of antibody in the patient's serum. Well-plates are coated with antigen, incubated with the patient's serum then washed. Any specific antibody present in the serum will bind strongly to the antigen fixed on the slide and is detected by further incubation with a fluorescein-labelled anti-human immunoglobulin.

MOLECULAR DIAGNOSTIC TECHNIQUES

Gene probes and *in situ* hybridization

Gene probes are derived from microbial nucleic acid sequences that are linked to an enzyme or labelled with a radioactive tag. Binding of the gene probe to complementary sequences in the clinical material can then be detected by autoradiography, by autoradiography if a radiolabelled probe is used or by an enzyme reaction causing a colour change with specific substrate, or another reaction such as chemiluminescence leading to detectable light. Potential advantages of the technique include high sensitivity and specificity. Viable organisms do not need to be present provided that there is sufficient nucleic acid to be detected, which has advantages and drawbacks.

In situ hybridization uses gene probes to identify complimentary microbial nucleic acid sequences in tissue samples. This technique can be helpful to identify infection on tissue samples and is a useful experimental tool to investigate the pathogenesis of disease and the mechanisms of colonization and spread of infection.[15]

Gene probes are not routinely used in the diagnostic microbiology laboratory but are used in histopathology. Gene probes have recently been utilized for the early detection of resistance genes in clinical isolates of *Mycobacterium tuberculosis*,[16] however they have been largely superseded by gene amplification techniques.

Gene amplification

A number of methods are now available to amplify microbial nucleic acid and the polymerase chain reaction (PCR) is the most widely used technique. Many pathogenic organisms have now been partially or completely sequenced and the results have revealed areas of highly conserved sequences. Oligonucleotides, typically around 15 bases in length, corresponding to these highly conserved regions can then be synthesized and used to amplify the intervening genome. The resulting amplification product is usually visualized by agarose gel electrophoresis.

Advantages of the technique include its extreme sensitivity and ability to detect as few as single gene sequences; the ability to quantify the number of organisms present and the detection of dead or non-viable organisms.[17] It is also possible to amplify and detect drug-resistance sequences. The PCR methodology is relatively straightforward and can now be fully automated.

Gene amplification techniques are being introduced into most microbiology laboratories and have become the gold-standard for the detection and monitoring of certain infections e.g. HIV, hepatitis C and cytomegalovirus. The use of these techniques in respiratory medicine is still rather limited due to the large number of potential pathogens present. However, multiplex PCR is a future possibility. This uses a cocktail of primers to amplify gene material from a range of potential pathogens each yielding a product of different size if the specific pathogen is present.

Current disadvantages of gene amplification techniques include the relatively high cost of equipment and reagents and great care must be taken to avoid contamination in view of the extreme sensitivity. The presence of a few genomes of microbial material does not necessarily imply causation of disease by that particular pathogen as it could simply be a colonizing or contaminating organism.

Contamination of samples particularly with upper airway organisms may be problematic, so that positive results from sterile sites including blood or pleural fluid are more informative. Rapid diagnosis of diseases caused by mycobacteria, *Chlamydia* and *Bordetella pertussis* could be extremely valuable.

OTHER INVESTIGATIONS

Immunodeficiency

The possibility of immunodeficiency should be considered in any child with severe or recurrent respiratory infections (Case studies 12.3 and 12.5). Relevant tests should be discussed with the immunology laboratory and may include quantification of major immunoglobulin levels and IgG subsets, specific antibody responses, complement levels, functional complement activity, neutrophil function and lymphocyte subsets (see Chapter 8). The possibility of vertically acquired HIV infection should also be explored (Case study 12.3).

Basic investigations such as a sweat test, CF genotype and non-infective causes of respiratory distress such as gastro-oesophageal reflux and aspiration should be considered. Nasal brush biopsy for ciliary functional and structural studies to exclude primary ciliary dyskinesia is required if the history is strongly suggestive.

Chronic infection and inflammation

It is important to remember that children with illnesses including cystic fibrosis, primary ciliary dyskinesia and bronchiectasis may have acute or chronic infection in the absence of obvious clinical signs. For example, a 5-year-old child with cystic fibrosis with an infective exacerbation will usually:

- state they 'feel fine'
- be apyrexial
- have a normal respiratory rate and no recession
- not have finger clubbing
- have no abnormal auscultatory findings
- not produce purulent sputum (if present they swallow it)
- be unable to perform reliable spirometry
- have minimal changes on chest X-ray.

A 'moist' sounding cough may be the only obvious feature. Recognition of this has led to active early treatment of infection in this age group and attempts to isolate *Pseudomonas aerginosa* from throat swabs, cough swabs and in some cases by bronchoscopy.

Diagnosis of pulmonary tuberculosis[18,19,20]

Two or more of the following are required:

- History of close contact with a known or suspected infectious case of TB. The contact history may be obvious but not always. The source case may not have been diagnosed, it may be somebody not considered to be a close contact or there may be a reluctance to tell medical details of other family members.
- Radiographic findings compatible with TB. Any chest X-ray abnormality is compatible with TB but hilar and paratracheal lymph node enlargement or miliary changes strongly suggest TB even in the absence of other clinical features.
- A positive tuberculin skin test. Criteria for a positive skin test are problematical and vary in different situations. In general, in situations where there is a clinical suspicion of TB 5 mm induration is positive for a 1:1000 strength (10 tuberculin units, 0.1 mL) Mantoux tests. This is also equivalent to a grade II heaf test. If the child has had a BCG this test will over-estimate, but there is evidence that a 0.1 mL of 1:10,000 (1 tuberculin unit) will give a better differentiation.[21]

In situations of immunosuppression, the skin reaction may be unreliable. An interpretation of the tuberculin skin test depends on various circumstances, the strength, the size of the reaction and the interpretation of the reader should be recorded. It is unusual to have a bacteriological diagnosis in children. They are rarely smear positive and are a low infection risk to their contacts. This is acceptable if there is a known source from whom samples can be cultured. However, if the child is the index case reasonable steps should be taken to confirm the diagnosis bacteriologically and document sensitivities.

Young children swallow their sputum. To obtain a specimen of sputum, the stomach contents should be aspirated through a nasogastric tube soon after the child wakes in the morning and before food is taken. If no gastric secretions are obtained, lavage should be performed through the tube using about 5 mL/kg of sterile distilled water (tap water may contain environmental mycobacteria). Aspirates should be sent to the laboratory on three consecutive days if it is clinically acceptable to wait before treating. Gastric aspiration is better than flexible bronchoscopy and bronchoalveolar lavage (BAL) for diagnosis of TB in children. *M. tuberculosis* is isolated from gastric aspirate in 30–40% of infants and young children with a clinical diagnosis of TB.

Smears are obtained using a fluorescent dye. This is thought to be faster and more sensitive than the Ziehl–Neelsen staining technique for acid-fast bacilli. The lowest concentration of organisms that can be detected in microscopy is approximately 10^4 organisms per mL.

M. tuberculosis may be identified by means of a PCR, but sensitivity is no better than culture and its primary use is as an epidemiological tool for tracing outbreaks of TB. Regardless of microscopy results, specimens should be cultured and susceptibility of the organism to anti-tuberculous drugs determined.

Imaging techniques to identify respiratory infection

The chest X-ray is still the standard initial radiological investigation for respiratory disease, but has been supplemented by ultrasound scanning, CT scanning and magnetic resonance imaging (MRI), for particular situations (Chapter 10).

ULTRASOUND SCANNING OF THE CHEST

Ultrasound can be helpful to detect the quantity and characteristics (loculation for example) of pleural fluid or pleural thickening. Ultrasound also allows the guided aspiration of pleural effusions and percutaneous biopsy of localized fluid or solid lesions arising from the chest wall, pleura, peripheral lung or mediastinum. Culture and histology of the specimens obtained can help to establish the diagnosis of infection.[22]

COMPUTERIZED TOMOGRAPHY (CT)

CT scanning has revolutionized the investigation of respiratory disease and is particularly helpful in the diagnosis of diffuse pathological processes including pneumonitis and interstitial fibrosis.[23] High resolution CT scanning (HRCT) is now the investigation of choice for fibrosing alveolitis and bronchiectasis and may be helpful in establishing the cause of recurrent purulent chest infections. Dilated bronchi in patients with bronchiectasis are very obviously seen on HRCT [24] and the investigation can be used to identify patients with localized disease that could be amenable to surgery.

Certain infections may be associated with a characteristic appearance on CT scanning, including ground glass shadowing seen in *Pneumocystis carinii* pneumonia,[25] cavitating upper lobe lesions of reactivating tuberculosis, widespread diffuse deposits in miliary TB and invasive aspergillosis infection,[26] with characteristic lesions adjacent to blood vessels. The significant X-ray exposure from CT scanning should be taken into account, particularly when scanning young patients.

MAGNETIC RESONANCE IMAGING (MRI)

Magnetic resonance imaging has yet to find an established place in the routine investigation of respiratory infection but may occasionally be of value in defining mediastinal or hilar masses.[27]

CONCLUSIONS AND FUTURE PROSPECTS

The past decade has seen enormous advances in our ability to identify and treat respiratory pathogens, particularly viruses and atypical organisms. Molecular methods can now be used to diagnose many infections rapidly and with exquisite sensitivity. These techniques are only just being introduced into clinical practice and will need further evaluation. The need for rapid and accurate diagnosis is becoming greater with the increasing number of seriously ill and immunocompromised patients, the mounting problem of antibiotic resistance and the introduction of novel antimicrobial agents. The future will see continuing improvements in the speed and accuracy of diagnosis.

Case study 12.6: Lung abscess complicating acute pneumonia

A 3-year-old girl called Una presented following a 4-day history of pyrexia and cough. Her initial X-ray revealed left upper lobe consolidation and she was treated with intravenous penicillin and erythromycin. Her temperature continued to spike up to 39°C over the next 7 days. Her haemoglobin fell from 12 to 8.5 g/dL and her CRP and white cell count were markedly raised. A repeat X-ray showed fluid levels within the left upper lobe. A CT scan confirmed multiple abscesses. A history of vomiting with possible aspiration at the beginning of the child's illness might have been relevant.

Penicillin has been an appropriate choice of antibiotic for the therapy of lung abscess caused by aspiration of oropharyngeal flora. Because of the lack of response to penicillin in this case, metronidazole was added to cover the possibility of ß-lactamase-producing anaerobes from the oropharynx. High dose flucloxacillin was added to cover possible infection with *Staphylococcus aureus*.

The child's temperature fell over the next 3 days and a further 2 weeks of IV antibiotics were given followed by 6 weeks of oral antibiotic therapy.

Comment: If this child's clinical condition had not improved rapidly following the change of antibiotics and a supportive blood transfusion, an ultrasound or CT guided diagnostic needle aspiration of the lung abscess was planned. Sensitivity and specificity of this procedure are high. In one study from the Far East, 33 out of 35 needle aspirations of lung abscesses, in older patients, were successful. Two developed a pneumothorax, both of which resolved spontaneously without insertion of a chest tube. Ninety-four percent were demonstrated by ultrasound. One or more microorganisms were recovered from 31 of the 33 patients. The corresponding pathogen was recovered from only 3% of blood cultures, 11% of sputum and 3% of alveolar fluid cultures.[30] Limited information is available on the use of BAL.

Occasionally, surgical intervention is considered to provide adequate drainage (or rarely lobectomy) for a child with a lung abscess. Indications include failure to respond to anti-microbial therapy and the severity of the illness, for example a child who is critically ill.

Case study 12.7: Paroxysmal cough

Kolya, a previously well 6-year-old boy presented with a 10-week history of intense coughing spasms. No abnormalities were found on physical examination and spirometric results were within the normal range. The coughing spasms were initially associated with an inspiratory whoop and had become less frequent. A presumptive diagnosis of whooping cough was made and no investigations ordered.

Almost no other acute infectious illness causes a cough that lasts for more than 6–8 weeks in children. The only conditions that can occasionally lead to confusion are a hacking cough in asthma, T.B., bronchitis due to *Chlamydia pneumoniae* and cystic fibrosis. Adenovirus can cause a pertussis-like syndrome. Laboratory tests that support the diagnosis of whooping cough become more difficult to interpret after the first few weeks and diagnosis at this time is largely clinical. Investigations available to support the diagnosis are discussed below.

Laboratory investigations
Lymphocytosis where the lymphocyte differential count is above 70% or more in an apyrexial or slightly pyrexial child with a typical cough is suggestive. It does not distinguish other causes of pertussis-like syndromes such as adenovirus infection. Cultures of nasopharyngeal specimens for *Bordetella pertussis* are positive in 80–90% of cases during the catarrhal and early paroxysmal phases.

Heininger and colleagues[31] found the rate of isolation of *pertussis* in the first 2 weeks was 59%, with cough persisting for 4 weeks. This increased to 80% if cough was associated with a whoop. Isolation rates fall markedly after 21 days of cough.

The best results are obtained when sterile cotton swabs on thin metal wire are introduced in the nasopharynx through the nostril. Nasopharyngeal secretions are smeared on slides for fluorescent microscopy and culture is undertaken.

No single serological test has a high sensitivity and specificity. Direct fluorescent antibody assays have false positive and false negative results, therefore culture confirmation should be sought in all suspected cases.

PCR assays are rapid, specific and sensitive for demonstrating *B. pertussis* in nasopharyngeal secretions, especially during the first weeks of illness.

Adenovirus and *Chlamydia pneumoniae* should be considered as these may also mimic pertussis syndrome. Pertussis may be associated with concomitant infection with respiratory viruses, including adenovirus and parainfluenza infection.

Case study 12.8: 'Atypical' pneumonia

A 7-year-old girl, Martine, presented to hospital with a 7-day history of malaise, cough and increasing respiratory distress. She had been prescribed a cephalosporin by her family doctor 3 days prior to admission. A generalized wheeze was heard and decreased breath sounds over her right lower lobe. Chest X-ray revealed right lower lobe consolidation. The following day mild inspiratory crackles were also detected.

Erythromycin was added to cover the possibility of a *Mycoplasma pneumoniae* infection and symptoms gradually improved over the next two days. Investigations (see below) were considered unnecessary.

Early in an infection with *M. pneumoniae* auscultation may be normal. However, at some stage well over half of patients have crackles on auscultation, and a significant number have wheeze or bronchial breathing.

Case study 12.8: 'Atypical' pneumonia (continued)

Chest X-ray findings can be unilateral, but are very variable, including: a reticular and interstitial pattern, patchy or segmental consolidation, pleural effusion, and hilar adenopathy. M. pneumoniae is resistant to cell wall-active antibiotics such as cephalosporins and penicillins. Erythromycin or one of the newer macrolides are the treatment of choice.

Comment: The use of laboratory investigations to diagnose M. pneumoniae is often unhelpful during the acute illness. White blood count usually normal. ESR or plasma viscosity is often raised. Direct Coombs' test may be positive, as may serological tests for syphilis and ANA.

M. pneumoniae can be cultured from the throat and nasopharynx in infected children but must be transported and inoculated in special media (i.e. SP4 media). In sputum, the sensitivity of antigen detection has been found to range from 40–80% and specificity of 64–100%.[32] The sensitivity was below 20% with nasopharangeal aspirates, but almost 100% specific.

Non-specific cold agglutinins consisting mostly of immunoglobulin M (IgM) appear by end of the first week and disappear by 2–3 months. A bedside test is available but lacks specificity and sensitivity. A low positive antibody titre may result from various respiratory or collagen vascular diseases.

Direct methods such as PCR are not widely available, therefore serological tests (complement fixation) are mainstay for diagnosing Mycoplasma infection. Sera from patients in acute and convalescent stages are run in pairs and a fourfold change in antibody titre is diagnostic of infection. A titre greater than 1:32 in a single serum sample is also considered diagnostic. Negative tests do not exclude reinfection. Sensitivity and specificity have been reported as 90% and 94% respectively.[32]

Antibody responses may not be apparent in immunocompromised children or infants under 12 months. Absence of an IgM response does not necessarily indicate absence of infection, especially in adults.

Case study 12.9: Acute infantile bronchiolitis

Carl, a 3-month-old infant presented with a 4-day history of coryza and increasing respiratory distress. On examination he was cyanosed in air with moderate respiratory distress and grunting, fine inspiratory crepitations and a temperature of 37.5°C. A presumptive diagnosis of bronchiolitis was made. Although the vast majority of cases of bronchiolitis in infancy are due to the respiratory syncytial virus the same clinical picture can result from infection with other viruses including, parainfluenza viruses, influenza viruses, rhinoviruses and adenoviruses.

Described below are the investigations available to help in the diagnosis of specific viral infections.

Respiratory syncytial virus (RSV): Immunofluorescent detection of RSV antigen in exfoliated nasopharyngeal cells or enzyme-linked immunoassays of nasopharyngeal secretions are the methods of choice. Sensitivities are 90% or more compared with cell culture. Serological tests are relatively insensitive and the diagnosis is delayed. Culture requires several days of incubation.

RSV can be found in the upper respiratory tract for up to six days prior to respiratory distress and may continue to be shed for 1 to 20 days. Immunocompromised children may shed virus for 45 days or longer.

Parainfluenza virus: Rapid immunofluorescence has a high specificity (>90%). Sensitivity ranges from 60–80%. Enzyme-linked immunoassays may be used. Primary culture takes longer. The diagnostic testing for influenza virus is similar to parainfluenza virus.

Case study 12.9: Acute infantile bronchiolitis (continued)

Adenoviruses: Asymptomatic shedding from throat or GI tract is common in young children therefore isolation from throat or stool supports but does not confirm diagnosis. Paired acute and convalescent serological studies may help confirm diagnosis but should be two weeks apart. Immunofluorescence and immunoenzyme assay have sensitivities of only between 30 and 60% but are quite specific. Diagnosis confirmed by detection of virus in tissues including lung aspirate or biopsy specimen

Coronaviruses: Enzyme-linked immunosorbent assay to detect human virus antigens and PCR have been used in research studies.

Rhinoviruses: No rapid diagnostic test available; diagnosis depends on culture of agent in tissue culture. PCR has been used on a research basis.

ACKNOWLEDGEMENT

Thanks to Dr Wren Hoskyns for his helpful comments on tuberculosis.

REFERENCES

1. Press S. Association of hyperpyrexia with serious disease in children. *Clin Pediatr* 1994: **33**: 19–25.

2. Rust M, Albera C, Carratu L, *et al.* The clinical use of BAL in patients with pulmonary infections. *Eur Respir J* 1990; **3**: 954–9.

3. Ahluwalia G, Embree J, McNichol P, Law L, Hammond GW. Comparison of nasopharyngeal aspirate and nasopharyngeal swab specimens for respiratory syncytial virus diagnosis by cell culture, indirect immunofluorescence assay and enzyme-linked immunosorbent assay. *J Clin Micro Biol* 1987; **25**: 763–7.

4. Overal J. Is it bacterial or viral? Laboratory differentiation. *Pediatr Rev* 1993; **14**: 251–61.

5. de Blic J, Scheinmann P. Fibreoptic bronchoscopy in infants. *Arch Dis Child* 1992; **67**: 159–61.

6. Dorca J, Manresa F, Esteban L, *et al.* Efficacy, safety and therapeutic relevance of thoracic aspiration with ultra thin needle in non-ventilated nosocomial pneumonia. *Am J Respir Crit Care Med* 1995; **151**: 1491–6.

7. Chaudhary S, Hughes WT, Feldman S, *et al.* Percutaneous transthoracic needle aspiration of the lung: diagnosing *Pneumocystic carinii* pneumonitis. *Am J Dis Child* 1977; **131**: 902–7.

8. Sokolowski JW Jr, Burgher LW, Jones FL, Patterson JR, Selecky PA. Guidelines for percutaneous transthoracic needle biopsy. *Am Rev Respir Dis* 1989; **140**: 255–6.

9. Bozeman PM, Stokes DC. Diagnostic methods in pulmonary infections of immunocompromised children: bronchoscopy, needle aspiration, and open biopsy. In: *Patrick CC. (ed). Infections in immunocompromised infants and children*, Edinburgh: Churchill Livingstone, 1992.

10. Rohner P, Ninet B, Metral C, Emler S, Auckenthaler R. Evaluation of the MB/BacT system and comparison to the BACTEC 460 system and solid media for isolation of mycobacteria from clinical specimens. *J Clin Micro Biol* 1997; **35**: 3127–31.

11. Genewein A, Telenti A, Bernasconi C, *et al.* Molecular approach to identifying route of transmission of tuberculosis in the community. *Lancet* 1993; **342**: 841–4.

12. Sarkkinen H. Respiratory viruses. In Wreghitt TG, Morgan-Capner P, (eds.) *ELISA in the clinical microbiology laboratory.* London: Public Health Laboratory Service, 1990: 88.

13. Ray CG, Minnich LL. Efficiency of immunofluorescence for rapid detection of common respiratory viruses. *J Clin Microbiol* 1987; **25**: 355–7.

14. Grandien M, Pettersson CA, Gardner PS, Linde A, Stanton A. Rapid viral diagnosis of acute respiratory infections: comparison of enzyme-linked immunosorbent assay and the immunofluorescence technique for detection of viral antigens in nasopharyngeal secretions. *J Clin Microbiol* 1985; **22**: 757–60.

15. Hogg JC, Irving WL, Porter H, Evans M, Dunnill MS, Fleming K. *In situ* hybridization studies of adenoviral infections of the lung and their relationship to follicular bronchiectasis. *Am Rev Respir Dis* 1989; **139**: 1531–5.

16. Telenti A, Persing DH. Novel strategies for the detection of drug resistance in *Mycobacterium tuberculosis*. *Res Microbiol* 1996; **147**: 73–9.

17. Hayden JD, Ho SA, Hawkey PM, Taylor GR, Quirke P. The promises and pitfalls of PCR. *Rev Med Microbiol* 1991; **2**: 129–37.

18. Migliori GB, Borghesi A, Rossanigo P, *et al.* Proposal of an improved score method for the diagnosis of pulmonary tuberculosis in childhood in developing countries. *Tuber Lung Dis* 1992; **73**: 145–9.

19. American Academy of Paediatrics Committee on infectious diseases: update on tuberculosis skin testing of children. *Pediatrics* 1996; **45**: 282–4.

20. Klein M, Iseman MD. Mycobacterial infections. Chapter 34, pp. 702–36. In: Taussig LM, Landau LI (eds.). *Pediatric Respiratory Medicine*. London: Mosby, 1999.

21. Hoskyns EW, Simpson H, Monk P. Use of the 1 tuberculin unit (TU) Mantoux test in the assessment of tuberculous infection in children following neonatal BCG vaccination. *Thorax* 1994; **49**: 1006–9.

22. Izumi S, Tamaki S, Natori H, Kira S, *et al.* Ultrasonically guided aspiration needle biopsy in disease of the chest. *Am Rev Respir Dis* 1982; **125**: 460–4.

23. Corcoran HL, Renner WR, Milstein MJ. Review of high-resolution CT of the lung. *Radiographics* 1992; **12**: 917-39.

24. McGuinness G, Naidich DP, Leitmen BS, McCauley DI. Bronchiectasis: CT evaluation. *AJR* 1993; **160**: 253–9.

25. Bergin CJ, Wirth RL, Berry GJ, Castellino RA. *Pneumocystis carinii* pneumonia: CT and HRCT observations. *J Comput Assist Tomogr* 1990; **14**: 756–9.

26. Kuhlman JE, Fishman EK, Burch PA, *et al.* CT of invasive pulmonary aspergillosis. *AJR* 1988; **150**: 1015–20.

27. Link KM, Samuels LJ, Reed JC, Loehr SP, Lesko NM. Magnetic resonance imaging of the mediastinum. *J Thorac Imaging* 1993; **8**: 34–53.

28. Stokes DC. Respiratory infections in the immunocompromised host. Chapter 40, pp. 664–681. In: Taussig LM, Landau LI. (eds.) *Pediatric Respiratory medicine*: London: Mosby, 1999.

29. Dichter JR, Levine SJ, Shelhamer JH. Approach to the immunocompromised host with pulmonary symptoms. *Hematol Oncol Clin North Am* 1993; **7**: 887–912.

30. Yang PC, Luh KT, Lee YC, *et al.* Lung abscesses: US examination and US-guided transthoracic aspiration. *Radiology* 1991; **180**: 171–5.

31. Heininger U, Cherry JD, Eckhardt T, *et al.* Clinical and laboratory diagnosis of pertussis in the regions of a large vaccine efficiency trial in Germany. *Pediatr Infect Dis J* 1993; **12**: 504–9.

32. Kleemola M, Raty R, Karjalainen J, *et al.* Evaluation of an antigen-capture immunoassay for rapid diagnosis of *Mycoplasma pneumoniae* infection. *Eur J Clin Microbiol Infect Dis* 1993; **12**: 872–5.

CHAPTER THIRTEEN

GASTRO-OESOPHAGEAL REFLUX *AND* ASPIRATION

M. R. Green

- Background
- Why look for evidence of gastro-oesophageal reflux?
- How to do it
- Interpretation of results

- How to integrate results into management
- Clinical research issues
- References
- Further reading

BACKGROUND

Gastro-oesophageal reflux represents the involuntary passage of stomach contents back into the oesophagus. This is a normal physiological process throughout life but in circumstances where the severity and/or frequency of gastro-oesophageal reflux is increased, it may become pathological. Dysfunctional motility in the upper gastro-intestinal tract creates disordered co-ordination in the oesophagus in addition to alterations in the lower oesophageal sphincter pressure and delays in gastric emptying time. In such circumstances the normal symptoms of gastro-oesophageal reflux including posseting and vomiting may be present to a marked degree and complications may result (see Table 13.1).

Like most functional problems related to immaturity, in the vast majority of children physiological gastro-oesophageal reflux is self-limiting and has settled by 18 months of age.

A minority of infants and children may have severe gastro-oesophageal reflux without manifest symptoms related to the gastro-intestinal tract. Pathological gastro-oesophageal reflux has been cited as a contributory factor in many respiratory illnesses including those listed in Table 13.1.[1] It has been well described that more than 70% of children suffering acute life-threatening events (ALTE) have pathological acid gastro-

Table 13.1: Symptoms and complications of gastro-oesophageal reflux

Infants
Posseting
Vomiting
Oesophagitis leading to:
irritability
feeding difficulties
haematemesis
abnormal posturing (Sandifer's syndrome)
Failure to thrive
Aspiration pneumonia (recurrent)
Apnoeas/acute life-threatening events (ALTE)
Cyanotic spells
Recurrent croup
Cough
Wheeze
Stridor
Older children
Above plus:
Abdominal pain (epigastric)
Nausea
Dysphagia
Anaemia
Oesophageal strictures

oesophageal reflux and it is postulated that reflux episodes may produce profound vagally mediated responses.[2,3] It is possible that stimulation of laryngeal receptors precipitated by the arrival of refluxed matter in the pharynx produces an apnoeic response which overwhelms the usual airway protective responses including arousal, swallowing and cough. There have now been many reports of a causal association between gastro-oesophageal reflux and respiratory disease following the observation of improved pulmonary function in children particularly with asthma or stridor following anti-reflux medical therapy or surgery. It may be of relevance particularly when the symptom in question is resistant to standard medical therapy. Gastro-oesophageal reflux may also be a factor in prolonging oxygen dependency in bronchopulmonary dysplasia and worsening chest disease in cystic fibrosis.[4,5]

The demonstration of acid gastro-oesophageal reflux in infancy and childhood relies on a suggestive history and there is really only one useful diagnostic investigation. The gold standard is oesophageal pH monitoring which is unfortunately invasive. In this technique pH levels are monitored usually in the lower oesophagus on a continual basis over a period of 18–24 hours. The method is entirely specific for acid reflux (defined as lower oesophageal pH of less than 4.0) but does not identify alkaline reflux (defined as oesophageal pH of greater than 7.5). The role of alkaline shift in the oesophagus in the development of pathology has not been defined. In infancy less than 10% of a 24-hour period would be spent with a lower oesophageal pH of less than 4 and this figure drops to 5% in children over one year of age. This figure is known as the Acid Reflux Index and is the usual figure cited in these studies but, as will be described later on, many other factors should be taken into account when interpreting results. The respiratory symptoms associated with so called 'silent' reflux appear to be particularly related to nocturnal episodes. About 94% of children whose respiratory symptoms ceased with medical anti-reflux therapy had a mean duration of episodes of sleep reflux of over four minutes, whilst in all those in whom the respiratory symptoms were unrelated to reflux the duration was less than four minutes.[6]

The mechanisms for the generation of respiratory disease are not entirely clear but almost certainly include direct aspiration as well as neural reflex arcs. Reflex theories, other than direct aspiration, have been postulated because of the difficulties of correlating reflux episodes seen on oesophageal pH monitoring and clinical respiratory events. There is often a marked time-lag and therefore the evidence for a causal association lies largely on the observation of clinical improvement following anti-reflux manoeuvres.[7,8,9,10]

WHY LOOK FOR EVIDENCE OF GASTRO-OESOPHAGEAL REFLUX?

In most cases of overt but uncomplicated gastro-oesophageal reflux investigation is not warranted. It is entirely appropriate in these circumstances to employ standard treatment based on the reported severity of symptoms, including those cases where there is evidence of possible oesophagitis and mild failure to thrive. However when the response to treatment is poor or when there are more worrying complications, such as those listed in Table 13.1, then the most useful investigation is oesophageal pH monitoring which will confirm the diagnosis and give some indication of severity.

The question of when to, and indeed whether or not to, perform pH monitoring in children with respiratory symptoms is less clear. However, in view of the association between silent gastro-oesophageal reflux and many chronic respiratory symptoms oesophageal pH monitoring should be mandatory in infants presenting with significant apnoeic spells or acute life-threatening events. The other more obvious circumstance is infants presenting with recurrent pneumonias which may result from aspiration. The other 'softer' symptoms where the picture is not so clear include persistent cough, wheeze and stridor, particularly when resistant to treatment. These complaints are of course much more common in clinical practice than the acute events and therefore present more of a challenge. In these circumstances the confirmation of pathological gastro-oesophageal reflux, particularly when this occurs largely at night, is useful evidence that the symptoms in question are not purely respiratory in origin. It is then appropriate to consider adding anti-reflux treatment and to use reported symptoms and objective measurements where appropriate in order to judge the response. Case studies 13.1 and 13.2 illustrate typical clinical scenarios and approaches to their management.

Case study 13.1: Chronic lung disease of prematurity

James was delivered by elective caesarean section at 28 weeks' gestation. He was ventilated for two weeks and thereafter remained in incubator oxygen until his final discharge on continuous home oxygen therapy at the age of 5 months. He had always been a difficult feeder but became increasingly so over his first 3 months at home. His oxygen requirements did not decrease. He then developed periods of acute distress and irritability often related to feeds and his parents interpreted this as indicative of abdominal pain.

At review plans were made to perform an upper gastro-intestinal endoscopy which confirmed a macroscopic and histological oesophagitis. 24-hour oesophageal pH monitoring confirmed significant acid reflux with a reflux index of 15%. He was commenced on anti-reflux therapy with an H_2 antagonist and a prokinetic agent. Over the subsequent 6 weeks his periods of apparent distress settled and he began to feed much better. Two months after the commencement of anti-reflux therapy he no longer required additional oxygen.

Case study 13.2: An infant with stridor

Priya, a 3-month-old child who was born at term by the normal vaginal route, is referred to Outpatients because of inspiratory stridor. Her parents had noted this within a few days of birth, but had now brought it to medical attention as it seemed to be worsening.

The clinical diagnosis was one of laryngomalacia and review was arranged for 5 months of age. By this time her parents reported that the stridor had become continuous and that she was no longer feeding as well. She had also had occasional choking episodes during feeding. The ENT surgeon planned a laryngoscopy and bronchoscopy and asked for an oesophageal pH probe to be sited after these procedures but before anaesthesia was reversed. Lipid-laden macrophages were demonstrated on the tracheal aspirate and the oesophageal pH monitoring confirmed significant reflux with an acid reflux index of 18%. The episodes were frequent and often prolonged during the day and night.

Following 6 weeks of anti-reflux treatment her symptoms were much better and her stridor was now described as intermittent and mild, a pattern which was consistent with benign laryngomalacia.

There may be no history of posseting or vomiting even when the respiratory symptoms worsen. It is therefore suggested that in any child with chronic wheeze or cough or upper airway symptoms oesophageal pH monitoring is considered if the response to standard treatment is not as one would expect.

HOW TO DO IT

This section will concentrate on the technique of oesophageal pH monitoring but some other investigative methods which are of relevance will be briefly mentioned.

The contrast swallow and meal is often falsely interpreted as an indicator of pathological reflux. This investigation is useful to demonstrate the anatomy of the upper bowel, but no inference can be made about the presence or absence of gastro-oesophageal reflux. The administration of barium to an often screaming infant is not a normal situation and therefore if reflux is seen during the brief screening period of a barium swallow, one does not know whether this represents simple physiological reflux or whether it has been induced by the distress caused by the examination.

Isotope milk scans may be helpful especially when oesophageal pH monitoring is not available. They may demonstrate both direct aspiration and aspiration associated with reflux of stomach contents.[11] If bronchoscopy is being performed as part of the investigation of respiratory symptoms some workers, particularly in the United States, will look for the presence of lipid-laden macrophages as presumptive evidence of reflux and aspiration of milk feeds.[12] Both methods lack sensitivity.

One should always take the opportunity to consider performing oesophageal pH monitoring when one is undertaking upper GI endoscopy under general anaesthesia. Endoscopy is particularly relevant where there is clinical evidence of possible oesophagitis and enables one to confirm this macro- and microscopically. Other complications such as Barratt's oesophagus and oesophageal stricture formation in older children may be revealed. These are much more likely in children with neurological handicap when permanent postural problems and lack of muscle tone and co-ordination may contribute to the gastro-oesophageal reflux. In these children medical therapy is more likely to fail and definition of the anatomy is essential prior to surgery.

ESPGAN, the European Society of Paediatric Gastroenterology and Nutrition, have described the desired approach to oesophageal pH monitoring in some detail.[13] Ideally this study should represent a situation as close as possible to the normal physiological state. It is essential therefore that the recording equipment is portable and that the study is ambulatory. Treatment with H_2 blockers or proton pump inhibitors should be stopped 3 to 4 days before the study and prokinetic agents should be stopped 48 hours beforehand, with antacids being omitted from 24 hours prior to the study. It is possible to use electrodes with an internal reference, but these are of larger bore and most often in infants we will use an antimony electrode with an external reference which is taped onto the anterior chest wall with liberal quantities of electrode gel. It is essential that the probe is calibrated in both pH 1.0 and 7.0 before use and then the catheter is introduced via the nose to a position in the lower oesophagus. Strobel's formula (5 + 0.252 × length of child in cm) is used to calculate the distance from the nostril to the lower oesophageal sphincter (LOS). This is reasonably reliable in infancy but less so in older children. For this reason it is important to confirm the position of the electrode, the tip of which should be ideally lying over the third vertebral body above the diaphragm during both phases of respiration. The electrode position may be confirmed by fluoroscopy or standard chest X-ray or at endoscopy if the two procedures are being combined. If combined oesophageal manometric measurements are

being made then these can be used to confirm the electrode position by pulling back from the determined position of the LOS. In similar fashion the position can also be confirmed by inserting the catheter into the stomach and waiting for the pH reading to stabilize. Then the probe may be withdrawn slowly watching the pH display to determine when the probe tip is passing back into the oesophagus.

During the recording an accurate diary should be kept by the child's carer noting the time of any particular symptoms or events as well as body position, sleep and administration of feeds or medicines. At the end of the recording the data is down-loaded into a standard software programme which will produce a printout of the continuous pH recording as well as various statistics. The accepted definition of a reflux episode is a lower oesophageal pH of less than 4.0 for more than 15 seconds. The Acid Reflux Index describes the total percentage of the recording time spent with a lower oesophageal pH of less than 4.0.

INTERPRETATION OF RESULTS

There are a number of important parameters to consider as well as the calculated Reflux Index before planning clinical management based on the results of the pH study. These include the number of prolonged episodes (defined as a pH of less than 4.0 for more than 5 consecutive minutes) and also determination of the longest episode. It is essential to view the whole tracing, preferably hour by hour on screen prior to printing, together with the diary. This will enable careful matching of pH to clinical events and also alert the user to periods of disconnection which otherwise might go undetected and be interpreted by the software as evidence of gross acid reflux. The frequency of brief episodes is also then clearly displayed.

Accurate documentation of feeding is essential. Ingestion of fruit juices will lower the oesophageal pH transiently and these episodes may be falsely interpreted as evidence of reflux. Recordings made in infants who are taking frequent milk feeds should be interpreted with caution. In these circumstances the gastric pH will be higher than normal for a greater proportion of the recording time and so genuine reflux episodes may be missed. The period of recording prior to the next feed may give useful clues if the trend shows a gradual drifting in the pH.

The Acid Reflux Index should be less than 10% during infancy and less than 5% in children over one year of age. A figure of 5–10% represents mild reflux, 10–20% moderate, and more than 30%, severe reflux. At this end of the spectrum it becomes increasingly unlikely that the child will respond to medical therapy and the threshold for progressing to anti-reflux surgery is much lower as illustrated in Case study 13.3.

Case study 13.3: Recurrent pneumonia and quadriplegia

May, a ten-year-old girl with profound spastic quadriplegia is admitted for assessment. Over the past two years her parents have had increasing difficulty persuading her to eat and she has vomited on a daily basis. She also has frequent choking and coughing episodes associated with feeding. Three months ago she was admitted with her third episode of right-sided pneumonia in seven months. Nasogastric feeding was therefore instituted at that stage, but the vomiting has persisted and she has become increasingly irritable during tube feeds. Her weight and skinfold thicknesses are all well below the third centile.

With this clinical picture one should be suspicious of reflux oesophagitis and even without the overt vomiting one needs to be aware of aspiration of feeds either directly during swallowing or following reflux of gastric contents.

A contrast swallow without the nasogastric tube demonstrated normal anatomy, but tracheal aspiration during swallowing. There is poor bolus formation of both liquid and more formed contrast media and propulsion beyond the oropharynx is interrupted by unco-ordinated oesophageal contractions. Free gastro-oesophageal reflux into the upper oesophagus is also noted. Upper GI endoscopy under general anaesthesia confirmed the presence of oesophagitis both macroscopically and microscopically. An oesophageal pH probe was sited whilst still under anaesthesia. The trace is shown in Figure 13.1. It shows frequent and prolonged episodes of acid reflux during both day and night with an index of more than 50%.

Whilst nasogastric feeding will avoid direct aspiration into the airways it will not prevent reflux of stomach contents with the risk of aspiration. In order to provide this child with adequate nutrition it is clearly appropriate to consider gastrostomy. However it is recognized that the gastric dilatation associated with delivery of feeds directly into the stomach predisposes to gastro-oesophageal reflux. It was therefore decided to perform a gastrostomy together with fundoplication, a procedure which then allowed adequate nutritional manipulation without the risk of aspiration, either directly or during reflux episodes. The complications of chronic acid reflux, including oesophagitis and stricture, are also then avoided. A common surgical procedure is a Nissen's fundoplication in which the gastro-oesophageal junction is tightened using a 360° diaphragmatic sling. It may be performed laparoscopically.

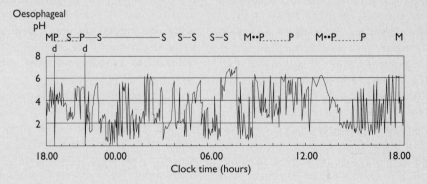

Figure 13.1: 24-hour lower oesophageal pH recording from Case study 13.3.

How to integrate results into management

The vast majority of mild uncomplicated reflux needs no specific treatment and will settle spontaneously with time. It may be useful to suggest positioning the child at roughly 30% from the horizontal, especially after feeds, but the clinical evidence that this makes any sustained difference is not strong, particularly when respiratory symptoms are foremost. Similarly feed thickeners and antacids may help at the mild end of the spectrum. In older children it is always worth giving some dietary advice including avoidance of spicy foods, caffeine and fizzy drinks.

In more overtly symptomatic children, and certainly in those with respiratory symptoms where pathological reflux is demonstrated on oesophageal pH monitoring, then prokinetic agents are warranted. Cisapride acts by enhancing the release of acetylcholine in the myenteric plexus resulting in an increase in motility and antroduodenal co-ordination. It is the only drug of its class, but has recently been withdrawn because of cardiotoxicity. Where there is evidence of complications then gastric acid suppression agents (either H_2 antagonists or a proton pump inhibitor) should be used. If there is failure of symptomatic response on appropriate doses of medical therapy then at that stage surgery should be considered as in Case study 13.3 which describes a common problem in clinical practice, an appropriate approach to investigation and management based on the results.

Clinical research issues

Gastro-oesophageal reflux and respiratory symptoms are both common problems in paediatric practice. The aim of investigation and treatment is to reduce the danger of permanent lung damage or of more acute events related to presumed gastro-oesophageal reflux. There is a growing body of evidence describing the problems of silent oesophageal reflux and in a number of circumstances, particularly in asthma resistant to normal treatment, it is possible to demonstrate clinical improvement following anti-reflux therapy. However definition of the precise relationship between gastro-oesophageal reflux and respiratory symptoms and disease remains elusive. The development of newer prokinetic agents which may be more effective in reflux associated with neurological handicap will transform nutritional and general management for these children.

References

1. Burton DM, Pransky SM, Katz RM, Kearns DB, Seid AB. Pediatric airway manifestations of gastroesophageal reflux. *Ann Otol Rhinol Laryngol* 1992; **101**: 742–9.

2. Veereman-Wauters G, Bochner A, Caillie-Bertrand MV. Gastroesophageal reflux in infants with a history of near-miss sudden infant death. *J Pediat Gastroenterol Nutr* 1991; **12**: 319–23.

3. See CC, Newman LJ, Berezin S, *et al.* Gastroesophageal reflux induced hypoxaemia in infants with apparent life-threatening events. *Am J Dis Child* 1989; **143**: 951–4.

4. Booth IW. Silent gastro-oesophageal reflux: how much do we miss? *Arch Dis Child* 1992; **67**: 1325–7.

5. Newell SJ, Booth IW, Morgan ME, Durbin GM, McNeish AS. Gastro-oesophageal reflux in preterm infants. *Arch Dis Child* 1989; **64**: 780–6.

6. Jolley SG, Herbst JJ, Johnson DG, Matlack ME, Book LS. Esophageal pH monitoring during sleep identifies children with respiratory symptoms from gastroesophageal reflux. *Gastroenterology* 1981; **80**: 1501–6.

7. del Rosario JF, Orenstein SR. Evaluation and management of gastroesophageal reflux and pulmonary disease. *Curr Opin Pediat* 1996; **8**: 209–15.

8. Blecker U, de Pont SM, Hauser B, Chouraqui JP, Gottrand F, Vandenplas Y. The role of 'occult' gastroesophageal reflux in chronic pulmonary disease in children. *Acta Gastroenterol Belg* 1995; **58**: 348–52.

9. Krishnamoorthy M, Mintz A, Liem T, Applebaum H. Diagnosis and treatment of respiratory symptoms of initially unsuspected gastroesophageal reflux in infants. *Am Surg* 1994; **60**: 783–5.

10. Tucci F, Resti M, Fontana R, Novembre E, Lami CA, Vierucci A. Gastroesophageal reflux and bronchial asthma: prevalence and effect of cisapride therapy. *J Pediat Gastroenterol Nutr* 1993; **17**: 265–70.

11. Heyman S, Kirkpatrick JA, Winter HS, Treves S. An improved radionuclide method for the diagnosis of gastroesophageal reflux and aspiration in children (milk scan). *Radiology* 1979; **131**: 479–82.

12. Nussbaum E, Maggi JC, Mathis R, Galant SP. Association of lipid-laden alveolar macrophages and gastroesophageal reflux in children. *J Pediat* 1987; **110**: 190–4.

13. Working group of ESPGAN. A standardized protocol for the methodology of esophageal pH monitoring and interpretation of the data for the diagnosis of gastroesophageal reflux. *J Pediat Gastroenterol Nutr* 1992; **14**: 467–71.

FURTHER READING

1. Walker WA, Durie PR, Hamilton JR, Walker-Smith JA, Watkins JB (eds). *Pediatric gastrointestinal disease.* Philadelphia and Toronto: BC Decker Inc.

CHAPTER FOURTEEN

QUALITY *OF* LIFE

D. Wensley

- Introduction
- Measurement tools and how to use them
- Research – the future

- References
- Further reading

INTRODUCTION

Assessment of the impact of disease and its treatment on individual patients is especially important in chronic disease. Where cure is not a possibility, patients and their immediate families must come to terms with changes in life-style which may vary with time. Health professionals implicitly assume that improvements in symptoms mean that the patient has a better quality of life. This is a great over-simplification. Quality of Life (QoL) assessment incorporates not only the impact of illness and treatment on physical function, but also its effect on life-style and emotional well-being, features which are often overlooked. More than a measure of the extent of functional impairment, which may be obtained using other methods, quality of life deals with a higher order of complexity: the impact of functional impairment on other aspects of life, e.g. for children, the ability to go to school or play and the emotional effect of these restrictions.

Quality of life is increasingly used as an outcome measure in clinical trials to assess new treatments or regimes. The concept of quality of life and its place in clinical practice has not yet been fully explored. This chapter will consider measurement tools and how to use them and the application of quality of life measurement in paediatric respiratory medicine.

THE CONCEPT OF QUALITY OF LIFE

Quality of life assessment is a formal measure of individual well-being, arguably a measure of health.[1] Both healthy and sick populations can be assessed. In disease, information about the physical, social, occupational and psychological effects of illness is sought, which may otherwise be overlooked by more traditional methods.[2,3] QoL measurement offers the ability to gain the patient's perspective of the impact of disease, encompassing a wide range of health issues. Definition is complex (Box 14.1). The World Health Organization attempts to incorporate all aspects of measurement, whereas other commentators specify quality of life assessment in illness. For clinical purposes, impact of illness (disease-related quality of life) is of most relevance.

Box 14.1: Definitions of quality of life

'Quality of life is ... an individual's perception of their position in life ... in relation to their goals, expectations, standards and concerns. It is a broad ranging concept affected ... by the person's physical health, psychological state, level of independence, social relationships, and their relationships to salient features of their environment.'[30]

'represents the functional effect of an illness and its consequent therapy ... as perceived by that patient'[31]

Development of QoL questionnaires has made assessment a possibility. These are available for use with different sections of the population and different age groups (Box 14.2). Some questionnaires concentrate on particular areas of life which may be compromised, e.g. participation in work, others on more individual aspects such as personality. Paediatric assessment tools are limited in number and tend to consider all aspects of life in order to gain a more global picture (Table 14.1).

In paediatric respiratory medicine information about disease course is available from a number of sources. Assessing disease severity or the impact of treatment includes objective assessment such as lung function testing; clinical scores; use of rescue medication; number of unplanned visits to the GP or hospital and school absence. Other, more subjective assessments can be made such as symptom reporting, perhaps with a diary. Paediatrics offers the opportunity to supplement clinical assessment

---

Box 14.2: Types of Quality of Life instrument

Generic: general assessment of quality of life, applicable to any person healthy or not, e.g. Nottingham Health Profile.[32]

System specific: designed for use with a specific system condition in mind, questions can be more focused and ask about the specific impact of a condition and its treatment, e.g. St George's Respiratory Questionnaire.[33]

Utility: to assess the economic aspects of disease and cost effectiveness of treatment, e.g. Rand Health Insurance Measure.[34]

Disease specific: for use only with a particular disease, very specific and so cannot be generalized or applied to any other situation, e.g. Childhood Asthma Questionnaire,[24] Juvenile Arthritis Questionnaire.[22]

Table 14.1: Qol measurement tools for chidren with respiratory disease

Measure type	Name of assessment tool	Who competes	Age	Comments
Asthma (disease specific)	Childhood Asthma Questionnaire[24] Form A Form B Form C	Child and parent Child alone Child alone	4–7 8–11 12–16	Uses smiley faces Difficult concepts for youngest group
Asthma (disease specific)	Paediatric Asthma Quality of Life Questionnaire[36]	Child	6–17	Interview or self-administered Children seem to find some questions ambiguous
	Caregivers Quality of Life Questionnaire[13]	Parent	Parents	Caregivers complete questionnaire relating to the impact of asthma from a carer's perspective
Asthma	Usherwood[27]	Parent	Children	Primary care tool Proxy measure
Generic	Rand scale[34]	Adult	Children	Parent's perception of child functional limitation
Generic	Family Impact[37]	Parents	Parents	Parent assesses effect on family of illness

with information from both children and parents which may offer some objectivity. It has generally been accepted that parents are the main source of information and as such detailed parental questioning forms part of any assessment. Whilst a full history from a child may be unreliable[4] or inadequate because of problems with time perception,[5] information about current symptoms and feelings about disease state is often illuminating and can greatly supplement parental information. This may be especially true in the case of chronic diseases such as asthma and cystic fibrosis because their severity and time course are so variable. Patient perception is a critical aspect of disease course and much of the daily impact of the disease is subjective, as is decision to treat with increasing self-management at home (Chapter 24). Discrepancies between quality of life assessment have been demonstrated between patients and doctors,[3,6] and also parents and children,[7] especially adolescents.[8]

WHY SHOULD WE MEASURE QoL ?

Until the development of questionnaires, all non-clinical data available was considered to form quality of life. In highlighting the poor design of many studies stating quality of life as an outcome measure, Bowling argues that many studies mention quality of life (some 3–50% of her sample) whilst only 2–7% actually measured it. Availability of specific tools makes quality of life a realistic measure of outcome.[3]

To ensure it is valid, a questionnaire inevitably requires some means of comparison with other measures of disease severity. QoL questionnaires include other measures of symptoms or activity limitation as part of their design. However, there is evidence that they measure some other aspects of the disease which are not wholly represented by other means of assessment.[1] Objective improvements in physical function are important, but may not be relevant to the patient.[9] Although traditional clinical assessment can provide an indication of impact, the picture is incomplete; quality of life assessment incorporates different issues. Improvements in functional status may be accompanied by similar improvements in quality of life in some patients but not others, whose overall health is not much better.[1]

QoL assessment can be used to measure the impact of treatment. Since most questionnaires have been designed for repeated assessment, it is possible to measure QoL sequentially. Improvements in quality of life may enhance the patient's sense of well-being. Negative feelings about disease impact, when symptomatic control is good, offer the health professional the opportunity to elicit patient concerns and promote discussion to attempt to resolve the problems.

Clinical outcome measures are the main focus during exacerbations of disease when other issues seem less important. Encompassing other issues provides an overview of patient disease management at other times (Box 14.3). This knowledge may reduce the risk of exacerbations for some individuals, accepting that illness forms a part of their overall quality of life assessment. For patients, areas of concern other than the immediate effect of increased symptoms and may be especially important during exacerbations. Absence from school, cancelled social engagements or (for older children) loss of earnings can be critical issues.

Clinicians are considered to be poor assessors of patients' quality of life, perhaps because the criteria they use differ from those of the patient.[1] As discussed earlier, the case of children is more

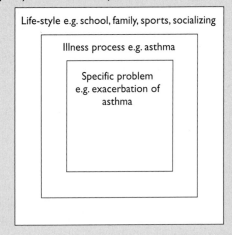

Box 14.3: Disease as the focus

Clinicians are consulted when symptoms are worsening and traditional measures of condition are poor. Consideration of impact at other times provides an insight into management strategies and aspects of quality of life which may enhance assessment.

Life-style e.g. school, family, sports, socializing

Illness process e.g. asthma

Specific problem e.g. exacerbation of asthma

complicated with parents seeming to have difficulty in assessing children's quality of life. Physical symptoms may be alleviated only at the expense of activities which give great pleasure, such as participation in sports activities or the ownership of a pet. Family and/or child may feel that whilst physically they feel better in terms of symptoms, their quality of life has deteriorated because of a direct effect of treatment decisions, removal of a family pet, for example. Knowledge of the child's feelings on the issue provides a basis for real negotiation rather than traditional 'doctor knows best' form of control (Case study 14.1).

Implications of drug and treatment side effects are another issue which is relevant here.[10,11] Clinical assessment may lead us to conclude that a patient is much improved. This fails to take into account the fact that they have had to alter their life-style or suffered side effects which may fail to show on a symptom diary. Treatment itself may impact indirectly on quality of life, for instance: ridicule at inhaler use at school; weight gain with glucocorticoid therapy; nasal distortion with use of nasal continuous positive airway pressure (CPAP) or nocturnal ventilation.

Accepting that non-compliance is a real issue for adolescents allows clinicians to truly negotiate (Case study 14.2). Whilst this approach may seem idealistic, it accepts that there are times when teenagers are reluctant to participate in treatment and that their personal view concerning the cost/benefit balance of treatment is different from that of health professionals.

Implications for the family of chronic illness or a deterioration should also be considered and some questionnaires are available to measure the QoL of carers of children with particular illnesses.[12,13]

The affect on the family as a whole, particularly in the case of younger children can be assessed by appropriate questionnaire e.g. the family impact scale (Case study 14.3).

A number of benefits may result from the effort to take the patient's perspective:

- Attempting to measure QoL may itself influence the clinician/patient relationship.[14]
- Patients who feel their opinion is being sought may be more likely to listen to the health professional.[14]
- Knowledge about the emotional impact of illness and the way people feel about disease progression or treatment may enhance care. The patient's expectations from treatment are usually far from the clinician's aims or the medical therapeutic model.[15]

Case study 14.1: Asthma

Paul has asthma. He is 13 years old and lives at home with his mother and sister. He is failing at school and finds it difficult to concentrate. He is small which has resulted in bullying. He participates in sporting activities, runs long distance for his school and county and is a keen swimmer.

In recent months his asthma has been difficult to control and running in cold weather has precipitated an acute attack. Introduction of long-acting β_2 agonists improved the situation slightly in terms of symptoms and lung function. It was suggested that he stop running in competition for a short time to reduce his heavy training schedule and to monitor his peak flow (PEF) regularly at home.

This would improve symptoms and PEF, and might lead to a reduction in medication. What would be the impact on Paul's quality of life?

Paul refused to stop running. After discussion, he agreed to monitor his PEF if he could continue to participate in competition and return for review 6 weeks later. If no improvement had occurred within this time, Paul agreed to miss a small number of races towards the end of the season. On return to clinic, Paul was somewhat improved and with discussion, it became evident that Paul had remembered to take his treatment more regularly since the previous review.

Case study 14.2: The impact of treatment in cystic fibrosis

Stephen has cystic fibrosis. He is 15 years old and lives with parents and two younger siblings who have no health problems. His respiratory health was good until 12 months ago when he began deteriorating.

When Stephen is well, daily treatment regimen involves:

- physiotherapy three times;
- nebulized therapy including bronchodilator three times; DNAse once and nebulized antibiotics twice;
- pancreatic supplement capsules at each meal time and with several snacks during the day;
- prophylactic antibiotics orally three times.

During an exacerbation, physiotherapy and antibiotics increase and Stephen's parents sometimes wake during the night to administer additional therapy. Stephen's parents are also able to administer intravenous antibiotics at home if necessary.

Stephen's physical condition is maintained by this regime. Skipping treatments leads to a deterioration in symptoms, a need for intravenous medication and extra physiotherapy, but for Stephen it is worth it at times when peer pressure means socializing is an easier option. Measuring QoL may increase Stephen's morale[35] and allow patient and physician to focus on susceptible times and negotiate treatment regimes to enhance compliance.[14]

Case Study 14.3: Impact on the family, chronic lung disease of prematurity

Sam is 2 years old. He was born at 28 weeks' gestation after an uneventful pregnancy and developed chronic lung disease of prematurity. He was discharged home at 16 weeks post-natal age. He has one older sister at school and his father and mother are a professional couple working full and part-time respectively.

Before Sam's birth, his mother worked 21 hours a week since her older child had started school. Sam has been oxygen dependent since birth and for the past six months has needed oxygen every night, but only during the day if he is unwell. His mother reduced her working hours when it became apparent that Sam would need extra care.

When Sam develops a cold every 6–8 weeks, his sleeping pattern is disrupted and he has increased oxygen requirements. His mother has access to the respiratory nursing service at the local hospital to check oxygen saturation levels, but doesn't want to 'bother the nurses'.

During each cold, Sam's mother is awake for most of three nights and his father has disturbed nights. Sam's sister is sometimes woken. His father has difficulty concentrating at work, and his mother is unable to work for two weeks, during which time Sam has day-time oxygen requirements and the nursery refuses to take him. After 14 days, 'normal' life is resumed for the family.

All family members are affected by these infections. Oxygen dependency means access to financial help, e.g. the Disability Living Allowance. This ends when the children no longer need oxygen. If Sam's mother does not return to work when he no longer needs oxygen, the family income will fall. The alternative, extended absences for child illness, will create a great deal of stress for the mother and raises a number of issues for her employers.

The effects on this family are physical, emotional and economic. This may not be true of all families with oxygen-dependent children and formal quality of life measurement may elicit these concerns.

- By paying attention to quality of life, patient satisfaction and hence adherence to therapy may be improved.[14] For instance, a simpler, less intrusive medication regime, may be more likely to be adhered to. The relationship between quality of life and compliance is complex and far from proven. Quality of life may improve without any significant changes in objective measures simply because the time involved in taking treatment is reduced.

Including QoL assessment in management is possible and many questionnaires are available. Questionnaires concerned specifically with paediatric respiratory care, are limited in number although well developed.

MEASUREMENT TOOLS AND HOW TO USE THEM

Health professionals carry out quality of life assessment informally during clinical assessment: 'How are you?' 'How have you been since I last saw you?' This lacks focus, is highly subjective on the part of the clinician and is far from standardized between clinicians and patients. Clinicians may not 'hear' the patient's reply. Assessment is complex and dependent on time available, effectiveness of measurement tool, application of results and need for full assessment. Formal assessment is possible using quality of life measurement tools. Despite criticism of the subjective nature of these tools, there is a great similarity between these measures even though they have been developed in different ways.[1]

Paediatric instruments are few, and some conditions (cancer, arthritis) are well represented. There are a number of tools for use in respiratory medicine especially asthma (Table 14.1), although some diseases are poorly served. There are no current validated tools for use in children with cystic fibrosis, although these are being developed.

In the case of young children, measurement of quality of life is complicated by the presence of a third party – the child's parents. Parents almost always accompany their children to consultations. This applies even to teenagers. Clinicians frequently choose to listen to parent's views (usually by habit rather than design), and the child's opinions are neither voiced nor heard. There may be big differences of opinion between parent and child[7,8,21] although some surveys have shown good agreement.[22] Children change as they develop and grow. Some questionnaire developers have recognized that issues differ in importance at different ages and stages of development, and have responded by producing alternative questionnaire forms for different age groups (e.g. Childhood Asthma Questionnaire[23,24]).

Some of the measures described require a formal training process prior to use by clinicians. This can be time consuming and expensive. Others are supplied with guidance notes and information for anyone wishing to implement them as part of their management strategy.

The choice of questionnaire depends on a number of factors.

- Validity and suitability (Box 14.4). A plethora of questionnaires are available and it is important to choose one which has been validated appropriately. Where all appropriate tools have undergone necessary development and testing, practical issues become important. Ease of application and number of questions are important considerations if quality of life is to be measured in a busy outpatient department, for example.

Box 14.4: The validity and suitability of the questionnaire

- Has it undergone thorough development the results of which have been published?

- Does it have face validity? Are the questions sensible to an intelligent audience,[2,38] does it make sense 'on the face of it', do questions make sense to the user. Face validity is important but not sufficient to justify using a particular QoL questionnaire.[38]

- Does it have content validity? Do groups of questions capture concepts relevant to the population? Are questions relevant to the developer's aims?[38] Is coverage comprehensive?[2] Each item should fall into at least one area under consideration. The number of items listed in each conceptual group should reflect the importance of that concept.[3]

- Does it have criterion validity? When used in conjunction with an existing (superior) measure, the results should be comparable.[38] Many developers compare questionnaires with other more general tools. A validity coefficient needs to be established in correlation with a previously validated questionnaire.[2]

- Is it suitable for my population? Was it developed for use in children or has it ever been used in children?

- For which age groups was it devised?

- Is it designed for cross-sectional (one off) or longitudinal (repeated) measures?

- What is the time frame? Can I reassess quality of life at the time I want to – does my follow-up routine fit the validated time frame of the questionnaire?

- How long does it take to administer?

- Relevance (Box 14.5). If a disease-specific measure is used, individuals are unlikely to have a problem understanding the relevance of the questions. A questionnaire with a large number of questions may be intimidating.

Box 14.5: The specific questions

- Are they comprehensible by children and parents?
- Are they brief and to the point?
- Do they appear biased?
- Is the questionnaire self- or interviewer-administered?

- Accessibility of the results (Box 14.6). There is usually a choice of responses. These should be clear and straightforward. During completion, individuals should not require clarification as this may result in the introduction of bias. For practical purposes, answers should be available and accessible immediately to allow patient and clinician to discuss any issues raised at the time of completion.

Box 14.6: The results

Who provides the answers – parent or child and is this what you want?
- Proxy – the parents answer the questions[27]
- Parent and child e.g. Childhood Asthma Questionnaire (CAQ) form A[23]
- Child alone e.g. CAQ forms B & C,[23] Paediatric Asthma Quality of Life Questionnaire[36]

How are answers entered?
- Categorical/point system (too many options are confusing)
- Visual analogue scales (young children cannot group the concept)
- Yes or no answers
- Computer or paper
- How are answers displayed?
- Complex processing and hence delay, or 'on line' review?

PROBLEMS AND PITFALLS

Administration may be aided by comprehensive background information. There is a great potential for introduction of bias, particularly when working with children, especially if active interviews are needed.

Comprehension problems may arise. Language differences can cause obvious problems, but even in English speaking countries word choice means parents and children may not understand a questionnaire has been developed elsewhere. Cultural differences may cause problems of comprehension or applicability of some questions. Literacy becomes an issue if the questionnaires are to be self-completed. Parents or children may be reluctant to admit to reading difficulties. If an interview is possible, it may be wise to offer the choice. Some developers have assessed their questionnaire in populations to determine the reading level needed e.g. PAQLQ[25]; whereas others have designed age-specific forms of their questionnaires e.g. CAQ.[23]

Quality of life questionnaires usually report the situation over a specific time period – say the previous week. Poor memory may make recall difficult, while young children may have difficulty with the concept of elapsed time.[5] One commentator suggests it is useful to consider some activity or event to act as a focus and aid memory.[26] Some questionnaires are designed to be answered by the parent,[27] which avoids this problem but relies on parental assessment which may itself be inaccurate.[8,21] The older the child, the less likely are the parents to be able to report accurately the impact of disease.

Some measures for use with whole populations have reference values to act as a guide. Disease-specific measures cannot by definition have reference values but within-subject changes over time can be used to assess effects or interventions.

Where children are to be asked directly this should be done in the absence of parents.[26] Some parents may be suspicious but only in this way are the child's views properly represented.

Children need to be reassured that whatever answer they give is the right one! They may be looking for reinforcement but neither prompts nor clues to the desirability of particular answers should be offered. Juniper recommends merely repeating the question if a child is hesitant or voices concern.[26] This takes time and patience. Hurried children may sense disapproval which may be reflected in their responses.

All measures offer some range of responses (Box 14.6). Adults and children may interpret these differently.[21] This should be considered if using proxy measures or those which parent and child complete together or if a comparison is to be drawn between parent's and child's answers.

Whilst it is relatively easy to carry out quality of life measurement as a means of assessing outcome, what to do with the results is another matter. Some measures have had such widespread use that they have normal values to which patient results can be compared and the result is a norm-referenced measure. Unfortunately in paediatric medicine, many of the current tools do not have reference values, either because thus far experience is limited or because, by definition, disease-specific questions cannot be answered by healthy people. For clinical care the main application of these tools is to assess change following an intervention, treatment or management change. The main impetus is to assess within-patient changes in quality of life following an intervention, irrespective of clinical outcome. Scores should be used to give a qualitative guide, and not interpreted as precisely as, for example, FEV_1 or PEF. Most measures incorporate symptomatic outcome as one of the areas within the assessment tool, so there is likely to be some degree of correlation between overall quality of life change and the clinical assessment. As questionnaires develop, some provide a guide to the size of change in score which is clinically significant to provide guidance for clinicians who wish to include it in their management strategy.[28,29]

RESEARCH – THE FUTURE

Further research is needed before QoL assessment can realistically become a routine aspect of clinical management, particularly in the case of children. Questionnaire development is complex and time consuming and it is preferable to use existing measures which have undergone extensive testing for use with the population to be assessed. Any changes made to existing questionnaires need to be thoroughly tested. Even small changes may influence the results in a dramatic way.

Does QoL assessment improve patient satisfaction? QoL would have to be measured; along with some measure of satisfaction with treatment and clinical outcomes assessed. In this way the whole picture would be available for interpretation.

Since quality assurance is an important aspect of care in modern health systems, this question is extremely important.

Does QoL assessment improve compliance? This question is frequently asked and many commentators believe that compliance and QoL are intrinsically related. If one improves a patient's QoL, are they more likely to comply? Non-compliance is a costly problem and any insight into improving this problem is important.

Does QoL assessment improve control? For instance, is there a positive feedback effect or does increased control arise from facilitating negotiation between doctor and patient?

REFERENCES

1. Jones PW, Quirk FH, Baveystock CM. Why quality of life measures should be used in the treatment of patients with respiratory illness. *Monaldi Arch Chest Dis* 1994; **49**: 79–82.

2. Fallowfield L. *Quality of life: the missing measurement in health care*. London: Souvenir Press, 1990.

3. Bowling A. *Measuring health: a review of quality of life measurement scales*. Buckingham: Open University Press, 1997, 1–159.

4. Marra CA, Levine M, McKerrow R, Carleton BC. Overview of health-related quality-of-life measures for pediatric patients: application in the assessment of pharmacotherapeutic and pharmacoeconomic outcomes. *Pharmacotherapy* 1996; **16**: 879–88.

5. Piaget J. *The language and thought of the child*, 2nd edn. London: Routledge, 1952.

6. Shim CS, Williams MH Jr. Evaluation of the severity of asthma: patients versus physicians. *Am J Med* 1980; **68**: 11–13.

7. Wong TW, Yu TS, Liu JL, Wong SL. Agreement on responses to respiratory illness questionnaire. *Arch Dis Child* 1998; **78**: 379–80.

8. Guyatt GH, Juniper EF, Griffith LE, Feeny DH, Ferrie PJ. Children and adult perceptions of childhood asthma. *Pediatrics* 1997; **99**: 165–8.

9. Jones PW. Quality of life measurement in asthma. *Eur Respir J* 1995; **8**: 885–7.

10. Orenstein DM, Nixon PA, Ross EA, Kaplan RM. The quality of well-being in cystic fibrosis. *Chest* 1989; **95**: 344–7

11. Bowling A. *Measuring disease*, 1st edn. Buckingham: Open University Press, 1995.

12. Enskar K, Carlsson M, von Essen L, Kreuger A, Hamrin E. Development of a tool to measure the life situation of parents of children with cancer. *Qual Life Res* 1997; **6**: 248–56.

13. Juniper EF, Guyatt GH, Feeny DH, Ferrie PJ, Griffith LE, Townsend M. Measuring quality of life in the parents of children with asthma. *Qual Life Res* 1996; **5**: 27–34.

14. McGee H. Quality of life: assessment issues for children with chronic illness and their families. In: Christie M, French D (eds). *Assessment of quality of life in childhood asthma*. UK: Hardwood Academic, 1994, 83–97.

15. Clark NM, Evans D, Zimmerman BJ, Levison MJ, Mellins RB. Patient and family management of asthma: theory-based techniques for the clinician. *J Asthma* 1994; **31**: 427–35.

16. Wright PS. Parents' perceptions of their quality of life. *J Pediatr Oncol Nurs* 1993; **10**: 139–45.

17. Osman L, Silverman M. Measuring quality of life for young children with asthma and their families. *Eur Respir J* (Suppl.) 1996; **21**: 35s–41s.

18. Juniper EF, Johnston PR, Borkhoff CM, Guyatt GH, Boulet LP, Haukioja A. Quality of life in asthma clinical trials: comparison of salmeterol and salbutamol. *Am J Resp Crit Care Med* 1995; **151**: 66–70.

19. Eiser C, Jenney ME. Measuring symptomatic benefit and quality of life in paediatric oncology. *Br J Cancer* 1996; **73**: 1313–16.

20. Duffy CM, Arsenault L, Duffy KN, Paquin JD, Strawczynski H. The Juvenile Arthritis Quality of Life Questionnaire – development of a new responsive index for juvenile rheumatoid arthritis and juvenile spondyloarthritides. *J Rheumatol* 1997; **24**: 738–46.

21. Wensley DC, Silverman M. *Parent's perception of childhood asthma*. 1998; NAC conference (Abstract).

22. Duffy CM, Arsenault L, Duffy KN. Level of agreement between parents and children in rating dysfunction in juvenile rheumatoid arthritis and juvenile spondyloarthritides. *J Rheumatol* 1993; **20**: 2134–9.

23. Christie MJ, French D. *Assessment of quality of life in childhood asthma*. Switzerland: Harwood Academic Publishers, 1994, 1–189.

24. French DJ, Christie MJ, Sowden AJ. The reproducibility of the Childhood Asthma Questionnaires: measures of quality of life for children with asthma aged 4–16 years. *Qual Life Res* 1994; **3**: 215–24.

25. Juniper EF, Guyatt GH, Feeny DH, Griffith LE, Ferrie PJ. Minimum skills required by children to complete health-related quality of life instruments for asthma: comparison of measurement properties. *Eur Respir J* 1997; **10**: 2285–94.

26. Juniper EF. Paediatric Asthma Quality of Life Questionnaire: Background information and interviewing tips (available with Questionnaire). Hamilton, Ont: McMaster University, 1996.

27. Usherwood TP, Scrimgeour A, Barber JH. Questionnaire to measure perceived symptoms and disability in asthma. *Arch Dis Child* 1990; **65**: 779–81.

28. Juniper EF, Guyatt GH, Willan A, Griffith LE. Determining a minimal important change in a disease-specific Quality of Life Questionnaire. *J Clin Epidemiol* 1994; **47**: 81–7.

29. Redelmeier DA, Guyatt GH, Goldstein RS. Assessing the minimal important difference in symptoms: a comparison of two techniques. *J Clin Epidemiol* 1996; **49**: 1215–19.

30. The WHOQOL Group. The World Health Organisation Quality of Life Assessment (WHOQOL): Position paper from the World Health Organisation. *Soc Sci Med* 1995; **41**: 1403.

31. Schipper H, Olweny C, Clinch JJ. Quality of life studies: definitions and conceptual issues. In: Spilker B (ed). *Quality of life and pharmacoeconomics*. Philadelphia: Lippincott-Raven, 1996.

32. Hunt SM, McEwen J. The development of a subjective health indicator. *Sociol of Health Illn* 1980; **2**: 231–46.

33. Jones PW, Quirk FH, Baveystock CM. The St. George's Respiratory Questionnaire. *Respir Med* 1991; **85**: 25–31.

34. Eisen M, Ware JE, Jr., Donald CA, Brook RH. Measuring components of children's health status. *Med Care* 1979; **17**: 902–21.

35. Cribb A. Quality of life – a response to K.C. Calman. *J Med Ethics* 1985; **11**: 142–5.

36. Juniper EF, Guyatt GH, Feeny DH, Ferrie PJ, Griffith LE, Townsend M. Measuring quality of life in children with asthma. *Qual Life Res* 1996; **5**: 35–46.

37. Stein R, Reissman CK. The development of an impact on family scale: preliminary findings. *Med Care* 1980; **18**: 465–72.

38. Jenney ME, Campbell S. Measuring quality of life. *Arch Dis Child* 1997; **77**: 347–54.

FURTHER READING

1. Bowling A. *Measuring health: a review of quality of life measurement scales*. Buckingham: Open University Press, 1997.

2. McSweeny, AJ , Creer TL. Health-related quality-of-life assessment in medical care. *Dis Mon* 1995; **41**: 1–71.

3. Hyland ME. The validity of health assessments: resolving some recent differences. *J Clin Epidemiol* 1993; **46**: 1019–23.

4. Pal DK. Quality of life assessment in children: a review of conceptual and methodological issues in multidimensional health status measures. *J Epidemiol Comm Health* 1996; **50**: 391–6.

5. Fallowfield L. *Quality of life: the missing measurement in health care*. London: Souvenir Press, 1990.

6. Spilker, B (ed). *Quality of life and pharmacoeconomics*. Philadelphia: Lippincott-Raven, 1996.

CHAPTER FIFTEEN

BEHAVIOUR *AND* PLAY

S. Storer and N. Dogra

- Introduction
- What is behaviour?
- Managing behaviour problems
- The importance of play

- Future directions
- References
- Further reading

INTRODUCTION

The link between psychosocial factors and asthma has always been controversial. In the past, asthma was thought by some to be a psychosomatic disorder. In contrast, today psychosocial factors are usually dismissed. The relationship between psychosocial factors and other respiratory illnesses is even more rarely considered.

Three sets of psychosocial factors may impact on the physical disorder:

- individual factors within the child such as psychological symptoms, coping styles or personality characteristics;
- parental characteristics;
- familial function, attitudes and relationships.

The behaviour of children is the most obvious manifestation of psychosocial factors and also the most likely to be amenable to modification. The respiratory team needs to consider the behaviour of children, the role of play in management and the way they impact on engagement with the patient and in turn on compliance. This chapter will focus on behaviour and play and their relevance in both assessment and management .

WHAT IS BEHAVIOUR?

Behaviour is an action or reaction in a specified way in a given context. Acceptable behaviour is determined culturally in the broadest sense. For example, a particular family may find a particular behaviour acceptable, another family from a very similar background may find the same behaviour unacceptable. Society as a whole sets expectations of acceptable behaviour and there is legislation to support this. Behaviours that are considered antisocial usually cause the greatest concern.

WHEN IS BEHAVIOUR A PROBLEM?

Disturbed behaviour usually represents a quantitative rather than a qualitative departure from normal. A particular pattern of behaviour is likely to be considered a problem because of its frequency, severity, duration, as well as on its impact on the child, the family and on others such as peers and school staff. The age and the individual characteristics of the child may be important factors to consider. A behaviour that is appropriate at one age can become a problem if it persists. For example temper tantrums may be acceptable at three but are usually not acceptable at ten.

Challenging behaviour may not be perceived as a problem if the family is coping, but a change in family circumstances (such as parental depression, unemployment, financial or marital difficulties) can mean the family's ability is compromised, so that the same pattern of behaviour becomes unacceptable.

An additional medical problem may be the final straw. For example, an unco-operative child may simply be a nuisance, but a child with severe asthma, or a teenager with deteriorating cystic fibrosis who refuses to take his medication is a source of anxiety for all.

The range of behaviours which may be considered problematic is wide. In a medical context, it includes aggression, defiance, destructiveness, deceitfulness, disruptiveness, impulsivity, unco-operativeness, sulking, stubborn behaviour and impatience. Secondary patterns of behaviour which may be especially challenging to health professionals include smoking and drug or excessive alcohol consumption and deliberate self-harm, often manifested as lack of adherence to a disease-management plan.

Any individual child's behaviour may be determined by many factors, each of which may need to be considered by health professionals. As children grow, the situation needs to be reviewed. This is especially true for those with chronic diseases. The relevant factors are:

- individual characteristics of the child;
- characteristics of the respiratory problems;
- family characteristics and interactions between family members;
- interactions of the family members with external agencies such as school, hospital (relationships with individual clinic staff), and primary care workers (especially the general practitioner).

ASSESSING BEHAVIOUR

A standardized approach to the assessment of difficult behaviour should be helpful. Establish:

- the nature of the behaviour and for whom is it a problem;
- pattern, frequency and duration;
- the impact of the problem on the child and his/her family;
- its impact on the health of the child either directly (e.g. anxiety and asthma attacks) or

indirectly (by effects on compliance with therapy or on family relationships).

As part of assessment and management it is often helpful to ask the child and parents to keep a diary of the problem behaviours. They are asked to record the *antecedent* events preceding particular problem behaviour, the *behaviour* itself, and the *consequences* of the behaviour: the ABC of behaviour. A good diary enables the extent of the problem to be clarified as well as identifying exacerbating factors. It may also enable the child and parent to see patterns of behaviour and how their own responses may interact to exacerbate the situation.

MANAGING BEHAVIOUR PROBLEMS

Behaviour therapy is commonly used. It may be useful despite the fact that it does not always address the underlying causes of disturbed behaviour but just tackles the effects.

There are essentially two approaches to behavioural therapy, the choice of which depends both on the causes of behavioural problems and the age of the child. Examples are provided in Case studies 15.1 and 15.2.

- **Behaviour therapy** refers to techniques based on *classical conditioning* and developed in order to extinguish maladaptive behaviours and substitute adaptive ones.
- **Behaviour modification** refers to techniques based on *operant conditioning* and developed to build up appropriate behaviour (where it did not previously exist) or to increase the frequency of desirable responses and decrease the undesirable.[1] By rewarding positive behaviour, negative behaviours will hopefully diminish and the positive ones (or desired ones) increase.

THE ROLE OF THE RESPIRATORY TEAM

If the problem behaviour is well defined and relatively simple a number of general strategies can be adopted by the respiratory team before specific behaviour therapy needs to be considered. These include:

Case study 15.1: Toddler treatment tantrums

John is a 3-year-old with persistent asthma. Every time he has to use his spacer and inhaler he throws a temper tantrum. His single 22-year-old mother has effectively stopped trying to give him his medication. He is generally wheezy by day and his sleep pattern is disrupted by cough and wheeze.

The approach of the respiratory team can be structured as follows:

Take a thorough history to establish:

- exact nature of the temper tantrums: is it a problem just with the spacer or are there other parenting issues?
- how the tantrums are managed
- role of John's father
- relationship between John's parents
- whether the parents undermine each other or contradict each other with respect to managing John
- parental mental health
- any other psychosocial factors that might be compromising parenting, such as recent bereavement, etc.

Manage the situation by:

- Asking the child and parents to keep a diary which may serve as an assessment and therapeutic tool. For instance, the diary entry might be: 'Before John had the temper tantrum he was playing with his lego. When the pieces didn't fit he got frustrated and threw them all over the room. It was time for his medicines and he became difficult. I got angry and shouted at him. He got upset and cried and I knew we weren't going to get his medicine in'.
- Guiding John's mother to understand that the key to management of behavioural problems is:
  - clear and realistic expectations
  - consistency of approach by everybody
  - positive reinforcement for required behaviour
  - firmness to ensure programme adhered to
  - agreed and planned reinforcements
  - making the management fun.

Such programmes can be monitored using:

- star charts
- certificates from health workers as a positive incentive.

Case study 15.2: A teenager with cystic fibrosis

Lauren is a 14-year-old girl with cystic fibrosis. She has few symptoms and recently decided that she did not want further clinic appointments. Lauren's parents are distressed by Lauren's unco-operative attitude, which also extends to other areas of parental control, and would like you to sort these problems out.

A member of the hospital paediatric team needs to establish:

- Whether Lauren understands the nature of cystic fibrosis, or whether she needs information at an appropriate level for her age. She may want to make decisions for herself on the management of her illness. She may want greater autonomy and freedom, and consider her parents overprotective.
- What Lauren's parents understand about cystic fibrosis and its impact on adolescence. Lauren's parents may feel that Lauren is not mature enough to make important decisions about her health. The issue of non-attendance may be the only way for Lauren to get herself heard by her parents. There may be marital difficulties and the messages given to Lauren are inconsistent so that she does not know what is expected.

In managing this situation, the following strategies may be helpful:

- To speak to Lauren on her own or, if she does not attend, to write to her, explaining that you want to hear her concerns.

Case study 15.2: A teenager with cystic fibrosis (continued)

- To be honest and sensitive to Lauren's needs but give her real choices.
- To support the parents in adapting to Lauren growing up.
- To encourage Lauren and her parents to compromise; it may be helpful to reward Lauren with greater freedom if she shows she can be responsible in particular areas; again clarity and consistency are important.
- To be patient; Lauren might be testing your patience as well as that of her parents; she may be struggling with the impact of her illness on her life and need time and space to think about these.

Case study 15.3: Invasive procedure

Adam is a 12-year-old boy who is having a long line insertion. He has previously been prepared for this procedure and negotiated the coping strategy of his choice. He is becoming increasingly unco-operative with staff and is often rude and aggressive towards them.

Staff need to establish:

- Whether Adam is frightened of the procedure; unsure of the procedure; does not understand the need for the procedure; does not understand his illness, does not feel involved in the decisions being made about him.
- Whether the parents discomfort at Adam's illness and concern about the long term are being conveyed inappropriately to Adam.
- Whether clinic staff views or attitudes are giving Adam unclear messages. Staff may feel that Adam should be used to procedure by now. There may be a tendency to treat him like an older or younger child but at the wrong level for him; Adam's messages may be unclear and confusing to staff; what is a routine procedure to staff is not so for Adam.

The situation may be managed by:

- Making Adam feel comfortable and welcome.
- Giving Adam time to express his fears or concerns.
- Not allowing Adam's behaviour to make staff impatient or unsympathetic; it is unlikely to be personal.
- Giving Adam clear simple instructions of what is going to happen, when and what is required of him.
- Giving him strategies to cope e.g. counting, and slow breathing just before the start of the procedure may help.
- Having a nurse concentrate on the child throughout the procedure giving support and encouragement while the doctor proceeds.
- Telling Adam when the procedure has finished.
- Giving Adam time and permission to reflect on the experience.

In this case compliance was increased by a clear understanding of the problem and by responding appropriately and sensitively to the situation using the principles discussed above.

Case study 15.4: A new spacer

Sanjay is a three-year-old boy admitted with his first attack of asthma. He has been prescribed medication via a spacer. Having received no play preparation and mixed messages about using the spacer, he is now showing signs of anxiety and distress each time medication is required.

The play specialist needs to assess Sanjay's level of cognitive development, the family dynamics and his understanding of the condition and treatment by observing his interaction, understanding and compliance, relating the observations to developmental theories such as those of Bruce, Piaget or Sheriden. This assessment will be carried out through a session of free and structured play in partnership with the parents.

A sensitive introduction to the spacer is required giving Sanjay the opportunity to explore it and use it in a non-threatening way, using stories, role play or puppets.

The play specialist will work towards slowly building on Sanjay's confidence, encouraging him to role play his fears

Case study 15.4: A new spacer (continued)

and anxieties and giving him a simple, factual account of what has happened and will happen during subsequent treatments.

Areas will be identified that Sanjay has difficulty understanding or performing such as blowing and sucking. Structured play activities can then enable Sanjay to to practice those techniques in a non-threatening way – blow painting, sucking a ping-pong ball with a straw – with his parents encouraging, supporting and participating in the activities so that they understand their role.

After discussion with the team, a plan of sequential play events, appropriate words and coping strategies will be written to ensure a consistent approach.

Several play sessions may need to be undertaken using preparation, diversion and post-procedural play, providing Sanjay with the opportunities and encouragement he needs so that compliance with treatment changes from a difficult situation to a positive experience.

Case study 15.5: Cannula insertion

Emma, an 8-year-old girl, was admitted to hospital with acute lobar pneumonia. Intravenous antibiotics were prescribed. How was play used to facilitate the insertion of an IV cannula?

With the information obtained using the Assessment Model (Figure 15.1) the play specialist chose an appropriate tool, in this case a blood doll. A sensitive approach gave Emma the opportunity to ask questions, make comments and handle the equipment to familiarize herself with it.

It was important to be aware of factors that would disrupt the process (Box 15.3).

In order to cope, Emma needs opportunities to make choices throughout the procedure (Figure 15.2).

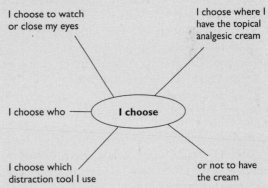

Figure 15.2: Choices.

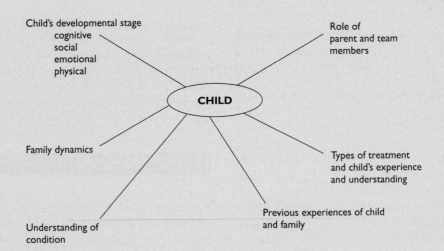

Figure 15.1: Assessment.

Case study 15.6: The first chest X-ray

Leroy is 5 and has been brought to the hospital for the first time by his father with a chest infection and is having difficulty with breathing. The medical team has requested an emergency portable chest X-ray. The play specialist who has introduced herself to Leroy and his father discusses with them all the people they will meet and investigations he is having.

A book describing having an X-ray is shown to Leroy and the use of the camera which takes a picture of the inside of his body and shows the doctors what is happening to him so that treatment can be given to make his breathing easier.

The play specialist has already discussed with him the coping strategies that they will use to support Leroy through the procedure, such as:

- looking at books
- breath holding and counting
- projected image on the ceiling.

After the procedure the doctor will show Leroy his X-ray and tell him what treatment he will be having and when he will have another X-ray.

- discussing the problems openly with the family;
- clear explanation of what the respiratory team's concerns are and why;
- the need to give the child or family a longer appointment to discuss the issues in a non-hurried sensitive way;
- seeing older children without their parents.

In older children there may have to be more negotiation about what is expected. Monetary rewards tend to be less successful than other rewards.[2]

SPECIALIST REFERRAL

If the respiratory team is unsure how to manage behavioural problems a stepwise approach may be helpful.

Step 1. Explore the problem in the way discussed above.

Step 2. Discuss the problem with specialist team members such as play specialists, this may be particularly useful for younger children but relevant to older children. The respiratory team may find alternative approaches useful.

Step 3. Discuss the case with a child psychiatrist or other children's mental health specialist. This consultation may enable the respiratory team to manage the case and also allow appropriate and necessary preparation if the case is to be referred to specialist mental health agencies.

Step 4. In complex cases where there are a number of issues such as individual difficulties, family pathology and/or developmental issues, referral to a mental health specialist may be appropriate. Ensure that the family understands the reason for referral and agrees with it. Psychiatric input may be useful in one of two ways: it may help reduce or limit disability and dysfunction attributable to illness by reducing symptoms (e.g. for asthma symptoms maintained by psychosocial factors); it may minimize secondary handicap or disability, such as that caused by overprotection by parents.

The psychiatrist may collaborate with the respiratory team providing advice and professional support, or take over case management. This will depend on how closely the respiratory problems and behavioural problems are linked.

THE IMPORTANCE OF PLAY

Play provides the child with the opportunities required to practice life skills and can be observed in all human cultures. It is now recognized that the development of children takes place through a series of sequential stages until

Box 15.1: Situations where play is helpful

- Structured and free play are used to **prevent regression** and aid the child to reach the recognized developmental milestones for his/her age. It offers the opportunity for fun, occupation and freedom of expression in a safe environment utilizing the child's experience and skills.

- **Preparation** through play for investigations such as radiology or lung function testing and treatments enables the team to meet the individual child's need to understand and explore their condition and requirements of treatment, so that compliance is maximized.

- **Distraction** is an agreed strategy between the adult and child which is used to maximize compliance throughout an investigation or treatment such as insertion of an intravenous line so that psychological distress is not inflicted upon the child.

- **Post-procedural** play provides the opportunity for the child to work through an experience and explore issues which have affected the child's understanding and compliance before, during and after investigations or treatments, especially if more interventions are likely to be needed.

Box 15.2: How to employ play in a health setting

Principles of preparation and post-procedural play	Tools of the trade
<ul><li>appropriate</li><li>timely</li><li>simple</li><li>factual</li><li>truthful</li><li>sequential</li></ul>	<ul><li>books, videos and tapes</li><li>doll play and puppets</li><li>role play</li><li>medical equipment and working models</li><li>play specialist or named person</li><li>to carry out task</li></ul>
Principles of distraction	**Distraction**
<ul><li>negotiate with child</li><li>appropriate</li><li>of interest to the child</li><li>simple</li><li>timely</li><li>does not hinder medical/nursing staff from task</li></ul>	<ul><li>interactive books and videos</li><li>pot of bubbles</li><li>hand-held computer game or solar projector</li><li>interactive toys appropriate for age task</li><li>play specialist or named person to carry out the task</li></ul>

maturity has been reached. Play enhances the emergence of personality, self-control and the ability to form relationships.[3]

Through play the child will be able to develop a rich and unique imagination alongside the need to explore situations and ideas.

Play is one of the methods children use to communicate their understanding of the environment around them and the relationships with the people they interact with. It is also a means of expressing their joys, anxieties, fears, and of exploring their self-image and place in the world.

PLAY AND HEALTHCARE

Play is a familiar aspect of life in hospital enabling the child to work through a new or repeated experience thereby minimizing the potential for developmental delay or regression (Box 15.1). Structured play is the means for the child to be helped to gain from experiences in a valid way, using therapeutic and educative tools.

The play specialist uses a variety of techniques to aid the child's understanding of the hospital experience, investigation, treatments and how these impact upon the child's' life.[4] The play

Box 15.3: Factors which disrupt the process

- interruptions or rush
- poor assessment of planning or misinformation
- poor co-operation within the team
- team not prepared; bad timing, excessive waiting around
- parental influence
- everyone talking to the child at the same time
- not listening to the child's views
- not being truthful with child
- bribes and threats
- failure to offer praise and encouragement

specialist can be thought of as a facilitator in the overall care of the child, minimizing the effects of hospitalization (Box 15.2).

In an outpatient setting, experienced health professionals who deal with growing children use play, toys and games to gain the confidence of children, reduce their anxiety and to teach them to cope with illness. Sometimes the situation demands the assistance of a specialist (Case study 15.4).

ISSUES OF PREPARATION AND POST-PROCEDURAL PLAY

The person allocated to prepare or to carry out post-procedural play needs to fully understand what will or has happened to the individual child, allowing the child the opportunity to explore and express their knowledge, fear and anxieties in their own way and time.

The whole team needs to agree on the facts and possible issues that will affect the child so that they all act and speak with one voice in negotiation with the child and family.

A number of factors can disrupt the process (Box 15.3).

FUTURE DIRECTIONS

The practice of using behaviour therapy and behaviour modification is well established in psychiatry and clinical psychology. The effectiveness of behaviour therapy has been proven although the

long-term benefits have been more difficult to establish. For play there is empirical knowledge that children benefit from its use in a variety of settings. Research into compliance has largely focused on aspects of treatment. The individual, familial, environmental and psychosocial factors have largely been neglected. Godding et al.[5] proposed and evaluated a model for joint consultation for high-risk asthmatic children and their families with a paediatrician and child psychiatrist as co-therapists. They found there were long-term benefits from this approach. Behaviour, play and compliance are complex issues and influenced by a number of independent and related factors. Any research into these areas needs to be multi-dimensional and to consider the role of the individual, the family, the environment and the illness itself. The field is open for research with sound methodology which can impact on clinical practice.

REFERENCES

1. Gross RD. *Psychology, the science of mind and behaviour*, 2nd edn. London: Hodder and Stoughton, 1992.

2. Dogra N, Parkin A, Trower T. *Child psychiatry module handbook*. Course Handbook, University of Leicester, 1996.

3. Brain J, Martin MD. *Childcare and health for nursery nurses*, 3rd edn. Cheltenham: Stanley Thornes and Hulton, 1989.

4. Save the Children. *A deprived environment for children, the case for hospital playschemes*. London: Save the Children, 1989.

5. Godding V, Kruth M, Jamart J. Joint consultation for high-risk asthmatic children and their families, with pediatrician and child psychiatrist as co-therapists: model and evaluation. *Fam Process* 1997; **36:** 265–80.

FURTHER READING

1. Campbell S, Glasper EA. *Whaley and Wong's children's nursing*. London: Mosby, 1995.

2. Pearce J. *Bad behaviour: how to deal with naughtiness and disobedience and still show you love and care for your child*. Thorsons Publishing Group, 1989.

PART TWO

CLINICAL MANAGEMENT

CHAPTER SIXTEEN

AIRWAY MANAGEMENT *IN* EMERGENCY SITUATIONS

D . L u y t

- Introduction
- Upper airway obstruction
- Anatomy of the upper airway

- Intubation of the trachea
- References
- Further reading

INTRODUCTION

Acute upper airway obstruction from whatever cause can be life-threatening, particularly in children where their smaller airway size imposes the risk of a greater degree of narrowing from swelling or secretions. Certain causes of acute upper airway obstruction such as epiglottitis and bacterial tracheitis carry a *very* high risk of total obstruction. In most instances the obstruction is not acutely life-threatening. Occasionally however the child may present with imminent upper airway obstruction where immediate action is necessary to establish and maintain a secure airway until a more permanent solution, either medical or surgical, is achieved.[1] It is essential that doctors rapidly and accurately assess the cause of and severity of upper airway obstruction and have a clear management plan for all clinical situations. They should be well versed with the anatomy of the paediatric upper airway and changes that occur with age and have a well rehearsed plan of action for establishing an artificial airway.

This chapter will address upper airway obstruction, its assessment and management, and the features of upper airway anatomy special to children.

UPPER AIRWAY OBSTRUCTION

The many causes of upper airway obstruction (see Further Reading) can most easily be classified by the duration of the history (neonatal onset vs later onset) and the rate of onset of symptoms (Table 16.1). Neonatal causes are generally classified anatomically, and post-neonatal causes by aetiology.

Physical examination does provide useful information about the site of obstruction (nasal, pharyngeal, laryngeal or subglottic) and its severity.

Emergency intubation to deal with or to prevent life-threatening airway obstruction is infrequent in acute laryngo-tracheobronchitis (1% of hospitalized cases), very rare in acute angio-oedema, and essential in all children with acute epiglottitis.

ANATOMY OF THE UPPER AIRWAY IN CHILDREN (FIGURE 16.1)

Children presenting with acute upper airway obstruction may require endotracheal intubation in conditions with a high risk of complete

Table 16.1: Contrasting features of croup, epiglottitis and foreign body (FB) aspiration

	Croup	Epiglottitis	FB aspiration
Age	6–18 months	2–5 years	> 6 months
Aetiology	Virus usually parainfluenza	H. influenzae	Food or toys
Associated URTI[†]	Present for 2–3 days	Absent	Absent
Onset	Insidious (over days)	Sudden (over hours)	Sudden (over minutes or hours)
Progression	Slow	Fulminant	Variable*
Stridor	High pitched Loud	Low pitched Soft	Variable* May wheeze
Barking cough	Severe	Absent or slight	Present, variable*
Hoarse voice	Present	Reluctant to speak Muffled voice	Variable*
Drooling	No	Frequent	No
Temperature	Low-grade	High	No
Toxic	No	Yes	No
Preferred posture	None	Sitting	Variable*
Demeanour	Noisy, happy	Anxious Sits still	Depends on degree of obstruction
Airway occlusion	Predictable	Unpredictable	Unpredictable*
Artificial airway	Uncommon	Always	Bronchoscopy

* Airway obstruction by FB is variable and unpredictable.

[†] URTI: upper respiratory tract infection.

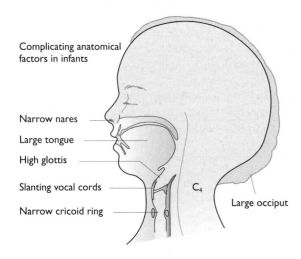

Complicating anatomical factors in infants

Narrow nares

Large tongue

High glottis

Slanting vocal cords

Narrow cricoid ring

C₄

Large occiput

Figure 16.1: Features of upper airway in infants (from Ref. 2).

obstruction *per se* (e.g. epiglottitis or bacterial tracheitis) or in conditions where the severity suggests a high risk of complete obstruction (e.g. grade 3 or 4 croup). Doctors treating children may well need to intubate a child as a life-saving procedure. They will need to be familiar with the anatomy of the paediatric upper airway,[2] and with the differences between infants and older children and adults (Box 16.1). A well rehearsed routine for safe intubation is essential.

CONSEQUENCES OF ANATOMICAL DIFFERENCES BETWEEN YOUNG CHILDREN AND ADULTS

These anatomical differences will have the following important consequences:

Airway size

A relatively small amount of mucosal oedema or obstruction can significantly reduce the paediatric airway diameter, increase resistance to airflow and increase the work of breathing (e.g. a 1 mm rim of oedema occurring in a 4 mm airway will increase resistance 16-fold).

Because of their higher metabolic rate, the oxygen demand per kilogram body weight in children is twice as high as that of adults (6–8 mL/kg per minute versus 3–4 mL/kg per minute). To

Box 16.1: Differences between young children and adults

Airway size
- Airway of an infant and child is much smaller.

Tongue
- The tongue is relatively larger in the infant.

Epiglottis
- Positioned at a 45° angle, away from the trachea into the pharynx, relatively large and is omega shaped in children.
- In adults the epiglottis is flat and lies in the longitudinal plane of the trachea behind the base of the tongue.

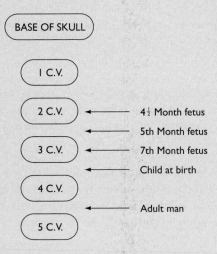

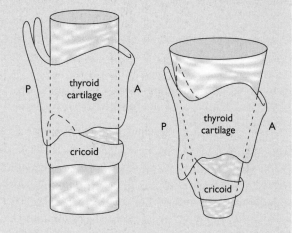

Figure 16.3: Funnel shape of larynx in infants (right) compared to the cylindrical shape of the adult larynx (from Ref. 2).

Figure 16.2: Relationship of the glottis to the vertebral column (after Weibley and Holbrook). CV: cervical vertebra.

Position of the larynx (Figure 16.2)
- More cephalad at the C-3 level in neonate rather than the C-4 to C-5 of the adult.
- Positioned more anteriorly in children.

Glottis: angulation and shape
- As the vocal cords have a lower attachment anteriorly, the relationship between the plane of glottis (the space between the vocal cords) and the long axis of the trachea angulates downwards posteriorly.
- In adults these two planes are at right angles to one another.
- Glottis is diamond shaped in infants as it is bounded in its posterior third by the arytenoid cartilages and the anterior two-thirds by the vocal cords.
- In adults the glottis is a narrow slit bounded by the vocal cords in entirety.

Narrowest point
- In children younger than 8 years of age, the narrowest portion of the airway is below the vocal cords at the level of the non-distensible cricoid cartilage (Table 16.2), and the larynx is funnel shaped (Figure 16.3).
- In older children and adults the narrowest point of the airway is at the glottic inlet and the larynx is the shape of a cylinder.

Box 16.1: Differences between young children and adults (continued)

Prominent occiput

- the infant ≤ 2 years old has a prominent occiput which, when supine, results in some neck flexion, affecting intubation (Figure 16.1).

Table 16.2: Internal circumference of the larynx and trachea in children

| Age of child | Internal circumference (in mm) | | |
	Glottis	Cricoid ring	Trachea
4 months	23–26	20	22–25
8 months	24	21	24
13 months	25	22	26
2 years	30	24	30
4 years	30–33	26	30–33
10 years	39	30	39

achieve this, the baseline work of breathing is higher in children and is stretched even further with airway obstruction.

The internal diameter or size of a child's airway determines the size of endotracheal tube (ETT) appropriate for intubation. Endotracheal tubes (ETTs) are sized according to their internal diameter in mm. ETTs available are sizes 2.5–6 uncuffed and 5–8 cuffed. ETTs with uniform internal diameter are preferred to tapered tubes. Shouldered ETTs may cause laryngeal injury. A cuffed ETT should have a high volume low pressure cuff and is generally indicated for children 8–10 years and older. In children younger than 8–10 years old the normal anatomical narrowing at the level of the cricoid cartilage provides a functional 'cuff'. If a cuff is present inflation is appropriate if a leak is audible when ventilation to a pressure of ≥30 cmH$_2$O is provided.

Table 16.3: Endotracheal tube placement (size and depth) in children

Age	Weight (kg)	Internal diameter (mm)	External diameter (mm)	Length (at lip) (cm)	Length (at nose) (cm)
Newborn	<0.7	2.0	2.9	5.0	6
Newborn	<1	2.5	3.6	5.5	7
Newborn	1.0	3.0	4.3	6	7.5
Newborn	2.0	3.0	4.3	7	9
Newborn	3.0	3.0	4.3	8.5	10.5
Newborn	3.5	3.5	4.9	9	11
3 months	6.0	3.5	4.9	10	12
1 year	10	4.0	5.6	11	14
2 years	12	4.5	6.2	12	15
3 years	14	4.5	6.2	13	16
4 years	16	5.0	6.9	14	17
6 years	20	5.5	7.5	15	19
8 years	24	6.0	8.2	16	20
10 years	30	6.5	8.9	17	21
12 years	38	7.0	9.5	18	22
14 years	50	7.5	10.2	19	23
Adult	60	8.0	10.8	20	24
Adult	70	9.0	12.1	21	25

The correct ETT size (Table 16.3) can be estimated by either choosing a tube with:

(a) *external diameter* approximately the diameter of the child's little finger, or
(b) *internal diameter* determined by the formula:

ETT internal diameter (mm) = (age in years/4) + 4

When preparing to intubate, ensure that one size smaller and one size bigger tubes are available. In clinical conditions where there is airway narrowing (e.g. croup) select the next smallest sized ETT.

The correct depth of oro-tracheal ETT insertion (mid-trachea) is determined by the formula:

ETT depth (cm) = (age in years/2) + 12

Depth must be checked clinically by auscultating the chest and by chest X-ray.

Tongue

Any enlargement of a child's tongue, particularly with posterior displacement, can result is airway obstruction. Controlling the position of this relatively large tongue with the laryngoscope blade may be difficult during tracheal intubation. As the relatively large tongue can obstruct one's view of the glottis, it can be pushed out of the line of sight by placing the laryngoscope in the right hand side of the mouth and sweeping the tongue to the left. If the large tongue is particularly problematical, the broader curved Macintosh blade rather than the narrower straight Miller blade might be helpful.

Epiglottis

The size and position of the epiglottis may obscure the glottic opening. The epiglottis can be moved from the line of view in one of two ways, depending which laryngoscope blade is used (Figure 16.4). With a curved Macintosh blade, the tip is inserted into the vallecula (the crypt between the base of the tongue and the epiglottis) and pulled forwards thereby pulling the epiglottis forwards and exposing the glottis. This procedure should be performed by moving the laryngoscope blade and handle in an upwards and forwards direction *together* and *not* by levering the blade on the upper teeth. When a straight Miller blade is being used

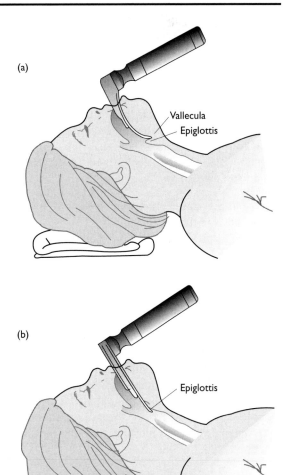

Figure 16.4: Positioning of the laryngoscope blade when using a curved (a) or straight (b) blade (from Chameides and Hazinski, Further Reading).

the tip of the blade itself is used to lift the epiglottis and thereby visualize the glottis. Here the tip rests beyond the vallecula.

Position of the larynx

The high anterior position of the larynx in infants makes the angle between the base of the tongue (in the oral axis) and the glottic opening (in the longitudinal axis of the trachea) more acute. These two axes are brought into alignment for glottic visualization by extension of the neck and anterior displacement (sniffing position) of the jaw.

Glottis – angulation and shape

As the high position of the larynx makes the glottic opening more anterior and cephalic, the ETT tip will tend to be directed towards the anterior wall of the larynx. This, together with the anterior slanting of the vocal cords, places the ETT at risk of being caught by the anterior commissure of the vocal cords.

If the ETT tip does get caught by the cords, advancing the ETT can be assisted by:

- cricoid pressure (Sellick manoeuvre)
- twisting the tube in its long axis
- gentle insufflation with a bag-valve device

Narrowest point

The ETT size will be determined by the size of the cricoid ring and not that of the glottic opening (glottis). An air leak observed at a peak inspiratory pressure of ≥ 30 cmH$_2$O should be present if the ETT size is appropriate. Furthermore, as the cricoid is triangular in shape and the ETT round, a 'tight fit' without a leak means that the pressure from the 'too big' ETT is too great along the walls of the triangle which can lead to pressure necrosis, scarring and subglottic stenosis.

Prominent occiput

The small infant with the large occiput requires the pillow under the neck and shoulders and not under the occiput.

INTUBATION OF THE TRACHEA

While often performed as an emergency (Table 16.4), the placement of an ETT must be approached in a deliberate and calm manner if trauma and patient instability are to be avoided. Therefore, regardless of the indication for intubation, airway control must be established immediately with the use of bag and mask ventilation (using 100% oxygen) whilst personnel, equipment and drugs are being readied. Intubation will be much safer in a stable well-oxygenated patient. This ideal may not always be achieved in practice!

Table 16.4: Indications for endotracheal intubation

Mechanical ventilation
Apnoea
Acute respiratory failure (Paco$_2$>7 kPa; Pao$_2$<6.5 kPa in Fio$_2$>0.5)
Elective/prophylactically e.g. post-operative, cerebral oedema
Airway protection
Coma (Glasgow Coma Scale < 8)
Bulbar palsy
Airway maintenance
Upper airway obstruction
Tracheal narrowing (bacterial tracheitis)
Pulmonary toilet

ECG monitoring and pulse oximetry must be performed during the procedure as ventilation will be interrupted. Intubation attempts must be brief. Those lasting more than 30 seconds can cause profound hypoxia. This is particularly so in infants.

PREPARATION

Whilst controlling the airway with a bag-valve-mask device (with 100% O$_2$) and attaching the

Table 16.5: Airways and laryngoscopes

Oropharyngeal airways	Sizes:
	00: newborn
	0: infant
	1: large infant 1–3 years old
	2: young childw 3–8 years old
	3: large child/small adult
	4: adult
Laryngoscopes	Blade sizes:
	0M: premature and newborn
	1M: infant and child up to about 3 years
	2M: child 3–6 years
	2M/2MAC: child 7–12 years
	3M/3MAC: child >12 and adult

M: Miller; MAC: Macintosh

patient to an ECG monitor and pulse oximeter, ensure that the trolley bearing the equipment necessary for safe successful intubation is available (Chapter 4, p. 39). Otherwise collect: suction equipment, oropharyngeal airways, laryngoscopes, endotracheal tubes, stylets and McGill's forceps (Tables 16.3 and 16.5).

PREMEDICATION

Laryngoscopy and intubation elicit physiological responses/reflexes which must be recognized and managed. These are: airway protective reflexes, (mediated via glossopharyngeal and vagal nerves, laryngospasm, cough, gag, sneeze); cardiovascular responses (sinus bradycardia by direct vagal stimulation or by hypoxia, tachycardia caused by anxiety and fighting as well as hypoxia, dysrythmias, especially if the patient becomes hypoxic). Premedication is used to blunt these responses. Abla-

tion of the airway protective reflexes requires the deep sedation or anaesthesia used for induction whilst cardiovascular responses, aside from the bradycardia produced by vagal stimulation (prevented with atropine), are largely prevented by avoidance of hypoxia. Premedication is as follows:

- Atropine: 20 µg/kg (minimum dose 100 µg), prevents vagally medicated bradycardia caused by intubation attempt, induces 'protective tachycardia' against hypoxia-induced bradycardia.
- Midazolam: 0.1–0.5 mg/kg as sedative; antegrade and retrograde amnesia occurs.
- Morphine: 0.1–0.2 mg/kg is primarily analgesic, but also causes mild sedation.

INDUCTION

Once the decision to intubate has been made, one must next decide whether sedation is

Table 16.6: Commonly used anaesthetic induction agents for intubation

Drug	IV dose (mg/kg)	Effect on ICP	Effect on BP	Advantages	Disadvantages and adverse effects
Thiopentone	2–5	Protective Decreases	Decreases	Rapid onset with short duration Reduces ICP and cerebral metabolism thus has protective effect on brain Anticonvulsant	Hypotension due to vasodilatation and myocardial depression Bronchospasm from histamine release, therefore not used in asthmatics No analgesic effect
Ketamine	1–2	Increases	Increases	Rapid sedation, analgesia and amnesia Use in hypovolaemic non-head injury patients as maintains BP Bronchodilatation useful in asthma and bronchiolitis Can be used IM (dose 5–10 mg/kg)	Increases ICP, increases secretions Short-term psychiatric effects such as nightmares are attenuated by premed with benzodiazepines e.g. midazolam
Propofol	1–2	Decreases	Decreases	Rapid onset sedation and amnesia Short duration of action Anticonvulsant	Hypotension
Etomidate	2–4	Decreases	Minimal	Anticonvulsant Little haemodynamic effect	Cortisol suppression

Table 16.7: Commonly used muscle relaxants for intubation

Drug	IV dose (mg/kg)	Advantages	Disadvantages and adverse effects
Succinylcholine Neonate Child Adult	 3 2 1	Rapid onset Short duration Can be used IM	Muscle contraction causes increase in serum K^+; contraindicated where risk with rise of K^+ (renal failure, burns, muscular dystrophy) Increased intracranial, intraocular and intragastric pressure Bradycardia, hypotension, asystole Muscle pain
Atracurium	0.5–1	Metabolism not influenced by renal or hepatic function	Slower onset than succinylcholine and rocuronium Histamine release: causes hypotension and bronchospasm Hypotension if injected rapidly
Rocuronium	0.6–1.2	Rapid onset Can be used IM	

required. Sedation is clearly not necessary in the child who has collapsed, but where the child is awake in an elective intubation, deep sedation is preferable. An awake or partially sedated child will be combative which can result in worsening of the hypoxia and in local trauma. An anaesthetic induction agent is chosen (Table 16.6) with or without a muscle relaxant (Table 16.7). Note that midazolam, morphine and fentanyl have not been included in the list of suggested agents because of their slow onset of action and inadequate sedation for intubation at recommended doses. Sedative agents recommended for different clinical scenarios are listed in Table 16.8. Muscle relaxants should be used with extreme caution. They should not be used where there is any doubt that an airway can be secured or that the patient can be artificially ventilated.

INTUBATION TECHNIQUE (FIGURE 16.5)

Endotracheal intubation can be divided into four basic manoeuvres:

- Visualization of the glottis (Figure 16.6) by alignment of the axes of the mouth, pharynx and trachea (Figure 16.7).

- Visualization of the glottis by displacement of soft tissues i.e. tongue and epiglottis.
- Insertion of the ETT via the mouth or the nose.
- Confirmation of ETT placement.

Many issues surrounding all three aspects of intubation have already been described.

Table 16.8: Sedative induction agents for selected clinical scenarios

Clinical scenario	Options
Normotensive / euvolaemic	Thiopentone, propofol
Mild hypotension / hypovolaemia with head injury	Thiopentone, etomidate
Mild hypotension without head injury	Ketamine, etomidate
Severe hypotension	Ketamine, etomidate
Severe asthma	Ketamine, propofol
Intractible fits	Thiopentone, propofol
Isolated head injury	Thiopentone, propofol, etomidate
Combative patient	Thiopentone, propofol

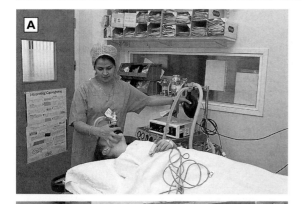

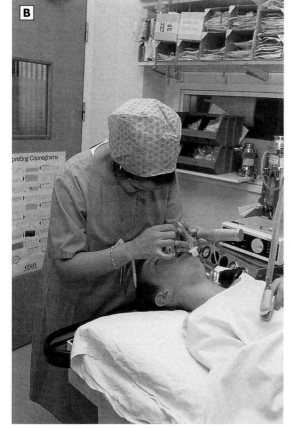

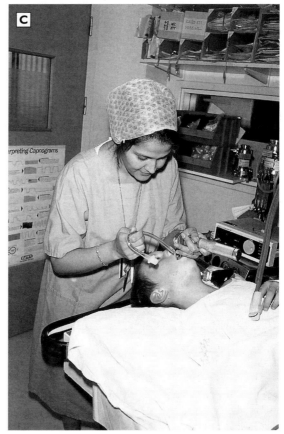

Figure 16.5: Endotracheal intubation: (A) pre-oxygenation, (B) visualization of the cords, (C) insertion of ETT.

Alignment of the axes of the mouth, pharynx and trachea (Figure 16.7) is best achieved by anterior displacement and simultaneous extension of the neck into the 'sniffing position'. Anterior displacement is achieved by placing a pillow under the patient's head. In infants and children less than 2 years of age, such displacement occurs naturally

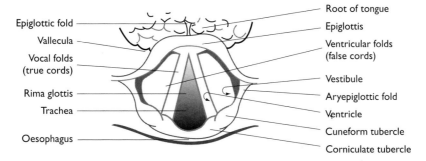

Figure 16.6: Operator's view of laryngeal anatomy.

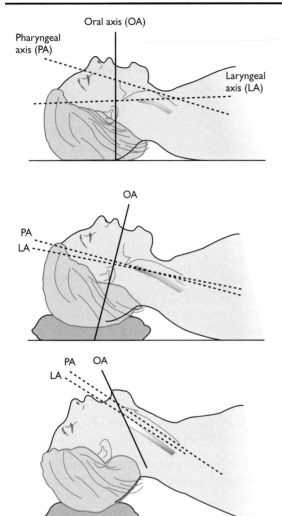

Figure 16.7: Alignment of airway axes for intubation (from Ref. 2). For an infant, a roll should be placed under the shoulders, not the occiput.

when the large occiput is placed on a flat surface with the child lying supine.

Displacement of the soft tissues is achieved as follows: The laryngoscope is held in the left hand. The blade is inserted into the right side of the mouth and the tongue is swept aside creating a channel in the mouth for visualization and insertion of the endotracheal tube. The epiglottis can be displaced in one of two ways depending whether one is using a straight Miller or curved Macintosh laryngoscope blade:

- Straight Miller blade: the tip of the blade is passed beyond the epiglottis which is then lifted out of the line of vision.
- Curved Macintosh blade: the tip of the blade is inserted into the vallecula (the crypt between the base of the tongue and the epiglottis) and lifted anteriorly thereby tilting the epiglottis from the line of vision. This is a lifting manoeuvre and should never be a rocking manoeuvre where the fulcrum would inevitably be the patient's teeth or gums.

The ETT must be inserted through the glottis under direct vision. This can be helped by passing the endotracheal tube from the right hand corner of the mouth and not in the line of vision down the barrel of the laryngoscope blade and cricoid pressure by an assistant.

In nasotracheal intubation (Table 16.9), the ETT is passed through the nasal cavity into the nasopharynx before the mouth is opened. Remember that the direction of insertion is in the plane of the hard palate, i.e. horizontally when standing or directly backwards when lying on one's back, i.e. not upwards in the plane of the bridge of the nose. Once the tip of the ETT is visualized with the laryngoscope in the hypopharynx it is grasped with the Magill forceps about 1 cm from its tip and the tip is then lifted over the posterior lamina of the cricoid cartilage and directed inferiorly through the vocal cords as the tube is gently advanced through the nose by an assistant.

Table 16.9: Pros and cons of nasotracheal intubation

Advantages
Patient comfort
Follows the normal direction of the airway
Eliminates the problems associated with biting the ETT
Easier to secure to nose and upper lip
Facilitates mouth care
Less subglottic trauma – as ETT more secure in nose than mouth there is less movement and thus less trauma by the tip in trachea
Problems
Epistaxis, trauma to nasal mucosa
Adenoid trauma
Pressure necrosis of nares
Sinusitis or otitis media
May require a smaller ETT than oral intubation

Confirmation of ETT placement should be sought immediately after intubation the position of the ETT by:

- auscultation of symmetrical breath sounds over each lateral chest wall high in the axillae;
- documentation of absence of breath sounds over the stomach;
- observation of symmetrical chest movements; and
- end-tidal CO_2 trace where available.[3]

MANAGEMENT OF THE INTUBATED CHILD

Stabilization of the ETT is the next step. The ETT is immediately secured to the patient's face. There are various techniques, as illustrated in Figure 16.8.

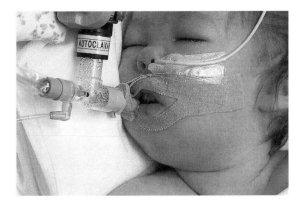

Figure 16.8: Fixation of the endotracheal tube.

Sedation is maintained with or without paralysis (dependent on clinical assessment) by continuous infusion in intubated patients (Table 16.10).

Humidification is essential as airway drying leads to heat and moisture loss.[4, 5] Dehydration of the respiratory tract causes epithelial damage, particularly of the trachea and upper bronchi, and impaired function of the mucociliary elevator with sputum retention and atelectasis.

Suction: Flexible (end-hole) suction catheters are used to clear the ETT and avoid blockage. Frequency of suctioning with or without prior installation of saline will depend on the volume and viscosity of secretions. The tip of the suction catheter should not be advanced beyond the tip of the endotracheal tube as sucking against the respiratory tract epithelium will traumatize it. Patients should be monitored during suctioning (heart rate and oxygen saturation) and each attempt should be no longer than 3 to 5 seconds.

FAILED INTUBATION

Failure to intubate a child is due either to complete obstruction (epiglottitis, foreign body) or to a difficult airway.

Complete obstruction should ideally be potentially suspected and, as mentioned, where possible pre-empted, i.e. intubation in the operating theatre with expertise and facility for emergency cricothyrotomy or tracheostomy. Percutaneous

Table 16.10: Suggested infusion chart for maintenance of sedation and paralysis

Drug	Dosage (μg/kg/min)	Infusion concentration (mg/kg)	Infusion rate = Dose
Sedatives			
Midazolam	10–30	3 mg/kg in 50 ml	1 mL/h = 1 μg/kg/min
Ketamine	10–40	20 mL undiluted (10 mg/ml)	0.06 mL/kg/h = 10 μg/kg/min
Morphine	10–30*	1 mg/kg in 50 ml	1 mL/h = 20 μg/kg/h
Fentanyl	1–8*	0.1 mg/kg in 50 ml	1 mL/h = 2 μg/kg/h
Paralysing agents			
Atracurium	10–40	30 mg/kg in 50 ml	1 mL/h = 10 μg/kg/min
Cis-atracurium	10–40	30 mg/kg in 50 ml	1 mL/h = 10 μg/kg/min
Vecuronium	1–3	3	1 mL/h = 1 μg/kg/min

*Infusion rates given for opioids is in μg/kg/**hour**.

cricothyrotomy kits (Melker Emergency Cricothyrotomy Catheter Sets, Cook® Critical Care) are available. The airway catheter has a standard 15–22 mm adapter for an appropriate ventilatory device. These kits should be available on emergency or 'crash' trolleys as the traditional method of passing a large bore needle does not permit adequate ventilation.

Difficult airways may be encountered at any time. Any clinician involved in paediatric airway management must be prepared to manage a child in whom endotracheal intubation cannot be accomplished in the absence of complete airway obstruction. After failed intubation, attempt to continue to monitor oxygen saturation and heart rate; continue to oxygenate via bag-valve-mask ventilation; ensure that the patient is sedated and paralyzed; repeat intubation attempts may be made after the patient is adequately prepared.

Other options available after repeated failed attempts include laryngeal mask airways[6, 7] and intubation bougies. The firm but flexible plastic bougie can be placed in the normal way into the trachea as an introducer or guide.[8] The endotracheal tube is immediately threaded over the bougie into the trachea.

Rapid sequence intubation (RSI)[9]

RSI is defined as the use of appropriate drugs to facilitate intubation and reduce the risk of complications of aspiration, hypoxia and increased intracranial pressure. RSI is an *organized* approach to *emergency* intubation comprising rapid sedation and paralysis with minimal or no prior positive-pressure ventilation. It basically involves preparation, pre-oxygenation, sedation, paralysis and intubation. Bag-valve-mask ventilation is avoided, unless hypoxia develops, to limit gastric distension in a situation where there is already a perceived increase risk of aspiration of gastric contents. RSI is used where a patient has a full stomach and needs immediate intubation. The use of anaesthetic induction agents and muscle relaxants abolishes the airway protective reflexes and places the patient at significant risk of aspiration of regurgitated stomach contents.

Patients regarded as having a full stomach include any with:

- recent oral intake
- bowel obstruction
- swallowed blood
- increased intra-abdominal pressure.

Significant pressure placed over the cricoid cartilage by an assistant to occlude the oesophagus prior to administration of sedatives can reduce the regurgitation of stomach contents. Pressure is maintained until the ETT is in place.

REFERENCES

1. Anderson CTM, Saltzmann JA. Congenital and acquired airway pathology and management: why is Leslie blue? *Semin Anaesth* 1989; **4**: 315–37.

2. Berry FA, Yemen TA. Pediatric airway in health and disease. *Pediat Clin N Am* 1994; **41**: 153–80.

3. Bhavani-Shankar K, Moseley H, Kumar AY, Delph Y. Capnometry and anaesthesia. *Br J Anaesth* 1992; **39**: 617–32.

4. Shelly MP, Lloyd GM, Park GR. A review of the mechanisms and methods of humidification of inspired gases. *Intensive Care Med* 1988; **14**: 1–9.

5. Hedley RM, Allt-Graham J. Heat and moisture exchangers and breathing filters. *Br J Anaesth* 1994; **73**: 227–36.

6. Brimacombe J, Berry A, Verghese C. The laryngeal mask airway in critical care medicine. *Intensive Care Med* 1995; **21**: 361–4.

7. Lopez-Gil M, Brimacombe J, Alvarez M. Safety and efficacy of the laryngeal mask airway. A prospective survey of 1400 children. *Anaesthesia* 1996; **51**: 969–72.

8. Gataure PS, Vaughan RS, Latto IP. Simulated difficult intubation. Comparison of the gum elastic bougie and the stylet. *Anaesthesia* 1996; **51**: 935–8.

9. Gerardi MJ, Sacchetti AD, Cantor RM, *et al*. Rapid-sequence intubation of the pediatric patient. *Ann Emerg Med* 1996; **28**: 55–71.

FURTHER READING

1. Mackway-Jones K, Molyneux E, Phillips B, Wieteska S (eds). Advanced Life Support Group. *Advanced pediatric life support. The practical approach.* London: BMJ Publishing Group, 1996.

2. Chameides L, Hazinski MF (eds). *Pediatric advanced life support manual.* Dallas: American Heart Association, and American Academy of Paediatrics, 1994; 4.1– 4.20.

3. Silverman M, McKenzie S. Respiratory system. In: *Forfar and Arneil's Textbook of paediatrics.* London: Campbell and Macintosh, 1992.

4. Morriss FC, Stone J, Butler LM. Intubation. In: Levin DL, Morriss FC (eds). *Essentials of pediatric intensive care.* St. Louis: Quality Medical Publishing, 1990: 888–96.

5. Rivera R, Tibballs J. Complications of endotracheal intubation and mechanical ventilation in infants and children. *Crit Care Med* 1992; **20**: 193–9.

CHAPTER SEVENTEEN

VENTILATORY SUPPORT *IN THE* CRITICALLY ILL CHILD

S. Nichani

- Background
- Positive pressure ventilators
- Future directions
- References

BACKGROUND

Mechanical ventilatory support is one of the most important supportive modalities used in treating critically ill patients. An essential element of cardio-pulmonary resuscitation, it can be life-saving during a variety of acute and chronic diseases.

The respiratory muscles share with other major muscle groups the characteristic that excessive work leads to fatigue. The application of mechanical ventilation allows the physician to temporarily reverse respiratory failure and sustain life.

Although ventilatory support is essential in cardio-pulmonary resuscitation, the supportive nature of this intervention should be stressed since only rarely will mechanical ventilation have a direct therapeutic effect and specific treatment is generally required to reverse the cause of respiratory failure and return the patient if possible to the pre-morbid status. The flip side is that mechanical ventilation may unnecessarily prolong the distress of terminal disease and the benefits of its use should be weighed against the disadvantages.

INDICATIONS

The most common reason cited for providing ventilatory support is 'respiratory failure'. Respiratory failure is defined as the inability of the breathing apparatus to maintain normal gas exchange. However a more useful classification of diseases best managed using mechanical ventilation is one based on underlying pathophysiology.

One such classification groups diseases into four categories:

1. Those such as severe infectious pneumonia, pulmonary oedema, pulmonary haemorrhage and adult respiratory distress syndrome which cause hypoxia unresponsive to supplemental oxygen.
2. Those such as obstructive airways disease with respiratory muscle fatigue, acute or chronic neuromuscular disorders, respiratory depressant effects of medicinal or recreational drugs where alveolar ventilation is inadequate to clear the carbon dioxide production.
3. Those rendering patients unable to protect and maintain patent airways either because of a decreased level of consciousness or an increase in airway secretions, e.g. situations of raised intra-cranial pressure.
4. Acute medical and post-surgical states wherein mechanical ventilation is used as adjunctive therapy to reduce the work of breathing, e.g. following open heart surgery or acute myocarditis.

BROAD CLASSIFICATION

Mechanical ventilators are specialized pumps, which perform the task usually done by the respiratory muscles and diaphragm, i.e. provide an external source of energy to move gas into the lungs and allow in the most part for passive exhalation. This permits both oxygenation and ventilation (carbon dioxide elimination).

The lungs can be artificially ventilated either by reducing the ambient pressure around the thorax (negative pressure ventilators) or by increasing the pressure within the airways (positive pressure ventilators).

PHYSIOLOGICAL BACKGROUND TO MECHANICAL VENTILATION

Mechanical ventilation interacts with normal physiology in various ways, some of which are listed below.

- The total ventilation required to maintain a normal arterial carbon dioxide ($Paco_2$) depends on the CO_2 production and the effective alveolar ventilation. There is an inverse relationship between minute ventilation and $Paco_2$. Hyperventilation reduces the concentration of CO_2 in the alveolar gas whereas during ventilatory failure, there is progressive retention of CO_2.
- At normal breathing frequencies, the pressure required to inflate the lungs, has two components, namely, that required to drive gas along the airways and that required to inflate the alveoli.
- When the lungs are exposed to a constant airway pressure, they fill to a volume that is determined by the applied pressure and the compliance (change in volume per unit change in pressure) of the lungs, a high pressure or a high compliance resulting in higher volumes being generated. The flow rate during the period of filling will depend on the difference in pressure between the alveoli and the source of pressure but also on the airway resistance.
- When a patient is supine, the blood flow is affected by gravitational forces and is distributed preferentially to the dependent part of the lung, although recent research suggests that there is an increased blood supply to the dorsal part of the lungs regardless of the position of the patient, i.e. whether the patient is supine or prone.[1]
- When the patient is supine, the pressure exerted by the abdominal contents forces the diaphragm into the chest reducing the functional residual capacity (FRC) and causing ventilation to be distributed to the anterior or non-dependent zones of the lung. Simultaneously, as blood flow goes to the dorsal part of the body, there is ventilation perfusion mismatch (V/Q). The reduction in FRC, can be reversed by the application of positive end expiratory pressure (PEEP) and the V/Q mismatch, could be improved by turning the patient prone. Airway resistance in the normal subject, is 1–2 cmH$_2$O /L/S (0.1–0.2 kPa/L/S). Airway resistance is increased by increased bronchial muscle tone, mucosal oedema and airway secretions. Patients with increased airway resistance often have hyper-inflated lungs, which may decrease the efficiency of the diaphragm and other respiratory muscles. The presence of an endotracheal tube also increases the resistance by a factor of about 5–10 times.[2] Since the resistance to laminar flow of gas through airways is inversely related to the fourth power of the radius of the airways, airway resistance increases with decreasing lung volumes.

POSITIVE PRESSURE VENTILATORS

BASIC DESIGN

Positive pressure may be defined as any pressure greater than atmospheric pressure. Designed to facilitate movement of gas into the lungs, mechanical ventilators have evolved from simple oxygen powered breathing devices to sophisticated microprocessor controlled systems with high speed electrically actuated gas control valves, capable of providing a variety of ventilator modalities.[3]

Compressed air and oxygen are delivered into the ventilator from high pressure sources; they are then mixed by blenders. Flow after the blender is controlled by two high speed electrically operated proportional gas control valves controlling both inspiratory flow and oxygen tension. The inspiratory flow rate is measured continuously by a flow meter placed just after the inspiratory valve and the valve is then servo controlled to produce the desired flow pattern, inspiratory time and tidal volume or pressure. A second valve on the expiratory side can be used to control expiratory time and flow and can be linked to airway pressure so that it can be used to maintain a given level of PEEP.

Pressure and flow sensors monitor the airway pressure and flow of gas into the patient.

TYPES OF MECHANICAL VENTILATORS

Ventilators can be classified according to their functional characteristics. Two aspects of function are considered: (i) the way in which the ventilator controls the pattern of gas flow in and out of the patient (the driving mechanisms); and (ii) the mechanisms which cause the ventilator to cycle between the two phases of respiration (the cycling mechanism).

Driving mechanisms:

- *Flow generators*: in this type of generator, the ventilator generates a fixed pattern of flow that is maintained despite changes in airway compliance and resistance.
- *Pressure generator*: is a ventilator that generates a pressure and the flow generated depends on the resistance and compliance that is encountered as the gas flows into the lungs.

In modern ventilators, increased flexibility has been provided by controlling the flow from a high-pressure source with rapidly acting inspiratory and expiratory valves. By using pressure and flow sensors in the breathing system, the machine can function either as a flow or a pressure generator, depending on the controls.

The second characteristic of the ventilator is the method of cycling from one phase to the other. Time, volume, pressure and flow rate are inter-related variables that are used to describe mechanical ventilation.

- Time cycled mechanical ventilation: is terminated after a pre-selected inspiratory time elapses.

- Pressure limited time cycled mechanical ventilation: a pressure limit is pre-selected to a specific value with this mode of ventilation. Once the pressure limit is reached, the airway pressure is held at that level until the ventilator time-cycles off.
- Volume cycled mechanical ventilation: is terminated after a pre-selected tidal volume has been ejected from the ventilator. It guarantees minute ventilation and changes in lung compliance are reflected by the pressures generated. This allows one to monitor and quantify compliance changes. It is simple to understand and easy to apply, but necessitates close monitoring and high pressures produced may result in damage to the lung (barotrauma) and may also have deleterious cardiovascular effects.
- Pressure cycled mechanical ventilation: is terminated when a pre-selected pressure is reached regardless of the tidal volume, inspiratory flow rate or inspiratory time. However, the tidal volume generated will decrease if the airway resistance increases or the lung compliance decreases.
- Flow cycled mechanical ventilation: is terminated when the inspiratory flow rate delivered by the ventilator decreases to a critical value.

THE BREATHING APPARATUS

Consists of the endotracheal tube (which is the main resistor), a set of breathing tubes, one to carry inspiratory gases to the patient and one to take the expiratory gases away from the patient. The tubing should be transparent, have a low resistance, be flexible and should not be expanded significantly by increased internal pressure. The incoming gas is humidified by a humidifier, which should have a low resistance and a small volume. It should be capable of delivering fully saturated gas at 37°C to the patient without condensation of water vapour in the inspiratory tubing along with a provision for the drainage of water that condenses in the expiratory tube.

CLASSIFICATION OF VENTILATORY SUPPORT

Controlled mechanical ventilation (CMV)

This is a full support mode in which the ventilator performs most or all of the work necessary to maintain adequate minute ventilation. Full support modes are often advantageous in the acutely ill patient who requires guaranteed minute ventilation. CMV delivers a pre-selected ventilatory rate, tidal volume or pressure and inspiratory flow rate which are independent of spontaneous effort on the part of the patient. The inspiratory pressure generated varies inversely with compliance and directly with resistance if the ventilator is volume cycled. Conversely for a pressure-cycled ventilator, the tidal volume generated depends on the compliance of the patient's lungs. The pressure-limited mode is used more frequently in paediatric and neonatal intensive care than in adult intensive care because unanticipated changes in lung mechanics are relatively small.

This ventilatory pattern is continued independently of patient effort and between ventilator breaths, the inspiratory valve is closed such that no additional breaths can be taken.

INDICATIONS
CMV is generally used to support patients without spontaneous respiratory effort. It ensures that a patient will receive a specified number of breaths at a designated pressure or volume independently of spontaneous efforts.

LIMITATIONS
Difficulties may arise when the patient is capable of spontaneous respiratory efforts since this can lead to patient ventilator dysynchrony. This occurs when the patient's breathing cycle is out of phase with that of the ventilator, i.e. the patient may be trying to exhale during the inspiratory cycle.

INITIAL SETTINGS
The clinician sets the respiratory rate, fraction of inspired oxygen concentration (FiO_2), peak pressure or tidal volume, inspiratory time, end expiratory pressure and the pressure and volume alarms.

Synchronized intermittent mandatory ventilation (SIMV)

The difference between CMV and SIMV is the fact that in the SIMV mode, the ventilator synchronizes breaths with the patient. Mandatory breaths are delivered at specified intervals. Prior to a programmed breath, the ventilator waits a predetermined period. The ventilator will supplement any breath initiated during this period such that the patient receives a full assisted breath. If no patient breath occurs, the ventilator delivers an unassisted breath. Between mandatory breaths, the patient is able to breathe spontaneously. This occurs as a consequence of a sensing device which detects a patient initiated breath as a fall in airway pressure below a specific airway pressure or a change in flow due to the patient taking some gas from the fresh source of gas that is available.

INDICATIONS
The SIMV mode can be used as a primary mode of ventilation because it provides backup ventilation or as a weaning mode. The major design advantage of SIMV is the opening of the inspiratory valve between ventilator breaths, which provides a source of gas and allows for spontaneous, synchronized patient breathing. This thus allows better synchrony between the patient and the ventilator.

LIMITATIONS
Patient asynchrony is still a possibility, e.g. if a patient is being underventilated by the machine and is breathing spontaneously at a higher rate, he/she may attempt to exhale during the mandatory breaths and may not receive effective ventilation.

SETTINGS
As it is usually used as a weaning mode, it is set at a rate lower than the patient's own rate, either by setting the pressure or the volume, depending on the type of ventilator.

Pressure support ventilation (PSV)

Pressure support ventilation (PSV) is patient triggered (initiated), flow cycled pressure ventilation where each spontaneous inspiratory effort is augmented by an operator-specified amount of positive pressure.[4] As long as the patient's inspiratory effort is maintained, the pre-selected airway pressure remains constant with a variable flow of gas from the ventilator. Inhalation cycles off when the patient's inspiratory flow demand decreases to a pre-determined percentage of the initial peak inspiratory flow rate. Expiration is passive and respiratory rate and tidal volume are determined by patient effort and respiratory system compliance respectively. Parameters set by the operator are inspiratory pressure, FiO_2 and end expiratory pressure.

INDICATIONS

PSV is used to wean patients from ventilatory support. Mechanical ventilation of more than 72 hours can cause respiratory muscle de-conditioning.[5]

One of the advantages of PSV is thought to be that it allows for respiratory muscle conditioning during weaning.

INITIAL SETTINGS

The pressure support level is set at half the peak pressure being generated on the current support mode.

The pressure support is then reduced to allow the patient to do more of the breathing, its main function being to help overcome the inspiratory load imposed by the breathing circuit and the endotracheal tube. When adequate gas exchange is achieved with pressure support of about 5 cmH_2O, extubation can usually be attempted.

Continuous positive airway pressure (CPAP) and positive end expiratory pressure (PEEP)

These are positive pressure modes, the former being employed individually and the latter in conjunction with positive pressure ventilation. CPAP refers to the addition of both positive inspiratory and expiratory pressures during spontaneous breathing while with PEEP, a pre-determined amount of positive pressure is applied at end exhalation to a mechanical ventilation cycle.

The benefits of applying positive pressure ventilation result from its ability to open closed alveolar units thereby recruiting lung volume and improving gas exchange.

INDICATIONS

The primary indication is hypoxaemia secondary to diffuse lung injury as occurs in ARDS and interstitial pneumonitis.

PEEP can be added to any volume or pressure cycled mode to help improve oxygenation.

CPAP can be administered in the non-intubated patient by using an airtight mask, which fits either over the nose or mouth or just over the nose.[6]

LIMITATIONS

The most frequent potential complication is haemodynamic due to a reduction of venous return. The other potential problem is that masks are uncomfortable to wear which makes patient compliance a potential problem. Also, in order to maintain CPAP, the rate of gas inflow must be greater than the patient's spontaneous inspiratory flow rate.

INITIAL SETTINGS

Positive pressure should be prescribed depending on the initial clinical setting, e.g. a child with obstructive airway disease like bronchial asthma requires minimal or no PEEP due to the significant positive end expiratory pressure being part of the underlying pathophysiology of obstructive airway disease.

On the other hand, a patient with ventilation perfusion mismatch as seen in ARDS, will benefit from greater than normal PEEP which could be increased in small increments, 2–3 cm H_2O at a time for a trial period of 10–15 minutes looking closely for haemodynamic change.

Unconventional modes of mechanical ventilation

Inverse ratio ventilation (IRV): refers to mechanical ventilation in which the inspiratory : expiratory (I:E) ratio is set at greater than one. This is achieved either by prolonging the inspiratory time or slowing the inspiratory flow rate. The end result will be physiology that is thought to be beneficial, i.e. a prolonged inflation cycle to allow for opening of alveolar units with long opening time constants which can then participate in gas exchange and increased time for gas diffusion.

INDICATIONS

The best studied clinical indication for considering use of IRV is diffuse lung injury with hypoxaemia in patients who are non-responders to CMV/SIMV with PEEP. It has been suggested that IRV can provide adequate oxygenation at lower peak airway and mean airway pressures than either CMV or SIMV.[7] In theory, this would reduce the risk of barotrauma and the potential for haemodynamic compromise.

LIMITATIONS

Because of limited experience with IRV, the full spectrum of potential limitations associated with its use are not fully appreciated. This mode usually requires heavy sedation, often with paralysis, because of the non-physiologic character of its tidal volume cycling.

INITIAL SETTINGS

IRV is used in clinical practice almost solely in the pressure-cycled mode. The operator must therefore specify the airway pressure profile and Fio_2. Tidal volume and flow profile are determined by the patient's respiratory system mechanics.

Airway pressure release ventilation (APRV)

In this mode of ventilation, the patient breathes spontaneously from a CPAP system with a release valve in the expiratory limb. A standing pressure (usually between 5–10 cmH$_2$O) is applied to the patient's airway either through an endotracheal tube or a facemask. When the expiratory valve opens, circuit and airway pressures drop from the CPAP level to near ambient pressure and this allows lung volume to decrease. Closing the valve restores airway pressure back to the CPAP level. Thus each mechanical breath is created by brief interruption and restoration of CPAP.

Maintaining CPAP recruits lung units and promotes oxygenation and carbon dioxide elimination is achieved by the periodic emptying of the lungs to atmospheric pressure at a frequency of 2–10 times per minute.

A variation on this theme is biphasic positive airway pressure ventilation (BIPAP) in which the pressure is not quite reduced to atmospheric pressure in the emptying phase. This helps to keep alveoli open.

These modes of ventilation are essentially time cycled, pressure controlled ventilation with low pressures and respiratory rates superimposed on spontaneous breathing.

INDICATIONS

APRV is thought to be a feasible alternative to conventional ventilation to augment mechanical ventilation in patients with acute lung injury of mild to moderate severity. It has been suggested that APRV can maintain blood oxygenation at lower peak and mean airway pressure than is possible using conventional ventilation. Also by allowing for spontaneous respiration, respiratory muscle conditioning can be maintained even in the setting of moderately severe lung injury.

This mode of ventilation has not yet made inroads into the practice of paediatric intensive care.

LIMITATIONS

Like IRV, APRV has been used infrequently in clinical practice especially in children and the full spectrum of potential complications is not yet known.

INITIAL SETTINGS

The clinician is responsible for setting airway maintenance pressure (peak airway pressure), airway pressure release level, ventilator rate and Fio_2. Initial settings for airway maintenance pressure range between 20–35 cmH$_2$O and for airway pressure release level between 2 and 10 cmH$_2$O.

High frequency ventilation (HFV)

This is a non-conventional mode of ventilation which involves the use of small tidal volumes delivered at respiratory rates ranging from 60 to 2400 (1 to 40 Hz) breaths per minute. The tidal volumes are equal to or smaller than the anatomic dead space. Compared with conventional ventilation, HFV offers several potential advantages, which include lower airway and intra-thoracic pressures, reduced intra-pulmonary pressure swings and decreased fluctuations in alveolar pressure, resulting in reduced cardiovascular impairment and reduced pulmonary barotrauma.

MECHANICS OF HIGH FREQUENCY VENTILATION

Gas exchange during HFV does not occur by convection alone as during conventional ventilation but is thought to involve several processes including:

1. Direct alveolar ventilation by bulk flow
2. Non-convective mixing due to pressure fluctuations from cardiac pulsations, and
3. Taylor-type dispersion which is the formal mathematical model of blowing smoke down a tube. If one imagines a puff of smoke travelling down a glass tube, the small volume will curl down the tube and then at some point disperse
4. Molecular diffusion.

There are three types of HFV:

- High frequency positive pressure ventilation (HFPPV).
- High frequency jet ventilation (HFJV).
- High frequency oscillation (HFO).

HFPPV: uses a conventional volume or pressure limited ventilation modified by the use of a low compliance ventilator tubing with minimum compressible volume. This allows the delivery of adequate tidal volumes with varying inspiratory times. The ventilator frequency varies from 60 to 150 breaths with tidal volumes between 3–5 mL/kg. Unfortunately, with increasing respiratory frequency, tidal volume may be compromised. This may result in alveolar hypoventilation even though the minute ventilation is normal or increased.

HFJV: is characterized by the delivery of brief, fast burst of gas through a small cannula either via an endotracheal tube or directly into the trachea.[8] The respiratory rate varies between 60 and 600 insufflations per minute with a short inspiratory time. A valve device applied to the expiratory limb supplies PEEP. Maintaining adequate humidification has been a problem with this mode of ventilation and there have been reports of necrotizing tracheobronchitis following the use of HFJV.[9]

HFO: utilizes a piston pump that produces to and fro oscillation around a continuous distending pressure.[10] Both the inhalation and exhalation are active as the gas mixture is forced into and out of the lungs. This is accomplished by a reciprocating device (piston pump and acoustic speaker cones) that generates a sinusoidal wave at the airway opening.[11] Frequencies range between 60 and 3600 cycles per minute (3 to 18 Hz). The mean airway pressure can be adjusted from 3 to 45 cm of H_2O, the oscillatory pressure from 0 to 90 cmH_2O, the I/E ratio from 30% to 70% and the bias flow (fresh gas) up to 24 L/min. A steady flow of fresh humidified gas crosses the oscillating gas stream so that the oscillating gas is continuously refreshed.

CO_2 clearance is variable but is roughly related to the frequency and to a square of the tidal volume. Oxygenation depends on the mean airway pressure and the Fio_2 The type of HFV used most commonly in neonatal and paediatric intensive care is HFO.

Recently, it has been used successfully in the management of severe neonatal respiratory distress syndrome[12] as well in the management of paediatric patients with severe respiratory distress syndrome.[13]

This mode should be used with caution in children with obstructive lung disease, due to potential for worsening hyperinflation by the significant continuous distending pressure that is inherent to HFO.

Negative pressure ventilation

The term is used to denote a method of producing lung expansion by intermittently reducing the absolute pressure around the chest wall.

The ventilator consists of either a chamber that encloses the thorax or a chamber (tank) that encloses the whole body below the neck. The pressure in the chamber is reduced cyclically by using a large volume displacement pump: this causes the lungs to expand and contract. Negative pressure ventilators are pressure cycled, allowing the operator to specify the respiratory system pressure while tidal volume, inspiratory and expiratory flows are determined by respiratory system impedance.

Tank ventilators: are no longer in use in paediatric intensive care as they are cumbersome, consisting of a large rigid container, which surrounds the whole of the patient's body except the head and neck. Other limitations are that it may not be able to generate sufficiently negative sub-atmospheric pressures to treat patients with acute lung disease and there are also difficulties in carrying out medical and nursing procedures through the portholes in the wall of the machine. The advantage is that this mode is non-invasive and laryngeal function is preserved.

Jacket ventilators: during the last few years, there has been a resurgence of interest in this type of ventilator. This is due to improvements in the design of the shell and the pump. The shell extends from the manubrium to the lower abdomen. By padding the edges with foam rubber and covering them with an airtight material, it is possible to make a light, airtight shell. The efficiency of the ventilator has been improved by replacing the large bellows unit, which generated the sub-atmospheric pressure, by specially designed rotary pumps. These have a high flow capability so that they can achieve a pre-determined sub-atmospheric pressure despite small leaks.[14] Since tidal volume is linearly related to the sub-atmospheric pressure, this ensures that ventilation is reasonably well maintained as long as there is no gross leak.[15] Most cuirass devices provide controlled ventilation but a patient trigger mode is also available. The most recent innovation available is the Hayek Oscillator which has a lightweight flexible chest enclosure which is attached to a piston pump which can provide negative pressure as well as ventilation up to high frequencies.[16]

INDICATIONS
Cuirass ventilators are often used to augment ventilators in patients with chronic respiratory insufficiency in either a continuous negative pressure mode or intermittent negative pressure mode to facilitate weaning. If the underlying condition is not progressive, the long-term prognosis is also improved.[17]

DISADVANTAGES
The patient has to sleep supine or slightly inclined to the side and pressure sores may develop where the shell presses on the skin.

RESPIRATORY THERAPY

Optimal ventilatory support requires the clinician to recognize the diversity of respiratory failure. Identifying and understanding each patient's underlying pathophysiology combined with a thorough knowledge of the ventilatory options, are often the most vital elements in the treatment of the critically ill child. The critical care physician should tailor ventilatory support to each patient's pathophysiology rather than employ a single technique for all patients with respiratory failure.

Also, regardless of the cause of respiratory insufficiency, the following priorities should be observed in ventilating children:

1. Strive for an adequate Pa_{O_2} (about 50 mmHg; 6.7 kPa) using the minimum amount of oxygen, an adequate amount of PEEP and avoid the use of over exuberant pressures to maintain that level of oxygenation.
2. Allow the Pa_{CO_2} where appropriate to rise such that the pH drops to 7.25 as long as there is no hypoxaemia or cardiovascular compromise. This helps avoid dangerously high pressures which can lead to significant lung damage.
3. Tracheo-bronchial toilet should be provided in the form of tracheal suction, physiotherapy and regular change in position of the child.
4. Encourage diaphragmatic activity as soon as possible.
5. Provide optimal patient comfort and safety.
6. Have a low threshold to provide inotropic support to the heart which is faced with an increase in afterload due to pathology in the lungs.

In patients with normal lungs, almost any ventilator can be used successfully. Heavy, stiff lungs which are found in patients with cardiogenic pulmonary oedema, life-threatening pneumonia or acute lung injury are characterized by low FRC, decrease in compliance, ventilation perfusion mismatch and an increase in dead space. In these cases, ventilation should be aimed at correcting the low FRC. Adequate PEEP may be life-saving. In the presence of obstructive lung disease, special consideration should be given to the high FRC, abundant secretions and increased airway resistance. The patient should be ventilated with a low rate, allowing a higher CO_2 and avoiding barotrauma by keeping volumes and pressures under control.

CHOICE AND USE OF VENTILATORS

In a *volume cycled ventilator*, the initial tidal volume should be set at about 10 to 12 mL/kg (normal tidal volume for a child is about 5 to 8 mL/kg) to overcome the mechanical dead space of the ventilator, the increase in dead space due to the underlying pathology, i.e. 'pathological dead space' and the compression volume of the ventilator. If the resultant inspiratory pressure exceeds 35 cmH$_2$O, 7 to 10 mL/kg would be a reasonable starting point. If the child does not have obstructive lung disease, the resultant lower minute ventilation can be compensated by increasing the respiratory rate. If mild to moderate CO$_2$ retention results, this is usually well tolerated provided the patient is not hypoxic.[18]

The objective of therapy is to provide an acceptable Pao$_2$ without using excessive pressures[19] to maintain adequate oxygen delivery to the tissues of the body. The modern day ventilators should be able to measure exhaled tidal volume, peak inspiratory and mean airway pressures, thereby being able to pick up changes in lung mechanics, acting as a safety mechanism against excessively high inspiratory pressures.

In a *pressure cycled ventilator*, the cycling mechanism is controlled by a pre-set pressure. The inspiration ends when the pressures near the mouth reach the preset value; consequently, both the lung compliance and resistance influence the tidal volume. If resistance increases or the compliance decreases, the pre-set pressure is reached before an adequate tidal volume is reached. The flow should be sufficient to achieve the desired peak inspiratory pressure.

The true test of the *effectiveness of mechanical ventilation* lies in its clinical and physiological effects on the patient. The patient must be examined immediately after placement on the ventilator for adequate and bilateral chest wall expansion. Lateral assessment of the child's thorax gives the best assessment of its excursion.

The Paco$_2$ is directly related to minute ventilation, which is determined by rate and tidal volume. Oxygenation is governed by airway pressure and Fio$_2$. As a general rule, deviation from physiological parameters for rate and inspiratory time should be avoided, although modes like inverse ratio ventilation are used in the management of intractable hypoxia due to acute lung injury. I : E ratios ranging from 2:1 to 4:1 are set on the ventilator. Improvement in oxygenation may occur by forcing open collapsed alveoli.[20]

In cases of severe obstructive airway disease, such as status asthmaticus, a ventilatory pattern characterized by a relatively short inspiratory time and prolonged expiratory time combined with low respiratory rates results in less physiological dead space and expiratory gas trapping and minimizes autoPEEP which is produced as a result of inadequate exhalation due to the obstructive lung disease.

The Paco$_2$ can be allowed to increase because if it doubles, i.e. from 40 to 80 mmHg (5.3–10.5 kPa), the pH will fall from 7.4 to 7.1. A buffer such as Tham (Tromethamine) can be administered if needed to raise the pH level and protect the heart from potential adverse effects.[21]

Mean airway pressure relates intimately to ventilation, arterial oxygenation, cardiovascular function and ventilator induced barotrauma and the use of this index should be encouraged as a guide to severity and therapy.

DRUG THERAPY

Sedation and analgesia

Any patient on a ventilator should be provided with sedation and analgesia, the degree varying depending on the clinical condition. If the patient is 'fighting' the ventilator so that co-ordination does not exist between the ventilator and the patient, the sedation and analgesia should be increased within reasonable limits to try to prevent that or alternatively, neuromuscular blockade should be used. The drugs used are usually a combination of opiate and benzodiazepine infusions.

Neuromuscular blockade

If sedation, analgesia and the selection of appropriate settings on the ventilator have failed to provide co-ordination of ventilation, control of ventilation with neuromuscular blockade may be employed to ensure adequate ventilation and minimize the likelihood of barotrauma. Neuromuscular blockade should be used with close monitoring because accidental disconnection from the ventilator or extubation could be catastrophic in these circumstances.

COMPLICATIONS OF MECHANICAL VENTILATION

Haemodynamic consequences

Increase in intra-thoracic pressure due to mechanical ventilation impedes venous return resulting in decreased cardiac filling and a decrease in cardiac output. Continuous positive pressure is also associated with a decrease in peripheral organ perfusion such as changes in corticomedullary distribution of renal perfusion. Decreased venous return from the cranial cavity is seen when a PEEP greater than 5 cmH$_2$O is used, which could then result in an increase in intra-cranial pressure which is of obvious significance in a child with a head injury.

Pulmonary side effects

Excessive airway pressure is known to affect the alveolar epithelial and pulmonary epithelial permeability.[22]

Increased transmural pressures of the extra-alveolar vessels, decreased lymphatic flow and overdistention of the alveolar epithelium may increase the permeability to protein and water which leads to pulmonary oedema in turn exacerbating the underlying lung pathology and contributing to morbidity and mortality.

Airway obstruction

Airway obstruction can result from inflammation and oedema that is the reaction of the tracheal mucosa to the foreign body, i.e. the endotracheal tube. This can be lessened by the use of appropriately sized, tissue-compatible endotracheal tubes, proper fixation and meticulous attention to the presence of a gas leak around the tube. Factors that contribute to more distal airway obstruction include disruption of the mucociliary escalator by the presence of the endotracheal tube, repeated suction causing trauma and poor humidification of inspired gases.

Infection

Trauma from the presence of the tracheal tube and suctioning manoeuvres may cause inflammation, which in turn provides a nidus of infection. In addition, because the usual barriers to micro-organisms are bypassed, the tracheal mucosa becomes colonized with Gram, negative as well as other pathologic examinations organisms. Hospital acquired (nosocomial) infections have been identified in 15.5% of patients ventilated for longer than 2 days.[23]

Barotrauma

Repetitive overexpansion of the lung can lead to structural damage and oedema (Box 17.1). Recent experimental evidence suggests that the use of high airway pressures can also cause pulmonary capillary damage similar to that seen in the early stages of ARDS and that overdistention of the lung is the important factor.[24] There is a significant incidence of barotrauma in patients with obstructive airway disease in which air trapping is common, this in turn may lead to pneumothoraces, pneumomediastinum and pulmonary interstitial emphysema. Although PEEP is useful in recruiting collapsed lung units, it can cause overdistention of relatively normal lung units thereby predisposing to air leaks.

Box 17.1: Circumstances associated with pulmonary barotrauman

- Obstruction to expiration
  - Partial obstruction (ball valve of endotracheal tube)
  - Partial obstruction of a central or peripheral airway
  - Insufficient expiratory time due to lengthy inspiratory time or excessively fast respiratory rates
- Extreme alveolar volume or pressure
- Patient–ventilator inco-ordination
- Regional differences in inspired gas distribution
  - Segmental lung collapse
  - Inadvertent endobronchial intubation.

WEANING

Criteria for withdrawal from mechanical ventilation should be based on clinical, physiological and ventilation factors. Successful weaning depends on careful consideration of the general patient status, the presence of adequate ventilatory reserve and of favourable pulmonary mechanics.

The clear superiority of one mode of weaning over another has not been demonstrated clinically. Change in respiratory rate or effort, if any, still remains one of the most important predicting factors and a subjective assessment of a weaning trial by an experienced clinician.

EXTRACORPOREAL MEMBRANE OXYGENATION (ECMO)

A complex life-support machine which uses a modified heart-lung bypass machine provides temporary respiratory support and if necessary circulatory support to patients with potentially reversible cardio-respiratory failure. It aims to take over the function of the lung and or heart, allowing time for damaged organs to recover while minimizing iatrogenic injury. ECMO requires cannulation of major blood vessels, usually the internal jugular vein and carotid artery. Venous blood is drained from the right atrium and pumped through an extra corporeal circuit consisting of an artificial membrane lung, a heat exchanger and the pump itself.[25] Blood is returned to either through the arterial circulation via a cannula placed in the carotid artery or to the venous circulation (Chapter 21, p.247).

The most conclusive evidence for the use of ECMO in neonatal respiratory failure, comes from the UK collaborative randomized trial in which 59% of the neonates allocated conventional treatment died compared with 32% of the neonates allocated ECMO.[26] This has led to an increase in the use of ECMO in paediatric patients and also following cardiac surgery. Early results are encouraging. The indications are failure of maximal conventional therapy, severe barotrauma and acute deterioration.

FUTURE DIRECTIONS

The most exciting innovation has been the advent of 'liquid ventilation'. This technique consists of instilling a liquid called perfluorocarbon (which in everyday use, acts as a refrigerator coolant), into the lungs of patients with severe lung disease. This liquid acts as a physical surfactant, allows exchange of oxygen and carbon dioxide and is also thought to have an anti-inflammatory effect.[27] The technique which is being studied in humans is called partial liquid ventilation, wherein the functional residual capacity of the diseased lungs are filled with the perfluorocarbon (30 mL/kg), mechanical ventilation is continued as previously. The perfluorocarbon evaporates over a few hours and the liquid level which is usually visible in the endotracheal tube is topped up. There are trials about to begin in adult patients.

REFERENCES

1. Albert RK. The prone position in acute respiratory distress syndrome: where we are, and where do we go from here *Crit Care Med* 1997; **25**: 1453–4.

2. Bolder PM, Healy TE, Bolder AR, Beatty PC, Kay B. The extra work of breathing through adult endotracheal tubes. *Anesth Analg* 1986; **65**: 853–9.

3. McMahon MM, Blanch P, Desautels DA. *Clinical applications of ventilatory support*. New York. Churchill Livingstone, 1990, 401–10.

4. Chao DC, Scheinhorn DJ. Weaning from mechanical ventilation. *Crit Care Clin* 1998; **14**: 799–817.

5. Hall JB, Schmidt GA, Wood LDH. *Principles of critical care*. New York; London: McGraw-Hill, 1992, Vol 1.

6. Hotchkiss JR, Marinii JJ. Non-invasive ventilation, an emerging supportive technique for the emergency department. *Ann Emerg Med* 1998; **32**: 470–9.

7. Gurevitch MJ, van Dyke J, Young ES, Jackson K. Improved oxygenation and lower peak airway pressure in severe adult respiratory distress syndrome. Treatment with inverse ratio ventilation. *Chest* 1986; **89**: 211–13.

8. Klain M, Smith RB. High frequency percutaneous transtracheal jet ventilation. *Crit Care Med* 1977; **9**: 19A.

9. Carbon GC, Ray C Jr, Mirodouni KS, Howland WS, Guy Y, Groeger JS. Physiologic implications of high-frequency jet ventilation techniques. *Crit Care Med* 1983; **11**: 508–14.

10 &11.Butler WJ, Bohn DJ, Bryan AC, Froese AB. Ventilation by high-frequency oscillation in humans. *Anesth Analg* 1980; **59**: 577–84.

12. HiFi Study Group. Randomised study of high frequency oscillatory ventilation in infants with severe respiratory distress syndrome. *J Paediat* 1993; **122**: 609.

13. Arnold JH, Truog RD, Thompson JE, Fackler JC. High frequency oscillatory ventilation in pediatric respiratory failure. *Crit Care Med* 1993; **21**: 272–8.

14. Kinnear WJ, Shneerson JM. The Newmarket pump: a new suction pump for external negative pressure ventilation. *Thorax* 1985; **40**: 677–81.

15. Libby DM, Briscoe WA, Boyce B, Smith JP. Acute respiratory failure in scoliosis or kyphosis: prolonged survival and treatment. *Am J Med* 1982; **73**: 532–8.

16. Thomson A. The role of negative pressure ventilation. *Arch Dis Child* 1997; **77**: 454–8.

17. Scano G, Gigliotti F, Duranti R, Spinelli A, Gorini M, Schiavina M. Changes in ventilatory muscle function with negative pressure ventilation in patients with severe COPD. *Chest* 1990; **97**: 322–7.

18. Reynolds EM, Ryan DP, Doody DP. Permissive hypercapnia and pressure controlled ventilation as treatment of severe adult respiratory distress syndrome in a pediatric burn patient. *Crit Care Med* 1993; **21**: 944–7.

19. Kolobow T, Moretti MP, Fumigalli R, Mascheroni D, Prato, P, Chen V, Joris M. Severe impairment in lung function induced by high peak airway pressure during mechanical ventilation. *Am Rev Respir Dis* 1987; **135**: 312.

20. Herman S, Reynolds EO. Methods for improving oxygenation in infants mechanically ventilated for severe hyaline membrane disease. *Arch Dis Child* 1973; **48**: 612–17.

21. Galvis AG. Intensive care of respiratory tract disorders. In: Bluestone CD, Stool SE. *Paediatric otolaryngology*, 3rd edn. Philadelphia: WB Saunders, 1995.

22. Parker JC, Hernandez LA, Peevy KJ. Mechanisms of ventilator induced lung injury. *Crit Care Med* 1993; **21**: 131–43.

23. Kollef MH. Ventilator-associated pneumonia: A multivariate analysis. *JAMA* 1993; **220**: 1965.

24. Dreyfuss D, Saumon G. Barotrauma is volutrauma but which volume is the one responsible? *Intensive Care Med* 1992; **18**: 139–41.

25. Goldman AP. Extracorporeal membrane oxygenation. *Care Crit Ill Child* 1999: 552–3.

26. UK Collaborative randomised trial of neonatal extracorporeal membrane oxygenation. *Lancet* 1996; **348**: 75–82

27. Heard SO, Puyana JC. The anti-inflammatory effects of perfluorocarbons: let's get physical. *Crit Care Med* 2000; **28**: 1241–2.

CHAPTER EIGHTEEN

CHEST DRAINS: INSERTION *AND* MANAGEMENT

G. G. Peck and R. K. Firmin

- Introduction
- Chest drain insertion
- Clinical situations

- Conclusion
- References
- Further reading

INTRODUCTION

Chest drain insertion is indicated in children with pleural effusion, empyema or pneumothorax. Despite its apparent simplicity however, there remains great potential for iatrogenic damage. In this chapter we describe a method of drain insertion which can be used in patients from birth to adolescence. We will discuss indications for drain insertion (drainage of air, fluid and pus), drain management and specialist referral.

CHEST DRAIN INSERTION

The key to safe and successful drain insertion is the surface anatomy (Figure 18.1). The approach described minimizes the risk to important intra-thoracic organs, and will ensure supra-diaphragmatic/intra-pleural drain insertion if used correctly. Deviation from this approach has lead to chest drain trauma to every intra-thoracic organ, and additionally to the stomach, liver and spleen.[1] It is important to remember the extension of the abdominal viscera into the bony thoracic cavity. This is accentuated in neonates where the ribs are almost horizontal, and the liver is large.

Drains should be inserted in the 5th interspace just anterior to the mid-axillary line. This corre-

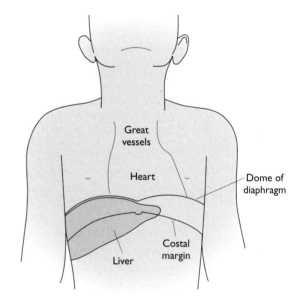

Figure 18.1: Surface anatomy.

sponds to a position just cephalad to a coronal plane through the nipple, and just posterior to the fold of the pectoralis major muscle (Figure 18.2).

INSERTION TECHNIQUE

Full aseptic technique is used. In the co-operative patient local anaesthesia may be used, but younger

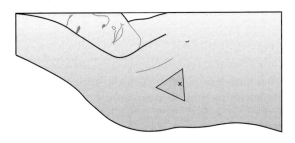

Figure 18.2: The triangle of safety.

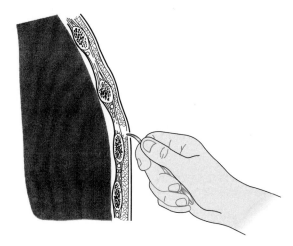

Figure 18.3: Forceps are inserted over the rib, with the curve downwards.

children may require heavier sedation or general anaesthesia. An appropriately sized drain is selected that will fit comfortably through the intercostal space. Drain sizes range from 8 F for a premature neonate up to 32 F for a large adolescent. A skin incision is made using a No.15 blade in the same direction as the intercostal space. The incision should be large enough to accommodate the drain without tension. A track is now developed through the fat and intercostal muscles to the parietal pleura by blunt dissection. This is accomplished by inserting a pair of curved artery forceps into the wound and spreading them, the forceps are then re-inserted at right angles and spread again.

Before the pleura is breached the drainage tube is readied and connected to the underwater seal. The forceps are now taken and held as shown in Figure 18.3, near the tip to prevent their sudden uncontrolled entry deep within the thorax.

The pleura is now breached by pushing the forceps over the lower rib, avoiding the intercostal bundle, using a slight twisting motion and following the curve of the instrument. A 'pop' is felt as the forceps enter the chest. The forceps are left in place and the grip is changed to the handle. The forceps are spread to enlarge the pleurotomy. The forceps are now removed and the drain is inserted through the track. In the larger patient a finger may be inserted into the pleural cavity to clear the drain track prior to insertion. Finger dissection should not be used to breach the pleura, however, as this can strip the parietal pleura off the inside of the chest wall resulting in extra-pleural but intrathoracic chest drain insertion.

The trocar should not be used to insert the drain. There are two methods that can be used to insert the drain through the track. In the first method the trocar is removed from the drain which is grasped near the end with the artery forceps. These are then pushed together into the pleural cavity, once inside the forceps are unclamped and the drain advanced. This method requires a larger wound, and is not easy to perform in smaller patients as the forceps tend to become stuck in the chest, and are difficult to withdraw past the drain.

The second method is easier and can be used in all patients. In this method the trocar is partially withdrawn from the drain (Figure 18.4) so that the sharp point does not protrude, but it still serves to stiffen the drain.

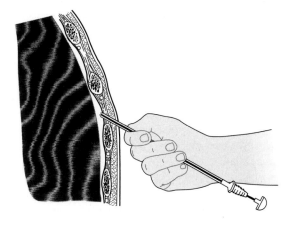

Figure 18.4: Drain with trocar pulled back gripped firmly near the end.

Having achieved entry into the pleural cavity the drain is advanced off the trocar. It is preferable to angle drains cephalic to drain air, and caudally to drain fluid. In practice drains will usually drain whatever is within the pleural cavity.

The drain is now secured with a non-absorbable suture and connected to the underwater seal. A horizontal-mattress suture can also be inserted at this time, to facilitate drain removal.

THE VENTILATED PATIENT

Positive pressure ventilation barotrauma is a common cause of pneumothorax.[2,3] Equally patients anaesthetized for drain insertion may also be receiving positive pressure ventilation. There is an important difference in the physiology of spontaneous and positive pressure ventilation. When the pleura is breached during spontaneous breathing, air enters the chest as the intra-pleural pressure is sub-atmospheric and the lung collapses. During positive pressure ventilation however, the situation is reversed. The airway pressure is positive and upon pleurotomy the lung is forced out through the wound. This is exacerbated by high PEEP. Severe lung damage can result from drain insertion in this setting.[1] It can be avoided by disconnecting the patient from the ventilator before the pleura is breached. This is especially important in hypoxic patients on high pressure ventilation. Whilst these patients can least tolerate missing one or two breaths, they are at highest risk of lung injury due to the disproportion between their airway pressures and atmospheric pressure, and they can least tolerate any chest drain injury to the lung.

CLINICAL SITUATIONS

PNEUMOTHORAX

Pneumothorax is the presence of free air within the pleural cavity. It may be spontaneous (primary) or secondary. Secondary causes include barotrauma as a result of mechanical ventilation (Case study 18.1), or asthma and direct lung injury during trauma. 'Spontaneous' pneumothoraces are also secondary, being the result of rupture of apical bullae.[2,4] Asthma is a rare cause of pneumothorax in children.[4]

Drains should be placed on 2–5 cm H_2O (0.2–0.5 kPa) of suction to keep the lung expanded. Suction should be discontinued approximately 24 to 48 hours after the drain has stopped bubbling (assuming the lung is fully re-expanded). The drain can usually be removed if there is no bubbling for 24 hours off suction, and the lung remains expanded. Under no circumstances should the chest drain ever be clamped as this can result in tension pneumothorax if there is a continuing air leak. If the air leak does not settle after several days on suction but the lung is re-expanded then conservative management can be continued. If the lung is not fully re-expanded then a further drain should be inserted and placed on suction. Additional chest drains should be placed by experienced practitioners. In ventilated patients it is sufficient to re-expand the lung and wait, usually the air leak will settle as the patient recovers and the airway pressures are reduced. In the ventilated patient who has had a protracted air leak, it is prudent to leave one drain in until extubation.

Case study 18.1: Neonatal pneumothorax

Baby Jones, a 1-day-old full-term infant was ventilated for group B-streptococcal sepsis. The oxygen saturation suddenly fell from 90% to 83%, the nurse started hand ventilation with 100% O_2, but the saturation continued to fall. At 60% the baby became bradycardic, hypotensive and poorly perfused. The ET tube was not blocked. On examination the right hemi-thorax was distended and the trachea and heart shifted to the left. Breath sounds were absent over the right lung.

The diagnosis is tension pneumothorax, radiological confirmation is not necessary and will delay the treatment required to save the baby's life. Emergency decompression should be performed by needle thoracocentesis.[5] A 21 G butterfly was inserted through the 2nd interspace in the mid-clavicular line to relieve the tension. A chest drain was then inserted using the technique described above, and connected to an underwater seal, with rapid clinical improvement.

In patients who are breathing spontaneously, a persistent air leak is more likely to indicate a broncho-pleural fistula. These patients should be discussed with a cardiothoracic surgeon if the air leak does not settle after a week of suction with full re-expansion of the lung. Again these drains should never be clamped, and the suction should never be interrupted as the lung must remain apposed to the pleura at all times if it is going to heal. A short period of partial collapse resulting from interruption of suction can destroy many days of progress.

Children with a spontaneous pneumothorax are at a higher risk of recurrence than their adult counterparts, due to a higher incidence of multiple and bilateral bullae.[2,4] They should be referred to a cardiothoracic surgeon if they have a protracted air leak, or present with a second pneumothorax.

PLEURAL EFFUSION

A pleural effusion is the presence of serous fluid within the pleural cavity. Haemothorax, or the presence of intra-pleural blood will also be discussed. The causes of pleural effusion in the antibiotic era were summarized by Alkrinawi and Chernick[6] who retrospectively examined 105 consecutive cases of pleural effusion. The mean age of patients was 7.2 years old. 61% of cases were para-pneumonic in origin. Other causes were malignancy (12.5%), renal causes (10.5%), trauma (8.5%) and miscellaneous (7.5%). Pleural effusion was 2.5 times more common in boys than girls. Of the largest group (para-pneumonic effusion) a pathogen was identified in 59%. This was bacterial in 84%, *Haemophilus influenzae* type B and *Staphylococcus aureus* being the two most common organisms. A viral pneumonia was the cause in 13%, and *Candida* in the remainder. This study also examined the biochemistry of the pleural fluid. There was no correlation between exudate, transudate and aetiology as often described in adults.[7]

Over two-thirds of para-pneumonic effusions can be managed by thoracocentesis alone, but the remainder require intercostal drainage[6] (Case study 18.2). Ultrasound of the chest may help to localize and quantify fluid and guide drainage.[8–10] Suction is not usually needed. Drains should be left in until they are dry or very nearly. This is especially true of post-operative chylothorax.[11]

When inserting drains for traumatic haemothorax large drains should be used to prevent them becoming obstructed by clot; 2–5 cm H_2O 0.2–0.5 kPa) of suction is also used. Old blood becomes de-fibrinated and will not clot and block the drain. However fresh haemorrhage, especially if profuse, retains normal coagulation. If bleeding is severe, accompanied by haemodynamic instability or does not settle then cardiothoracic surgical advice should be sought urgently.[5] Surgery may also be needed to remove large un-drained clots (clotted haemothorax) as these can act as a focus for infection and fibrosis. Again ultrasound is useful.

EMPYEMA

Empyema is still an important problem, despite the increasing use of antibiotics. It is the end result of para-pneumonic pleural effusion. Bacteria multiply in the effusion and pus is formed. Eventually an abcess forms with a fibrinous rim which encases the lung and restricts the parietal pleura. The latter condition is an indication for surgical

---

Case study 18.2: A parapneumonic effusion

Steve, a 5-year-old boy, presented with a 4-day history of left upper abdominal pain, fever and malaise. Examination of the abdomen was unremarkable, but the left chest was stony dull to percussion at the base with decreased breath sounds. Chest X-ray revealed a pleural effusion which was aspirated using a 20 G intra-venous cannula introduced below the upper limit of dullness to percussion posteriorly in the mid-scapular line. The haemo-serous fluid was sent for culture and cytology. Following aspiration an underlying pneumonia in the left lower lobe was evident. He was started on intra-venous cefuroxime and initially improved. Two days later the effusion had re-accumulated. A chest drain was inserted in the triangle of safety under general anaesthesia to evacuate the effusion. The drainage gradually decreased after the first 3 days and ceased completely after 7 days. The drain was removed on day 8. Pleural fluid grew *Staphylococcus aureus*.

intervention.[12,13] Early empyema will usually resolve if completely drained,[14] in conjunction with appropriate antibiotics.

The most common organisms are *Streptococcus pneumoniae* and *Staphylococcus aureus*.[12]

Drains for empyema rarely have to be placed on suction. The patient in Case study 18.3 had pus within the pleura but had not formed an abcess cavity, and resolution was therefore rapid and complete. Some patients with very early empyema can be managed by aspiration and antibiotics alone, however if any residual pus is left within the chest a drain should be inserted. Ultrasound can help to determine the presence, location and amount of any residual pus. If loculated empyema is demonstrated then each locule should be drained independently, this is an indication for specialist referral. Multi-loculated empyema (i.e > 2) is an indication for surgery, which can often be minimally invasive. Thoracoscopy,[15] mini-thoracotomy[16] or urokinase instillation[17] are useful if patients are referred early, avoiding postero-lateral thoracotomy.

Patients with severe empyema (defined by; pleural fluid pH < 7.2, glucose < 2.2 mmol/L scoliosis >10 degrees), evidence of lung entrapment or pleural thickening or presence of anaerobic organisms, require surgery to decorticate the pleural abcess. In these patients early operation reduces hospitalization from a mean of 12.4 days to 4.4 days, ($p < 0.001$).[12] Surgery should also be considered in patients who have not improved following a week of conservative treatment.

An intermediate group of patients develop a small abcess cavity focused around the drain site. These cavities do not communicate with the pleural space, and do not cause lung entrapment. However they do require prolonged tube drainage, often for several weeks, and will not resolve if the drain is left static. In these patients the drain is withdrawn a few centimetres every 4–5 days. Since the cavity does not communicate with the pleural space underwater seal drainage is not required, and drains can be cut off approximately 5 cm from the skin, transfixed with a safety pin and covered with a gauze dressing. This allows mobilization and play, and in some patients outpatient treatment. This type of empyema should be managed by a specialist.

CONCLUSION

In this chapter we have given a framework which should allow the generalist to manage the majority of children with air or fluid within the chest safely. We have also highlighted areas where early referral for specialist opinion and intervention is necessary in order to hasten recovery and limit morbidity.

REFERENCES

1. Peek GJ, Firmin RK, Arsiwala S. Chest tube insertion in the ventilated patient. *Injury* 1995; **26**: 425–6.

2. Poenaru D, Yazbeck S, Murphy S. Primary spontaneous pneumothorax in children. *J Pediat Surg* 1994; **29**: 1183–5.

3. Pollack MM, Fields AI, Holbrook PR. Pneumothorax and pneumomediastinum during pediatric mechanical ventilation. *Crit Care Med* 1979; **7**: 536–9.

Case study 18.3: Empyema

Zara, a 6-year-old girl, was referred with a 2-week history of malaise, cough with purulent sputum and fever which had been treated with oral amoxicillin. On examination there was tenderness, reduced respiratory excursion, dullness to percussion and reduced breath sounds over the right lower chest. Chest radiography revealed opacification of the right base, no pleural thickening and no scoliosis. Thoracocentesis was performed and thick pus was obtained. Pus was sent for culture and biochemical analysis; pH was 7.2 and glucose was 2.7 mmol/L. In view of the thickness of the pus, duration of the illness and low pH of the aspirated pus, a chest drain was inserted via the triangle of safety, under general anaesthesia. The empyema was completely evacuated over the following 7 days, and no loculi were demonstrated on ultrasound scan. She was treated with intravenous ceftriaxone; the pus eventually grew *Staphylococcus aureus* sensitive to ceftriaxone. Her fever settled rapidly after drainage of the empyema. The drain was finally removed after 9 days.

4. Davis AM, Wensley DF, Phelan PD. Spontaneous pneumothorax in paediatric patients. *Respir Med* 1993; **87**: 531–4.

5. Anonymous. *Advanced paediatric life support: The practical approach.* London: Advanced Life Support Group (BMJ Publishing), 1997.

6. Alkrinawi S, Chernick V. Pleural fluid in hospitalized pediatric patients. *Clin Pediat* 1996; **35**: 5–9.

7. Light RW, MacGregor MI, Luchsinger PC, Ball WCJ. Pleural effusions: the diagnostic separation of transudates and exudates. *Ann Intern Med* 1972; **77**: 507–13.

8. van Sonnenberg E, Nakamoto SK, Mueller PR, *et al.* CT- and ultrasound-guided catheter drainage of empyemas after chest-tube failure. *Radiology* 1984; **151**: 349–53.

9. Reither M. [Thoracic sonography in childhood]. [German]. *Radiologe* 1983; **23**: 49–52.

10. Hirsch JH, Carter SJ, Chikos PM, Colacurcio C. Ultrasonic evaluation of radiographic opacities of the chest. *AJR Am J Roentgenol* 1978; **130**: 1153–6.

11. Bond SJ, Guzzetta PC, Snyder ML, Randolph JG. Management of pediatric postoperative chylothorax. *Ann Thorac Surg* 1993; **56**: 469–72.

12. Hoff SJ, Neblett WW, Edwards KM, *et al.* Parapneumonic empyema in children: decortication hastens recovery in patients with severe pleural infections. *Pediat Infect Dis J* 1991; **10**: 194–9.

13. Khakoo GA, Goldstraw P, Hansell DM, Bush A. Surgical treatment of parapneumonic empyema. *Pediatr Pulmonol* 1996; **22**: 348–56.

14. Chan W, Keyser-Gauvin E, Davis GM, Nguyen LT, Laberge JM. Empyema thoracis in children: a 26-year review of the Montreal Children's Hospital experience. *J Pediat Surg* 1997; **32**: 870–2.

15. Kern JA, Rodgers BM. Thoracoscopy in the management of empyema in children. *J Pediat Surg* 1993; **28**: 1128–32.

16. Raffensperger JG, Luck SR, Shkolnik A, Ricketts RR. Mini-thoracotomy and chest tube insertion for children with empyema. *J Thorac Cardiovasc Surg* 1982; **84**: 497–504.

17. Handman HP, Reuman PD. The use of urokinase for loculated thoracic empyema in children: a case report and review of the literature. *Pediat Infect Dis J* 1993; **12**: 958–9.

FURTHER READING

1. *Advanced trauma life support course for physicians.* Chicago: American College of Surgeons, 1993.

2. *Glenn's thoracic and cardiovascular surgery.* Englewood Cliffs, New Jersey: Prentice-Hall, 1991.

3. Williams PL, Warwick R, Dyson M, Bannister LH (eds). *Gray's anatomy:* London: Churchill Livingstone, 1989; 661–858.

CHAPTER NINETEEN

TRACHEOSTOMY

C. O'Callaghan, A. Moir and H. Dunbar

- Introduction
- Tracheostomy technique
- Care of a child with a tracheostomy
- General activities
- Chest physiotherapy

- Long-term tracheostomy children
- Complications
- Acknowledgements
- References

INTRODUCTION

A tracheostomy is an artificial airway inserted surgically into the cervical trachea. The words tracheostomy and tracheotomy are used interchangeably though the latter refers to the surgical placement of the tracheostomy tube. The primary indication for a tracheostomy is to maintain a long-term artificial airway. The indications for a tracheostomy are listed in Table 19.1.

In this chapter we cover the technique of performing a tracheostomy, the care of a child with a tracheostomy and complications associated with their use.

TRACHEOSTOMY TECHNIQUE

The infant should be given a general anaesthetic in an operating theatre, with instrumentation of an appropriate size and a range of neonatal and paediatric 'plastic' tubes.

If at all possible, oral tracheal intubation to secure an airway should be performed, by an anaesthetist with paediatric experience.

Tracheostomy technique is important. Excision of a window of trachea from the anterior wall or creating a stellate incision, cutting the tracheal rings above and below and excising laterally to

Table 19.1: Tracheostomy may be required in the following situations

> **Upper airway obstruction**
> due to:
> 1 Laryngeal or pharyngeal cysts which cannot be removed to establish the airway.
> 2 Micrognathia or macroglossia.
> 3 Bilateral vocal cord paralysis.
> 4 Subglottic stenosis, now primary resection is preferable if the skill and resources are available.
> 5 Laryngeal oedema after burns.
>
> **Other conditions which may be treated by tracheostomy are:**
> 1 Epiglottitis.
> 2 Retropharyngeal abscess.
> 3 Facial or laryngeal trauma.
>
> However, oral/nasal endotracheal intubation by a skilled anaesthetist or paediatric intensivist and treatment of the underlying obstruction is now preferable.
>
> **Prolonged intubation:**
> - Bronchopulmonary dysplasia
> - Guillan–Barré syndrome
> - Coma with respiratory depression
> - Respiratory distress syndrome
> - Pulmonary toilet
> - Chronic aspiration
> - Neuromuscular diseases.

enlarge the opening in the trachea are no longer recommended. These techniques resulted in lack of anterior support of the tracheal wall and difficulties with decannulation. A standard operative technique for tracheostomy in infants and young children that has been developed is described below.[1, 2.]

There is a substantial advantage to visualize the larynx and trachea with a ventilating bronchoscope before intubation. This must only be done by an experienced endoscopic team. The infant is placed on the operating table with his/her head extended. A mechanism for warming the torso and head is essential for younger patients. A transverse skin crease incision is made, approximately half way between the cricoid cartilage and suprasternal notch. Subcutaneous fat is removed, the strap muscles parted in the midline, and the thyroid isthmus retracted to expose the anterior tracheal wall. A Proline stay suture is placed on either side of the midline, and tied in a long loop. The size of the tracheostomy tube is gauged, the anaesthetic connection checked and then a vertical incision is made through three to four trachea rings. Traction on the stay sutures will allow good visualization of the tracheal lumen (Figure 19.1), facilitating withdrawal of the endotracheal tube and insertion of the tracheostomy tube. The child is ventilated through the tracheostomy, the skin incision loosely closed and the tracheostomy tube secured with tapes and sutured to the skin. The stay sutures are taped to the appropriate side of the anterior chest wall with Mefix tape. The child should ideally be cared for by experienced paediatric nurses in the paediatric ITU for 24 hours. Humidification is essential, preferably warmed. In Leicester our policy is that children spend the first 48 hours in PICU. Practice varies in different localities depending on services available on the ward areas. The first tube change should be on the 5th to 7th post-operative day. We recommend that the first tube change is performed by ENT medical staff and thereafter by competent trained nurses/carers.

Every possible precaution should be taken to avoid accidental displacement of the tracheostomy tube in the first week. If this happens, oral endotracheal intubation may be the best way to establish the airway unless there is immediate expertise available in the retraction and manipulation of the stay suture to facilitate placement of the tracheostomy tube. Tracheal dilators are kept by the bedside for this purpose, but are only used by medical staff with experience. A tracheostomy tube one size smaller than usual is also kept by the bedside for emergency use if the insertion of the same size tube is not achieved after accidental decannulation. The child also is discharged home with a spare tube, one size smaller, in case parents are unable to reinsert the child's usual tube following accidental decannulation.

If accidental decannulation occurs and attempts to replace the original sized tube or one smaller has failed, then try the following: cut off the end of a suction catheter passed down into the stoma, is used to guide the tracheostomy tube along the catheter into the stoma. If this is also unsuccessful then ventilation can be achieved via the catheter or via mouth/nose to mouth or mouth to mouth dependent on the age of the child. It is important to combine this 'railroad' technique with a pulling up and out action of the stay sutures.

The replacement of metal tracheostomy tubes, that often caused secondary trauma, has reduced the incidence of post-tracheostomy stenosis. Excellent soft silicon rubber or polyvinyl tubes are now available with appropriate shapes for the anatomy of different sized tracheas.[3, 4, 5.] Using a standard protocol of home management following appropriate instruction and input, there should be a low incidence of complications. Post-tracheostomy stenosis should now be an uncommon problem.[6]

Extubation should be attempted as soon as the primary disease process has abated and the airway has been carefully evaluated from above by bronchoscopy. Unless the tracheostomy has been in place for longer than 2 weeks, the tracheostomy opening will usually close spontaneously within 48–72 hours after removal of the tube.[6]

Tracheal injuries in infants and children often result from iatrogenic causes. Intubation stenoses still occur although, with modern neonatal intensive care, these have reduced in number. Another major cause of tracheal stenosis requiring reconstructive procedures is an improperly performed tracheostomy.[7, 8, 9]

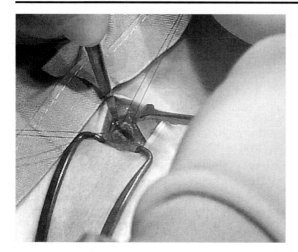

Figure 19.1: Photograph showing the midline incision through the tracheal rings with the stay sutures in place. The endotracheal tube is then withdrawn and the tracheostomy tube is inserted.

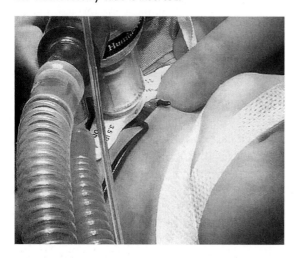

Figure 19.2: The tracheostomy tube has been inserted and the infant is now ventilated via the tube.

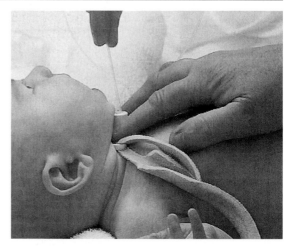

Figure 19.3: Suctioning of the tracheostomy tube immediately prior to the first tube change.

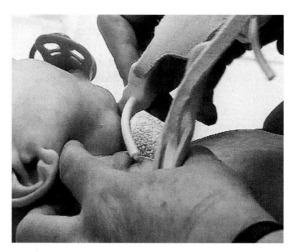

Figure 19.4: The tracheostomy tube has been removed and the new tube is about to be inserted. Note the tip of the obturator that is removed immediately after insertion of the tracheostomy tube, poking from the end of the tube.

CARE OF A CHILD WITH A TRACHEOSTOMY

A respiratory nurse specializing in the care of tracheostomies is essential, in association with medical staff, in the training of parents in tracheostomy care. Parents must be made familiar with the tracheostomy tube and also have a basic understanding of the anatomy and physiology of the upper airway and lungs. The use of a model is a great help. Before a child is discharged home it is our policy that two adult carers have been assessed and are competent in all areas of the care for the child. We use an educational programme (Table 19.2) to achieve this. Any other carers can be trained at home after the child has been discharged.

SUCTIONING

Suctioning is required only when necessary on the basis of clinical assessment when secretions are

Table 19.2: Education checklist for parents

> **You will be able to:**
> 1 Identify when to use suction.
> 2 Take care of the stoma.
> 3 Draw up saline and correctly put some saline into the tube.
> 4 Know how to use and care for the suction machine.
> 5 Select an appropriate size suction catheter.
> 6 Know the correct length of suction catheter to pass and how to apply suction.
> 7 Change the tracheostomy tapes.
> 8 Change the tracheostomy tube.
> 9 Use back-up suction facilities.
> 10 Recognize when the tracheostomy is partially or fully blocked.
> 11 Carry out resuscitation.

noted in the tracheostomy tube (heard within the tube) or when the child shows signs of respiratory distress.[10, 11] In children with no evidence of secretions, a minimum of suctioning, in the morning and at bedtime, to check patency of the tube is recommended (ATS guidelines).[18] If unable to pass the catheter down the tube, the tracheostomy tube should be changed and other causes of respiratory distress should be looked for, for example lower respiratory tract infection.

Parents are taught suction using a clean technique, suctioning to a pre-measured length into the tracheostomy tube. In Leicester measurement is achieved following a chart kept by the child's bed where exact measurements of length of tube, connector and 5 mm beyond the end of the tracheostomy tube have been calculated and the catheter is passed down this length. In other areas graduated catheters may be used. The suction procedure should not take longer than 10 seconds with suction applied on withdrawal of the catheter only. For neonates 10 seconds may be too long and 5–6 seconds may be more appropriate. However the ATS consensus statement[18] advocates a rapid technique completed in less than 5 seconds where suction is applied both while inserting and removing the catheter. Our experience suggests that use of a rapid technique increases the likelihood of having to repeat the procedure with the potential side effects due to this.

Each child is different and the need for suctioning must be assessed individually, dependent on clinical condition i.e. any changes in colour or consistency of secretions. If suctioning is being used more than that assessed as normal for a child then advice should be sought from a respiratory/tracheostomy nurse or paediatrician. Education about suctioning is often all that is required.

Normal saline instillation has been considered useful in achieving a cough or loosening secretions to aid the suctioning procedure. In Leicester no more than 2 mL of normal (0.9%) saline is used for any one suctioning episode. This is however, also age related, usually < 0.5 mL in a child under 5 years and 1 mL in a child 5–15 years with each suction attempt.[12,13] Nebulization of normal saline has also proved effective in the loosening of secretions in the immediate post-operative period. However the existing evidence does not support the use of normal saline instillation as being beneficial in removing secretions.[14]

Different types of suction catheters are used in different areas. Catheters vary in the types of suction holes they have, i.e. whether they are found distally, laterally or both on the suction catheter. This has implications for the distance to which the catheter needs to be passed beyond the tracheostomy tube. For example, a lateral hole catheter has to be passed 6 mm beyond the end of the tube to allow the lateral holes on the catheter to be effective. Whilst suctioning it is important that the catheter is put straight in and out of the tube and that there is no twisting or rotating of the catheter. This prevents potential complications involving the delicate tracheal epithelium.[17]

Suction pressures of 60–80 cm H_2O for neonates and 100–120 cm H_2O or equivalent are used for children.[10,11] Incorrect use of pressure can be directly related to the amount of tracheal damage. If pressure is too low clearing the child's airway will be ineffective. If pressure is too high it may cause atelectasis and mucosal damage.[15, 16]

A technique advocated in America, which requires more tuition but may have an advantage when the primary indication for the tracheostomy is pathology in the lower respiratory tract, is outlined below:

1 Give the child 4 or 5 breaths with a breathing bag (Ambubag).

2 Put a few drops of saline solution into the tracheostomy.

3 Use breathing bag to push both air and saline into the tracheostomy.

4 With left hand, carefully insert catheter 2 to 3 inches into tracheostomy tube or until child begins to cough.

5 Cover the suction port of the suction tube with thumb, sucking the secretions from the tracheostomy. Do not suck for more than 6 to 8 seconds as the child cannot get air whilst being suctioned. Remove the catheter.

6 Give the child a further 4–5 breaths with the breathing bag.

7 Allow the child to rest for 1 minute. If he or she continues to have secretions the procedure may be repeated until the tracheostomy is clear.

In general in the UK we do not advocate deep suctioning due to the potential complications that can occur especially to the carina. If the above technique is used, we would suggest using it only with ventilated patients and not those that are spontaneously breathing.

CLEANING THE TRACHEOSTOMY SITE

The post-operative tracheostomy site is an open wound that produces a serous discharge. The surrounding skin may be protected with a barrier cream such as zinc and castor oil. If *Staphylococcus aureus* colonization of the wound is a problem, topical antibiotics, with a steroid base are useful to eradicate the infection and inflammation. We suggest Terracortril (hydrocortisone and oxytetra-cycline) or mupirocin cream are used to treat the granulation externally. We have had positive results from the use of Terracortril cream used four times a day. Otherwise the granulation tissue is best treated with silver nitrate cautery. This technique is shown to the parents and can be repeated 1–2 times weekly until the granulation disappears. Some use silver nitrate as a first choice if the granulation is obstructive. If this is unsuccessful they may use triameinolone paste. When established the tracheostomy tract is a keratin lined fistula between the skin of the neck and the anterior tracheal wall. It is clean and secretion free unless there is inflammation in the respiratory tract.

The tracheostomy tube is held in position either by 1.25 cm cotton tape or a ready-made Velcro, felt tape. The latter is more comfortable and very easy to change; however there are some concerns that small children may pull the Velcro ties apart, leading to accidental decannulation. A common rule regarding the tightness of the tapes is that they should be tight enough to slip one finger beneath the tie. Tapes are changed when they become dirty, and are usually washed on a daily basis.

HUMIDITY

As the child no longer breathes through their nose, humidification of the inspired air is required. In the post-operative period, humidity is essential and is provided by a nebulizer or humidifier attached to a ventilator. We use warm humidification given via a Blease mixer and Fisher Paykel humidifier for approximately 48 hours post-operatively. Oxygen and air are titrated through the Blease mixer to keep saturations above 93%. Warm humidification, with or without oxygen, is maintained for 5–7 days. If oxygen is required after this time it is administered via an Aquapak and tracheostomy mask or humidifying barrel and oxygen attachment. Saline (0.9%) nebulizers are prescribed on an as required basis for the first week.

Warm humidification is gradually weaned and replaced with the use of frequent saline nebulizers and the use of a humidifying barrel (HME) 'artificial nose'. In the long-term humidity is reduced as much as the lower respiratory tract will allow. However, humidity is required at night particularly in the small infant, when secretions in a small lumen will appreciably increase the resistance to airflow. It is important that the correct type of HME is used dependent on the tidal volume of the child.

HOME EQUIPMENT CHECK LIST

- Mains powered suction unit, usually a Sam 12 unit.
- Portable suction unit with battery recharger.

- Suction catheters.
- Suction tubing.
- Tracheostomy tubes same size plus one of smaller size.
- Tracheostomy tube holders.
- Filter and humidifier barrel.
- Bronchoscopy mucous extractor for specimen collection and as back-up suction.
- Saline and syringes.

If nebulizer equipment is necessary then the child will be sent home with a portable nebulizer and relevant supplies.

If a child requires additional oxygen therapy and humidification, this will be supplied.

GENERAL ACTIVITIES

Infants and children should be allowed to undertake the same activities as their contemporaries but swimming is out. Children may take a bath or a shower. Care should be taken not to get water into the tracheostomy. If it does get in, suctioning of the tracheostomy may be needed. Avoid areas where there is heavy dust or pollen.

CHEST PHYSIOTHERAPY

General chest physiotherapy may be taught to parents when appropriate. It is not, however, a routine requirement.

LONG-TERM TRACHEOSTOMY CHILDREN

Small infants are usually looked after by their parents and close relatives, but older children become more independent and go to nursery or school. There must be a helper at the nursery or school trained to change the tracheostomy tube, administer suction and be fully aware of his or her responsibility.

The tracheostomy tube size must be increased to keep pace with the child's growth. At some point it may be possible to provide the child with a one-way, speaking valve on the tracheostomy tube. The child may breathe in through the tube, but forces expired air through the glottis thus facilitating phonation. Improved clearance of secretions may also be achieved. Some children with severe broncho- or tracheomalacia may benefit from the increased expiratory resistance provided by the speaking valve. The use of speaking valves must first be assessed by a speech therapist and nurse specialist trained in dealing with children with tracheostomies, as not all children can tolerate their use.

It is sensible to examine the airway with a bronchoscope at regular intervals to assess for complications and to evaluate the appropriate timing for decannulation.

Only a small percentage of children develop a persistent tracheocutaneous fistula that requires surgical closure. Very occasionally laryngeal or tracheal reconstruction is required before decannulation is successful.

COMPLICATIONS

Complications relating to a tracheostomy are listed in Table 19.3.

INFECTIONS

Concerns should be discussed with the specialist tracheostomy nurse or with medical staff.

Parents are taught to recognize and treat tracheostomy site infections and infections of the upper and lower respiratory tract. Erythema and drainage of the tracheostomy site are treated by increasing the frequency of tracheostomy site care to three times a day for 3 days. With persistent infection, parents are instructed to apply an antibiotic ointment containing neomycin, polymyxin or bacitracin to the site after cleansing.

With an upper respiratory tract infection, parents are instructed to provide prolonged periods of humidification to the tracheostomy hoping to keep secretions thin. More cleaning around the tracheostomy site may be required.

If an infection advances to the lower respiratory tract, medical staff should be notified and culture obtained. Signs suggesting a lower respiratory tract infection include changing colour of

Table 19.3: Complications of a tracheostomy

Early complications:
Haemorrhage
Accidental decannulation
Pneumomediastinum
Pneumothorax
Subcutaneous emphysema
Mucus plugging
Tracheitis
Chondritis of tracheal cartilage ring
Mediastinitis
Dysphagia
Aspiration
Pulmonary oedema

Delayed complications:
Granulation tissue in lumen or at stoma
Stoma stenosis
Tracheo-innominate artery fistula
    (Rare–not seen with plastic tracheostomy tubes)
Mucus plugging
Tracheitis
Tracheal stenosis
Tracheo-oesophageal fistula
Scar after decannulation
Dysphagia
Aspiration

the child's secretions to yellow or green, the onset of a fever or respiratory distress. Antibiotics are prescribed if there is any concern.

Chest physiotherapy should be instigated every 4 hours. Suction after chest physiotherapy should be done if needed. The tracheostomy site care should be twice daily, as needed, and humidity to the tracheostomy should be provided at all times.

BLEEDING FROM THE TRACHEOSTOMY

Parents are instructed that very slight bleeding, less than half a teaspoonful of blood, is probably due to irritation in the trachea, possibly from ambitious suctioning, excessive coughing or infection. Treatment includes regular use of saline during suctioning and increased humidity. In cold weather, with less humid air, drying of the tracheal epithelium may promote occasional bleeding. The tracheostomy nurse specialist should be contacted.

After the tracheostomy tract is healed, one rare but very severe complication is that of a tracheo-innominate artery fistula. While granulation tissue within the tract is usually the source of bleeding, granulation tissue on the anterior wall of the trachea suggests the possibility of such a fistula. Rupture of a tracheo-innominate fistula causes profuse and often fatal bleeding. It may be possible to control the bleeding temporarily by placing a cuffed endotracheal tube through the tracheostomy site and inflating the cuff in the hope that the pressure will prevent further bleeding. Thoracotomy and ligation of the innominate artery are then performed.

RESPIRATORY DISTRESS

Parents are taught the signs and symptoms of respiratory distress. Treatment includes suctioning using a clean technique with insertion of saline. If respiratory distress is not alleviated or if insertion of a catheter for suctioning is impossible, the tube is probably obstructed with a mucous plug. The parent should change the tracheostomy tube. Parents practice with a model first but should have changed the tracheostomy tube prior to going home. At least two extra tracheostomy tubes of the same size and one a size smaller, in case the stoma closes and will not accept the original tube, should be kept with the child at all times. If the child has a soft silicon tube, an extra tube with an obturator may be needed. Tracheal dilators are often mentioned in large texts. There are now three sizes available in the UK that can be used in all age ranges of children, but again we would stress that they are used with extreme caution and in experienced hands only.

ACKNOWLEDGEMENTS

We would like to thank Joanne Cooke, Tracheostomy Nurse Specialist, Hospitals for Sick Children, Great Ormond Street, London, for her helpful comments and suggestions on this chapter.

REFERENCES

1. McLaughlin J, Iserson KV. Emergency pediatric tracheostomy: A usable technique and model for instruction. *Ann Emerg Med* 1986; **15**: 463–5.

2. Miller JD, Kapp JP. Complications of tracheostomies in neurosurgical patients. *Surg Neurol* 1984; **22**: 186–8.

3. Aberdeen E, Downes JJ. Artificial airways in children. *Surg Clin North Am* 1974; **54**: 1155–70.

4. Galvis AG. Custom-made cuffed tracheostomy tubes for infants and small children. *Crit Care Med* 1986; **14**: 261.

5. Haller JA, Talbert JL. Clinical evaluation of a new silastic tracheostomy tube. *Ann Surg* 1970; 171–215.

6. Wetmore RF, Handler FD, Potsic WP. Pediatric tracheostomy. Experience during the past decade. *Ann Otol Rhinol Laryngol* 1982; **91**: 628–32.

7. Lynn HB, Van Heerden JA. Tracheostomy in infants. *Surg Clin North Am* 1973; **53**: 945–52.

8. Price DG. Techniques of tracheostomy for intensive care unit patients. *Anaesthesia* 1983; **38**: 902–4.

9. Tepas JJ. Tracheostomy in infants and children. *Ear Nose Throat J* 1983; **62**: 484–8.

10. Young CS. Recommended guidelines for suction. *Physiotherapy* 1984; **70**: 106–8.

11. Hodge D. Endotracheal suctioning and the infant: a nursing care protocol to decrease complications. *Neonatal Netw* 1991; **9**: 7–15.

12. Beeram MR, Dhanireddy R. Effects of saline instillation during tracheal suction on lung mechanics in newborn infants. *J Perinatol* 1992; **12**: 120–3.

13. Swartz K, Noonan DM, Edwards-Beckett J. A national survey of endotracheal suctioning techniques in the pediatric population. *Heart Lung* 1996; **25**: 52–60.

14. Blackwood B. Normal saline instillation with endotracheal suctioning: primum non nocere (first do no harm). *J Adv Nurs* 1999; **29**: 928–34.

15. Serra A, Bauley CM, Jackson P. *Ear, nose and throat nursing*. Oxford: Blackwell Scientific, 1986.

16. Shekleton ME, Nield M. Ineffective airway clearance related to artificial airway. *Nurs Clin North Am* 1987; **22**: 167–78.

17. Knox AM. Performing endotracheal suction on children: a literature review and implications for nursing practice. *Intensive Crit Care Nurs* 1993; **9**: 48–54.

18. American Thoracic Society, ATS 1999. Care of the child with a chronic tracheostomy. *Am J Respir Crit Care Med* 2000; **161**: 297–308.

CHAPTER TWENTY

ADMINISTERING TREATMENT — INHALED THERAPY

P. Barry

- Background
- Factors affecting drug delivery
- How to deliver drugs
- Assessing inhalation devices
- Assessing the published evidence
- Evaluating outcome
- Planning management
- Clinical research issues
- References
- Further reading

BACKGROUND

The aim of inhalational drug delivery is to deliver an appropriate amount of drug to the correct site of action in the lungs, with minimal overspill to other sites, in a reproducible, rapid and cost effective manner that is acceptable to the patient. The potential for drug administration by the inhaled route is great (Table 20.1), but this review will consider only those drugs which are used to manage respiratory disease.

The inhalational route has many advantages in the treatment of diseases of the respiratory tract. Medication may be delivered directly to its site of action, giving a faster onset of action and allowing lower doses of drug to be administered. Systematic absorption of drug is diminished, reducing

Table 20.1: Some indications and medications proposed for inhalational delivery

Asthma and chronic obstructive airways disease Bronchodilation: β_2 agonists, anticholinergics Prophylactic therapy: corticosteroids, cromoglycate Emergency treatment of acute asthma	**Treatment of hyperkalaemia:** Nebulized salbutamol (albuterol) **Immunization:** Measles vaccination

Cystic fibrosis
 Prevention/treatment of infection: inhaled antibiotics
 Reduction of sputum viscosity: DNAse
 Secretion hydration: amiloride
 Protease inhibition: α-1-antitrypsin
 Gene therapy: via liposomes or viruses
	Treatment of croup
	 Reduction of oedema:
	   – nebulized adrenaline (epinephrine)
	   – nebulized steroids
	
	 Inhalational drug delivery on intensive care
	 Treatment of bronchiolitis: ribavirin
	 Adult respiratory distress syndrome: surfactant
	 Prostacyclin, NO related vasodilators

Immune deficiency
 Prevention of *Pneumocystis carinii* pneumonia:
   Inhaled pentamidine
 	
 Dyspnoea: Inhaled opiates
	Pulmonary hypertension: nitroprusside, magnesium
	   sulphate
	 Bronchopulmonary dysplasia: corticosteroids

systemic side effects of the medication. However, the respiratory tract has a number of features that are designed to prevent particulate matter from entering the lungs, and inhalational therapy, especially for children who are unable or unwilling to co-operate, is difficult, variable and inefficient.

The costs of respiratory disease relate both to the direct costs of drugs and devices, the costs of hospitalization and medical care, and also to the indirect costs of loss of work and schooling, and the psychosocial effects of disease. Asthma drugs and devices account for 30–50% of the direct costs of asthma care. The price of different drug delivery devices varies greatly, and bears no relation to efficacy.

A large volume spacer and metered dose inhaler (MDI) is cheaper than a nebulizer, especially when capital costs are taken into account. In several studies MDI generated aerosols have been 50–75% less expensive than equivalent nebulizer therapy, including the cost of health professionals' time.

Cost comparisons in the past have not taken compliance into account. Patients seldom take all their medication as prescribed, with underuse of prescribed medications occurring approximately 50% of the time. Although there is no evidence that compliance is improved by changing to a different inhaler device, small, unobtrusive devices are often marketed on the basis that they are more acceptable to the patient, and will therefore be used more. There is increasing interest in drug delivery devices that can both monitor and prompt patient use. These devices are likely to prove more expensive, and the cost-benefit of using such devices (if indeed they do improve compliance and drug delivery) is unclear.

The drug treatment regimen for the majority of patients with asthma is straightforward and is documented in guidelines such as those produced by the British Thoracic Society.[1] The choice of drug delivery device is less clear. Clinicians and patients are frequently confused by the ever-increasing choice. For example, if a child with asthma, on prophylactic steroids, is seen in casualty, there is one chance in 125 of guessing the correct combination of inhalational device, drug and formulation that the child is using!

Close professional colleagues often choose different drug delivery devices for their patients. Confusion amongst junior medical and nursing staff as to which device and which strength of which inhaler has been prescribed is not uncommon. One can certainly sympathize with the problems of nursery staff and schoolteachers faced with a cupboard full of different inhalers. Asthma treatment may be improved by restricting the range of drug delivery devices used in any area. This approach may allow us to devote more time to counselling patients and focusing on compliance.

FACTORS AFFECTING DRUG DELIVERY

Effective drug delivery is dependent on a complex interplay of factors including the drug, the delivery device and the patient.

PARTICLE SIZE

The deposition characteristics of an aerosol in the airway depend largely on the particle or droplet size. Generally the smaller the particle the greater its chance of peripheral penetration and retention (Box 20.1; Figure 20.1).

Inhaled particles deposit in the body by five different mechanisms (Table 20.2), of which inertial impaction, sedimentation and diffusion are the most important. Interception and electrostatic attraction are less significant.

Box 20.1: Size and fate of inhaled particles

- Inhaled particles larger than 10 μm in diameter deposit mainly in the oropharynx.
- Particles between 5 and 10 μm show a transition from mouth to airway deposition.
- Particles smaller than 5 μm are more likely to be deposited in the lung, with a smaller particle size favouring more peripheral deposition, especially in patients with bronchoconstriction and in children.
- Particles smaller than 1 μm may be exhaled without depositing in the lung.
- Particles in the range 1–5 μm are often accepted as optimal for inhalational therapy, but these values are not universally accepted.

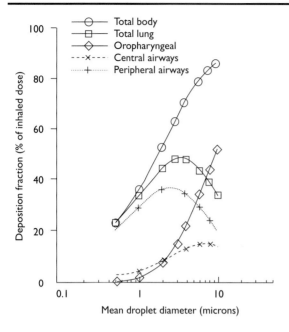

Figure 20.1 Effect of particle size on deposition in the airway (from Rudolph[2]).

PATIENT FEATURES (BOX 20.2)

Breathing pattern

Breathing pattern affects particle deposition in the airway. Fast inspiration encourages inertial impaction of drug in the upper airways and more central deposition. For instance, fast inspiration increases the threshold levels of response in bronchial provocation tests, possibly due to decreased lung delivery.

A breath hold or pause after inhalation increases lung deposition of drug by allowing longer for particles to deposit by sedimentation or diffusion.

Children may also not co-operate whilst receiving their medication, may breathe through the nose, and may have irregular breathing. Perversely, a toddler may decide to blow rather than inhale: this has disastrous effects on dry powder devices. These factors may explain the large variability in lung deposition and drug effects in children.

Breathing pattern is important when using nebulizers. Nebulizer output is fixed by the driving gas flow and the resistance of the nebulizer, and is constant throughout drug delivery. A child's inspiratory flow, by contrast, will vary accordingly to the respiratory pattern. Children who spend longer in expiration will tend to receive less aerosolized drug. Crying decreases lung deposition of nebulized drug (Case study 20.1).

In conventional jet nebulizers, the aerosol is carried in a volume of air dependent upon the driving gas flow. If this is, say, eight litres per minute, the patient will breath in approximately three litres of aerosol each minute (assuming an inspiratory : expiratory ratio of 2:3). *Entrainment of surrounding*

Table 20.2: Mechanisms of particle deposition

Inertial impaction	During inhalation, the airflow negotiates a series of bends in the airway. Aerosol particles may impact on the airway wall, dependent on their inertia, a product of their mass and velocity. Within the lung, maximum deposition by inertial impaction occurs at the carina, and to a lesser extent at other airway bifurcations.	
Sedimentation	Within the smaller airways and alveoli, where air velocity is low and the airway diameters are small, deposition is mainly by sedimentation or gravitational settling. This effect is enhanced by breath holding after inhalation.	
Diffusion	Brownian motion, particularly of sub-micron particles, may lead to deposition on the airway walls. Like sedimentation, this effect is greatest in the smaller airways, and is enhanced by factors that lead to prolonged residence times, such as breath holding after inhalation.	

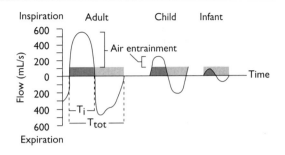

Figure 20.2 Air entrainment (from Collis[3]).

air occurs when the child's inspiratory flow rate exceeds the nebulizer output. Only the youngest children have inspiratory flows lower than commonly used nebulizer outputs (Figure 20.2), and for older children and adults aerosol will be diluted by entrained air. Thus the mass of drug inhaled with each breath remains constant throughout most of childhood, despite the fact that the body mass may increase five-fold. Some centres recommend age, weight or surface area correction of the concentration of drug placed in the nebulizer. Another approach is to nebulize the medication into a spacer or holding chamber, so that all of the child's inspiration consists of the aerosol cloud. Data from Salmon *et al*[4]. suggests that up to 1.5% of the dose of nebulized sodium cromoglycate will be deposited in the lungs of children from 6–36 months of age. Assuming that approximately 10% of a nebulized dose is deposited in the lungs of an adult, the dose per kilogram body weight can be calculated. For example, a 70 kg adult will receive 0.14%/kg (i.e. 10% $\div$ 70), whereas, using Salmon's data, young children will receive up to 0.15%/kg (i.e. 1.5% in a 10 kg infant). This suggests that although there may be poor drug deposition in infant lungs, this is compensated for by their small size, so that the final dose reaching the lungs per kilogram body weight may be very similar to that of an adult. This is supported by papers measuring the systematic availability of drug in children of different ages using nebulizers or spacers and suggests that the same nominal drug dose should be used in all age groups.

Upper airway

The adult nose is an excellent filter of inhaled particles, and nose breathing reduces the lung deposition of aerosols by half, most of the aerosol being deposited in areas of changing flow direction or turbulent flow in the anterior third of the nose. Little is known of the particle retaining properties of the nose in childhood.

Therapeutic failures may also occur if the patient inhales inappropriately through the nose rather than the mouthpiece. It is important to actually observe the child using his or her delivery device, and to be vigilant for some of the problems described in this chapter.

Age

There have been few clinical studies of deposition of nebulized aerosols in children. Some studies have suggested that the absolute lung deposition increases with age, but not all. Similarly the relationship between lung deposition and lung disease is not clear. In one study, children with normal ventilation scans had uniform deposition of labelled aerosol, whereas those with areas of reduced ventilation had corresponding areas of reduced deposition, but others have failed to confirm this. Total lung deposition from a simple jet nebulizer in older children is around 2.5% to 7% of the nominal dose, the same as in adults using similar nebulizers. The median deposition in infants aged 0.3 to 1.4 years, who breathed nasally during quiet sleep, was 1.3%. In some comparative studies children have more central drug deposition than adults.

Tal *et al.* studied a heterogenous group of 15 infants and children with respiratory disease aged between 2.5 months and 5 years. Technetium-labelled salbutamol was administered via MDI and Aerochamber spacer (Trudell Medical, Hamilton, Canada) plus facemask. Lung deposition varied from 0.2% to 5.1% (mean 2%, SD 1.4%), increasing with the weight of the child. The mean lung deposition was 0.2% per kilogram body weight, excluding one child noted to be crying during the study in whom the deposition was 0.036%. This compares with two adults in the same study who inhaled radiolabelled salbutamol from the Aerochamber with a mouthpiece, in whom lung deposition was 0.25%.

These deposition studies suggest that:

- the amount of aerosol inhaled may be independent of patient size after approximately 6 months of age;
- the amount of inhaled aerosol deposited in the lung does not appear to increase with age in children aged four or above;
- the situation in infants remains unclear, but the amount of drug deposited in the lungs per kilogram body weight may be similar for infants and adults;
- total deposition and deposition pattern may be altered by disease;
- the wide variation in deposition between individuals and possible differences due to the different drug delivery systems used must be borne in mind when interpreting studies of inhaled therapy.

Facemask or mouthpiece

The use of a facemask with a nebulizer or spacer device has been shown to be an effective method of drug delivery to children too young to use a mouthpiece. Potential problems with facemasks are that some of the drug will land on the face, some may be inhaled through the nose, or a seal may not be achieved, leading to leakage of the drug. Holding the facemask only 2 cm from the face may reduce drug delivery by 85% (Case study 20.2).

Case study 20.2: Croup

Eight-month-old Marie is admitted to the children's ward with fever, coryza and marked inspiratory stridor. A diagnosis of croup is made, and she is given a dose of nebulized budesonide. However, she becomes increasingly agitated and upset with the nebulizer and her mother is unable to do anything other than hold it six inches from her face. Her respiratory symptoms worsen over the next hour, but she is still tolerating sips of oral fluids. She is therefore given a dose of oral dexamethasone, and observed in the high dependency unit. Over the next two hours, her symptoms improve.

Nebulized budesonide is an effective treatment in the management of croup. However, oral or intramuscular dexamethasone is equally effective, may be tolerated better and is much cheaper.

There is one report (in abstract) on the use of fluticasone via a spacer device for the treatment of croup showing no benefit. It is possible that spacer devices may not deliver appropriate amounts topically to the area of obstruction. Further research is needed.

How to deliver drugs

Pressurized metered dose inhalers

The drug is dissolved or suspended in a propellant under pressure, and when activated, a valve system releases a metered volume of drug and propellant. These devices are cheap, convenient to carry and quick to use, but they are also difficult to use correctly. For optimum drug delivery, the metered dose inhaler requires a high degree of co-ordination and psychomotor skill, with inhalation, inhaler actuation and breath-holding all occurring in precise sequence (Box 20.3). The optimum metered dose inhaler technique is given in the box. Few patients can correctly use the metered dose inhaler, even after training, and less than fifteen percent of the emitted drug enters the typical patient's lungs. Metered dose inhalers should not be used alone in the treatment of children under 6 years of age, and because of co-ordination problems, are not the first choice device for older children.

The propellant in most metered dose inhalers is currently chlorofluorocarbons (CFCs). CFC-free pressurized metered dose inhalers may deliver different amounts of drug, and may taste and feel different to the patient than the inhalers they replace.

Breath actuated metered dose inhalers

These devices, such as the Autohaler (3M Riker) and the Easi-Breathe (Baker Norton) incorporate a mechanism, activated during inhalation, which

---

Box 20.3: The correct technique for using MDIs

- Shake the MDI
- Hold the MDI between the teeth
- Breath in deeply and slowly
- Activate the MDI during the first part of inhalation
- Complete the inhalation
- Hold breath for ten seconds.

Many adults have problems using inhalers, and repeated instructions and periodic checking of technique are important.

---

triggers the metered dose inhaler. In theory, this reduces the need for the patient or carer to co-ordinate inhaler actuation with inhalation. However, patients may stop breathing when the metered dose inhaler is actuated (the 'cold freon effect') or have a sub-optimal inspiration. Use of these devices for the delivery of β-agonists should be restricted to older children and adults. Evaluation of their efficacy in children under the age of 6 is limited. We are not aware of any trials that have been performed on the use of inhaled steroids from these devices in children or adults. Oropharyngeal deposition of steroids using these devices is still very high, and would be minimized by the use of a conventional metered dose inhaler and spacer instead.

The Easi-Breathe may be used with a short 'open tube' spacer (the 'Optimiser', available with beclomethasone and cromoglycate inhalers only). This addition may be expected to reduce extra-thoracic drug deposition, although there are no published evaluations of its use.

Intelligent devices, such as the Smartmist (Aradigm) have been developed which can deliver a drug bolus at a pre-programmed point in inhalation, defined by both flow and volume, and also store data on patient use and lung function. Cost may limit their use.

Metered dose inhalers with extended mouthpieces

The Spacehaler (Evans Medical) is a pressurized aerosol device that uses the same canister as a conventional metered dose inhaler. The actuator design, however, reduces the velocity of the aerosol cloud that emerges from the inhaler, reducing impaction of the aerosol in the oropharynx, and hence the amount of the non-respirable drug delivered to the patient. The device appears to be as effective in the delivery of salbutamol to adults as a metered dose inhaler and large volume spacer. Its advantage is that it is compact. There are no published studies of this device used by children or for the delivery of steroids.

The Syncroner (RPR), or 'open spacer' was designed primarily as a training aid. The spacer has an open section in its upper surface, and folds up like a clasp knife when not in use. When open the Syncroner places the metered dose inhaler

10 cm from the subject's lips, and if inhalation is not co-ordinated with metered dose inhaler actuation, aerosol cloud can be seen to escape from the top of the spacer, providing visual feedback to the patient of their poor technique. The spacer increases lung deposition and reduces oropharyngeal deposition of sodium cromoglycate compared with the metered dose inhaler. The Syncroner does not function as a holding chamber, and good co-ordination is still needed to use the device.

SPACERS

Spacer devices are becoming increasingly popular for the delivery of inhaled drugs in the treatment of asthma at all ages. They:

- reduce the problems of poor inhaler technique which may lead to treatment failure with metered dose inhalers;
- largely eliminate oral absorption of inhaled steroids;
- have been shown to be as effective as nebulizers in the treatment of acute severe asthma;
- can be adapted (using facemasks, for example) to treat patients of all ages.

There are two main types of spacer devices: 'extension devices' and 'holding chambers'.

Extension devices

These simply increase the distance the aerosolized drug has to travel before it is inhaled. Examples include the Optimiser (Baker Norton) and Integra (Allen and Hanburys) devices. The 'space' between the inhaler and the patient allows the aerosol to slow and propellants to evaporate, reducing the size of drug particles from metered dose inhalers, and trapping large particles in the device. These devices often do not have a valve and co-ordination is still required for optimal drug delivery. They are not suitable for young children and may be inappropriate for patients of any age who have difficulty in co-ordinating actuation of a metered dose inhaler and inhalation. Extension devices tend to deliver less drug than the larger holding chambers.

Holding chambers

These provide a reservoir of drug from which the patient breathes. Typically holding chambers also have the properties of extension devices, but in addition reduce the need for co-ordination between inhaler actuation and patient inhalation. *Valved holding chambers* allow the patient to breathe tidally from a reservoir of drug and are preferred especially for children. In practice, valves are not totally effective, allowing exhalate into the chamber, and on rare occasions may be difficult for the patient to open.

The size of the spacer may affect the amount of drug available for inhalation, and this will vary with the drug prescribed. Preparations may differ in their aerosol cloud speed and volume, and this may alter the amount of drug delivered from different spacers. The clinician should be aware that data about a spacer derived from studies with one drug may not apply to others. In general, small holding chambers deliver less drug than larger ones, although this may be less important in young children, as the breathing pattern rather than spacer size has the largest effect on delivered dose.

The addition of a facemask to holding chambers has revolutionized the treatment of children with asthma. Facemasks are available for an increasing number of spacers. Delivery of drug by a mouthpiece is more efficient, and patients should use this in preference to a facemask when possible.

The method of *spacer use* affects drug output, and inhaled drugs should be administered by repeated single actuations of the metered dose inhaler into the spacer, each followed by inhalation (Case study 20.3). There should be minimal delay between inhaler actuation and inhalation (Box 20.4). The technique is similar for infants (Box 20.5).

The valves of holding chambers may stick so it is important to ensure that the valve opens and closes with respiration. There appears to be little difference between two deep inspirations and five smaller breaths in the bronchodilator effect of β-agonists from large volume spacers, although rapid inhalation should be avoided.

Electrostatic charge accumulates on the walls of many polycarbonate and plastic spacers, attracting drug particles, which become charged when they are produced at the metered dose inhaler

Case study 20.3: A spurious dose of steroids

Christine is a busy 16-year-old, whose asthma has become progressively worse recently. Her GP has referred her as she is currently taking 1.25 mg of beclomethasone twice daily, via an MDI and spacer, with little relief, and has required a number of courses of oral steroids to control her symptoms.

In clinic, Christine has good inhaler technique, and understands the reasons for using a spacer. However, in order to take her medicine more quickly, she has been actuating the MDI into the spacer five times in quick succession before taking one big breath.

A short course of oral steroids controls her acute symptoms. Thereafter she is rapidly stepped down from her nominally high dose inhaled steroids by teaching her to take one actuation at a time, each followed by a breath. Within a month, her asthma is well controlled on 0.25 mg twice daily, probably the same inhaled dose as she had received with her poor spacer technique. There is, however, considerably less anxiety about the dose, and less expense.

Box 20.4: Using an MDI with a spacer

- Shake the MDI and insert it into the spacer
- Place the spacer mouthpiece in the mouth
- Activate the MDI into the spacer
- Breath in deeply and slowly
- If the child is able, hold breath for ten seconds
- Breath out, then take a second inhalation from the spacer*
- Wait about 30 seconds before taking a second dose.

*In one study, tidal breathing from the spacer was as effective as two single breaths.

Box 20.5: Spacer use in an infant

- Shake the MDI and insert it into the spacer
- Place the spacer facemask so that it covers the mouth and nose* creating a seal with the face
- When the child is settled, activate the MDI into the spacer
- Wait about 30 seconds before giving a second dose.

*The child may not tolerate the facemask being held against the face – if the mask is held a *little* away from the face the dose of drug delivered will be markedly reduced. Inhaled medications may also be administered to infants while they are asleep.

output may be achieved by washing a polycarbonate spacer in detergent and allowing it to drip dry in air, concern has been expressed that contact dermatitis may occur from the unwashed detergent. Simple washing in detergent and rinsing, prior to first use, followed by the repeated lining of the spacer walls with drug that occurs with routine use, and washing the spacer no more than monthly, may be considered an appropriate alternative.

DRY POWDER INHALERS

The use of conventional dry powder inhalers should be restricted to those over 6 years of age because young children tend to blow, not suck, which loses the drug and, in some devices, dampens the powder.

Dry powder inhalers use the patient's inspiration to disperse the drug into small particles. The effect of flow on the particle size output of drug from the inhaler varies between different types, and most need an inspiratory flow of at least 30 L/min to generate small particles. Most adults and children above 6 years of age are able to generate sufficient flow, but younger children may not be able to do so, even with extensive training. With some dry powder inhalers, the particle size of the emitted drug is determined by the inspiratory flow. The Turbohaler (Astra Zeneca) has high resistance, which may improve lung deposition if the patient can generate sufficient inspiratory flow, and has been found to give twice the lung deposition of a similar nominal dose from a correctly used metered dose inhaler. Dose reduction when changing from an MDI is recommended.

valve stem. This reduces the amount of drug delivered from the spacer. Washing polycarbonate spacers with detergent negates the effect of static charge with some drugs. Whilst the highest drug

To overcome the requirement for the patient to aerosolize the drug, power assisted DPIs are being developed, which use a mechanical piston or compressed air to force the powder into a spacer, from which it may be inhaled. It remains to be seen whether this has any advantage over the metered dose inhaler and spacer device.

NEBULIZERS

Indications for nebulized treatment in asthma have declined, especially in the community setting. Depending on which device is purchased, the patient may receive a four-fold difference in drug delivered without being aware. Nebulizers use either a compressed gas flow or ultrasonic power to break up solutions or suspensions of medication into droplets for inhalation. With many nebulizers, less than 10% of the prescribed dose reaches the lung.

The nebulizer does not rely on patient co-operation or co-ordination to work, although deposition is improved by the use of a mouthpiece rather than a facemask, by holding the facemask close to the patient, and by the patient breathing quietly, rather than crying or rapid breathing.

The output of drug suspensions, such as budesonide, from the majority of ultrasonic nebulizers is very low and they are not recommended for this task.

To reduce their inherent inefficiency, three types of nebulizers have been developed.

'Open vent nebulizers' incorporate an inlet that allows additional air to be drawn through the nebulizer. Examples include the Sidestream nebulizer (Medicaid, UK). The additional airflow pushes out more of the small particles, increasing nebulizer output and reducing nebulization time. If the extra vent was blocked, preventing additional flow of air through the chamber, a similar amount of drug would leave the nebulizer, but over a longer time. The main advantage of this device is halving of the delivery time. Because of the high flow of aerosol-laden air from the device, the dose received by younger children may be surprisingly small due to their low inspiratory flow and tidal volume.

'Breath enhanced, open vent nebulizers' have a valved inlet that opens during inspiration. On exhalation this valve closes, and expired air passes out of the device through a separate expiratory port. Examples include the Pari LC Plus (Pari, Germany) and Ventstream nebulizers (Medicaid UK). The amount of drug inspired may be doubled, but nebulization time is similar to that of the conventional jet nebulizer.

'Intelligent dosimetric nebulizers' monitor the breathing pattern of the patient and generate pulses of aerosol during early inspiration only. An example is the Halolite nebulizer (Medicaid, UK). As the patient's breathing pattern is known to affect the delivery of drug from nebulizers, this type of device may prove more efficient and reliable than conventional nebulizers. Early results are encouraging and further evaluation is awaited.

Nebulized drug delivery may be optimized by several simple manoeuvres:

- Administer the drug in an appropriate *fill volume*, since some drug is always retained in the nebulizer, and if the fill volume is small, very little drug is emitted. Conversely, large fill volumes lead to prolonged nebulization times.
- Drug and particle size output are determined by the *driving gas flow* or compressor output. Low flows or inadequately powered compressors generate large particles which may not reach the lungs. Check the nebulizer manufacturer's recommendations. In general, a flow of 6–8 L/min is needed, measured by a flow meter with the nebulizer attached.
- Most nebulizers stop releasing drug after 5 minutes, even though they may appear to be producing aerosol. Patients should be given a *set time* to continue nebulization.
- A *mouthpiece* is preferable to a *facemask* as lung deposition is increased. If tolerated, *nose clips* may improve drug delivery.
- Patients should undertake steady *tidal breathing*. Crying or fast inspiration reduces drug delivery.
- Compressors should undergo *regular servicing*, preferably by the medical physics department of the hospital that is supervizing the patient. Nebulizers should be cleaned according to the manufacturer's instructions. Care should be taken not to poke anything into the nebulizer jets, as this will alter emitted particle size.

ASSESSING INHALATION DEVICES

TERMINOLOGY

Particle size in this chapter generally refers to *aerodynamic particle size*, meaning the size of a spherical particle of unit density that settles with the same velocity as the particle in question. Clearly a very dense particle will have a different aerodynamic behaviour (an increased aero-dynamic size) to an equivalently sized but, less dense particle.

Aerosols produced by medical nebulizers and metered dose inhalers are heterodisperse, that is made up of particles of different sizes. For most therapeutic aerosols particle sizes are not normally distributed (the mean and median values are not the same, and the particle size distribution curve is not symmetrical about the mean). They usually conform to an approximately log-normal distribution. One way of describing such a distribution is in terms of the mass median aerodynamic diameter (MMAD) and geometric standard deviation (GSD) (Box 20.6).

Box 20.6: Aerosols – some definitions

An aerosol: a two phase system made up of a gaseous continuous phase, usually air, and a discontinuous phase of individual liquid or solid particles.

Mass median diameter (MMD): the diameter of a particle such that half the mass of the aerosol is contained in smaller diameter particles, and half in larger.

Mass median aerodynamic diameter (MMAD): the diameter of a sphere of unit density that has the same aerodynamic properties as a particle of median mass from the aerosol.

Geometric standard deviation (GSD): a dimensionless number which gives an indication of the spread of sizes of particles that make up the aerosol. An aerosol with a GSD of 1 is made up of particles of uniform size.

Heterodisperse aerosol: the aerosol is made up of particles of many different sizes. The GSD is >1.2.

Monodisperse aerosol: the aerosol particles are uniform size (or very nearly uniform). The GSD is <1.2.

METHODS OF DEVICE TESTING

The two most commonly used laboratory methods of pharmaceutical aerosol particle size determination are inertial impaction devices and laser-based light scattering devices (Table 20.3). Unfortunately neither method is ideal, and each has its own drawbacks. Their results may not be interchangeable. Ideally comparisons of the amount of drug contained in particles of various size from different inhalational drug delivery devices should use identical measurement techniques. *In vivo*, lung deposition may be estimated by radiolabelled aerosol deposition, or by pharmacokinetic methods (Table 20.3).

Pharmacokinetic studies suggest that absorption across the lung vascular bed is an important determinant of systemic bioactivity and adverse effects. On the basis of data from mouth rinsing and charcoal block studies it can be inferred that the systemic bioavailability of modern inhaled cortico-steroids is mainly determined by absorption across the lung vascular bed. Thus, a drug delivery system which improves lung deposition would, at the same time, be expected to increase lung bioavailability and hence overall systemic absorption.

ASSESSING THE PUBLISHED EVIDENCE

It is clear that the choice of delivery device, and its method of use, affect the amount of drug that may be delivered to the patient independently of such factors as age and severity of disease.

When assessing papers describing *in vitro* testing of inhalers, the reader should ask:

- Is the testing method appropriate to the device being tested? For instance, the choice of flow may be crucial in comparing different dry powder inhalers.
- Is the drug assayed, or some surrogate, such as a tracer? Have the authors demonstrated that the drug and tracer behave in the same way?
- Is the method described in detail? Even a one second delay between actuating an MDI into a spacer and sampling can reduce the amount of

Table 20.3: Methods of testing aerosol devices

Inertial impaction	Air is drawn through a nozzle towards an obstruction (impaction plate), at which the airflow is forced to make a 90° turn. Aerosol particles with sufficient inertia are unable to follow the airflow, and instead impact on the plate. *Cascade impactors* consist of a number of plates in series, each separating out sequentially smaller particles. Impacted drug is assayed specifically.
Advantages	Measure aerodynamic particle size. Measure size of particles containing drug only. Allow cumulative drug distribution to be calculated.
Disadvantages	High airflow may dessicate particles, making them shrink. Labour intensive. Requires specialized drug assays.
Laser diffraction	A laser beam passes through the aerosol cloud. Particles diffract the light at an angle inversely related to their diameter, and the diffracted light is detected by the machine. Light scattering theory is used to compute the volume of particles present in each band, and from this the particle size distribution.
Advantages	Easy to use, rapid results.
Disadvantages	Volume is measured, rather than mass or size, which are calculated. *Aerodynamic* particle size is not measured. All particles produced by the nebulizer that pass through the laser are measured, whether or not they contain drug. Metered dose inhalers are difficult to examine by laser diffraction.
Breathing simulation	The output of some devices is dependent on the patient's breathing pattern. This may be simulated and drug collected on a filter, or directed to a cascade impactor.
Advantages	Takes account of a biological variable.
Disadvantages	Measures drug availability at the airway opening, not in the lungs.
Gamma scintigraphy	Provides a graphical representation of the deposition of inhaled radioactive particles. Imaging may be two dimensional (planar) or may involve complex three dimensional imaging (i.e. SPECT scanning).
Advantages	Results include the effects of factors other than particle size, such as airway calibre, which are important in determining drug deposition.
Disadvantages	Measures radiolabel deposition, rather than drug. Qualitative rather than quantitative. Difficulties differentiating between sites of lung deposition. Concern over the use of radioactive substances for non-therapeutic purposes. Need for expertise and specialized equipment.
Pharmacokinetics	Serum or for some drugs urine concentrations of drug up to 30 minutes after inhalation reflect lung deposition. For instance, measurements of plasma salbutamol over the first 30 minutes following inhalation (prior to gastro-intestinal absorption) predominantly reflect lung absorption of drug. Lung deposition may be estimated from either the maximum concentration (C_{max}) or the area under the time/concentration curve.
Advantages	Results include the effects of factors other than particle size, such as airway calibre, which are important in determining drug deposition.
Disadvantages	Sensitive drug assay needed, capable of detecting, for instance, salbutamol (albuterol) concentrations to the order of 1 ng/mL.

drug recovered. Such differences in detail can make comparisons between studies very difficult.

For clinical studies involving inhalational therapy (or if planning a clinical trial), the reader should ask (or consider):

- Was data from patients using a variety of devices used in the analysis?
- In 'proof of principle' research, rather than pragmatic studies, were the devices used optimally? The administration of an apparently large dose of drug by multiple actuations of an MDI into a spacer prior to inhalation reduces drug delivery considerably.
- Were factors known to affect drug delivery, such as electrostatic charge, accounted for?
- Was the device used appropriate for the patient population? For instance some open vent nebulizers deliver little drug to small children at low tidal volumes. Reports suggesting a lack of efficacy of a drug using these devices may really be documenting a failure of drug delivery.
- Papers comparing drugs using different devices should be interpreted with extreme caution. The amount of drug delivered may vary by a factor of four depending on the devices used.

EVALUATING THE OUTCOME

Most patients are unable to use drug delivery devices correctly without tuition. The correct technique should be demonstrated when a particular device is prescribed, and it is worth taking some time with different devices to allow the family to choose one that the patient is happy with, rather than the 'best' one that the child may refuse to use. The patient should demonstrate his or her competence with the device, and inhaler technique should be checked at each consultation.

Written instructions on technique come with most devices, or can be adapted from the information given above. If the medication appears to be failing, device failure, failure of technique or lack of compliance with therapy must be considered in the diagnosis. Compliance with inhalational drug delivery may be affected by the choice of device. Many devices are marketed on the premise that their size, shape or appearance will improve compliance, although there is little evidence that this is so. This issue is dealt with further elsewhere.

PLANNING MANAGEMENT

There is much confusion in the choice and use of different inhalational drug delivery devices. Insufficient published information is available to allow clinicians to make an informed, independent, choice. Surprisingly, there is little regulation of drug delivery devices. A device manufacturer can make a new spacer or nebulizer device and place it on the market without providing information on the amount or variability of drug that it is likely to be delivered to the patient. Devices such as nebulizers may be bought over the counter by parents. Depending on their choice the amount of drug their child may receive may vary by up to four-fold. Many health care professionals falsely assume dose equivalence between devices.

There is however, broad agreement on the choice of inhaler to use for particular age groups (Table 20.4). The wider use of spacer devices has been supported by British guidelines on asthma management.[1]

The best engineered device will be ineffective if the patient will not use it. If asthma control is deteriorating, it is important to consider that device failure or non-compliance with therapy may be to blame (see Chapter 22). In some instances, re-education of the patient and parents may be all that is needed, but sometimes this will fail. In this case, a pragmatic decision must be made to prescribe the second choice therapy, adjusting the nominal drug dose appropriately.

Should patients be prescribed one device or two? Large volume spacers optimize therapy, but are bulky and obtrusive. They may not be used by children at school. Give a large volume spacer for steroids, kept in the bathroom or by the bed, as inhaled steroids are commonly administered in the morning and the evening. Keeping the spacer in the bathroom will encourage teeth brushing and mouth rinsing after using the device, reducing the incidence of steroid side effects. But give a

Table 20.4: The choice of inhalation device*

Age (years)	First choice	Second choice	Comments
0–2	MDI + spacer and facemask	Nebulizer	Avoid 'open vent' nebulizers
3–6	MDI + spacer	Nebulizer	Very few children at this age can use DPIs adequately
6–12 (bronchodilators)	MDI + spacer or breath actuated MDIs or DPI	–	If using DPI or breath actuated MDI, also prescribe MDI + spacer for acute exacerbations
6–12 (steroids)	MDI + spacer	DPI or breath actuated MDI	May need to adjust dose if switching between inhalers / Advise mouth rinsing or gargling
12+ (bronchodilators)	DPI or breath actuated MDI	–	
12+ (steroids)	MDI + spacer	DPI or breath actuated MDI	May need to adjust dose if switching between inhalers / Advise mouth rinsing or gargling
Acute asthma (all ages)	MDI + spacer	Nebulizer	Ensure appropriate dosing / Nebulize for a set period of time / Provide written instructions

MDI: Metered dose inhaler;
DPI: dry powder inhaler.
*Assumes all devices used optimally.

small, unobtrusive device (breath actuated MDI or DPI) for use with bronchodilators at school (Case study 20.4). The large volume spacer may also be used with a bronchodilator MDI for an acute exacerbation, when the DPI may be less effective.

CLINICAL RESEARCH ISSUES

Much of our understanding of inhalational therapy has come from *in vitro* studies of drug delivery devices. Further research is needed to determine the exact relationship between particle size and lung deposition, especially in children and patients with airways disease.

Case study 20.4: A device for use at school

James is a 6-year-old boy whose asthma has deteriorated since starting school. On three occasions he has been sent home after becoming acutely wheezy during games. Instructions to take his reliever inhaler prior to sports have not helped, and the school have asked his parents to get the doctor to 'do something about it'. On closer questioning, it becomes clear that James has been using an MDI alone for his reliever, as his friends say that 'spacers are for babies'. Although he breathes deeply and breath-holds, his MDI co-ordination is truly awful.

A compromise is reached in clinic. James agrees to use an MDI and spacer for his inhaled steroids at home, but is given a space age DPI for his reliever. Decorated with the appropriate pictures of space heroes, James is now happy, and his ability to play sports improves.

Compliance and spacer efficiency may be improved by 'smart' devices that both monitor and prompt patient use. Delivery devices that interact with the patient, measuring drug delivery and feeding this information back to the patient and doctor, may improve care, but cost may limit their use.

There is increasing interest in the delivery of innovative therapy (i.e. gene therapy) and of drugs for systemic effect, such as insulin. For this to work, devices that not only produce an accurate dose, but deliver it repeatedly, are needed. This will involve either removing the patient interaction with the device, or monitoring it and adjusting the dose released appropriately.

With increasing understanding of the variability of drug delivery from different devices, there is increasing awareness of the need for tighter regulation of devices. This should ideally be undertaken by a body independent of the device and drug manufacturers, and devices should be regulated in a similar way to the medicines that they deliver.

REFERENCES

1. British Thoracic Society. The British guidelines on asthma management. *Thorax* 1997; **52**: Suppl. 1.

2. Rudolph G, Kobrich R, Stahlofen W. Modelling and algebraic formulation of regional aerosol deposition in man. *J Aerosol Sci* 1990; **21**: S306–S406.

3. Collis GG, Cole CH, Le Souef PN. Dilution of nebulised aerosols by air entrainment in children. *Lancet* 1990; **336**: 341–3.

4. Salmon B, Wilson NM, Silverman M. How much aerosol reaches the lungs of wheezy infants and toddlers? *Arch Dis Child* 1990; **65**: 401–3.

FURTHER READING

1. Barry PW, O'Callaghan C. Therapeutic aerosols. *Medicine* 1999; **27**: 33–7.

2. O'Callaghan C, Barry PW. Inhalation devices for young children. *Paediat Perinatal Drug Ther* 1997; **1**: 59–65.

3. Barry PW, O'Callaghan C. Nebuliser therapy in childhood. *Thorax* 1997; **52** (Suppl 2): S78–88.

4. O'Callaghan C, Barry PW. The science of nebulised drug delivery. *Thorax* 1997; **52** (Suppl 2): S31–44.

5. Anonymous. Drug delivery systems in asthma. *Drug Therapeut Bulln* 2000; **38**: 9–14.

6. O'Callaghan C, Barry PW. How to choose delivery devices for asthma. *Arch Dis Child* 2000; **82**: 185–7.

7. Selroos O, Halme M. The effect of a volumatic spacer and mouth rinsing on systemic absorption of inhaled corticosteroids from a metered dose inhaler and dry powder inhaler. *Thorax* 1991; **46**: 891–4.

8. Partridge MR. Metered-dose inhalers and CFCs: What respiratory physicians need to know. *Respir Med* 1994; **88**: 645–7.

9. Pedersen S, Frost L, Arnfred T. Errors in inhalation technique and efficiency in inhaler use in asthmatic children. *Allergy* 1986; **41**: 118–24.

10. Tal A, Golan H, Grauer N, Aviram M, Albin D, Quastel MR. Deposition pattern of radiolabeled salbutamol inhaled from a metered-dose inhaler by means of a spacer with mask in young children with airway obstruction. *J Pediat* 1996; **128**: 479–84.

11. Iles R, Lister P, Edmunds AT. Crying significantly reduces absorption of aerosolised drug in infants. *Arch Dis Child* 1999; **81**: 163–5.

12. Bisgaard H. Patient related factors in nebulised drug delivery to children. *Eur Respir Rev* 1997; **7**: 376–7.

13. Cates CJ. Holding chambers versus nebulisers for beta agonist treatment of acute asthma (Cochrane Review). In: The Cochrane Library, Issue 1, 1999. Oxford: Update Software.

OXYGEN THERAPY

A . T h o m s o n

INTRODUCTION

The administration of oxygen is the most important therapeutic manoeuvre in the management of hypoxaemia and tissue hypoxia. This chapter deals with the administration of oxygen to children, together with assessment of oxygenation and oxygen therapy.

Important factors in *oxygen delivery* include:

- adequate pulmonary gas exchange
- adequate cardiac output
- adequate haemoglobin level
- adequate saturation of haemoglobin
- appropriate oxyhaemoglobin dissociation curve (i.e. temperature, pH and 2,3-diphosphoglyceride (2,3-DPG) levels).

EVALUATION OF OXYGENATION

ARTERIAL BLOOD GAS ANALYSIS

Radial artery sampling using a heparinized syringe is most often performed in children; 'arterialized' capillary sampling is inappropriate when peripheral circulation is poor. Measurements should be made at 37°C.

Several factors affect blood gas results:

- type of blood – 'arterialized' capillary corresponds closely to arterial blood as long as it has not been contaminated by blood from venules or over-exposed to air;
- body temperature – pH decreases and CO_2 increases with fever;
- type of breathing – mild hyperventilation in an anxious child, for example, will decrease CO_2 and increase pH.

TRANSCUTANEOUS MEASUREMENT

Accuracy is dependent on the tissue perfusion. The blood flow in the skin needs to be high. In order to achieve this the sensor heat should be at 43–45°C. There is a risk of superficial skin burns, so the sensor should be moved 2-hourly. In preterm and young infants transcutaneous oxygen measurement can give an accurate measurement of arterial oxygenation. However as the infant ages and skin thickens it is useful only as a trend indicator, and under-represents true PaO_2.

OXYGEN SATURATION (SaO_2) BY PULSE OXIMETRY

Transcutaneous SaO_2 measurement using pulse oximetry is very widely used in paediatrics. In general, there is good correlation with arterial blood samples. However, there are limitations of pulse oximetry that are easily understood with reference to the basic principles involved (see Further Reading).

The oxyhaemoglobin dissociation curve

Oxygen chemically combines with haemoglobin to form oxyhaemoglobin.

$$Hb + O_2 = HbO_2$$

This reaction can move in both directions. In conditions which favour a rightward movement of the reaction haemoglobin binds with oxygen in the alveoli. When the reaction moves to the left oxygen is released from oxyhaemoglobin to tissues. The relationship between Pao_2 and arterial oxygen saturation (Sao_2) is expressed as the oxyhaemoglobin saturation curve (See Chapter 00, Figure 00).

- On the steep slope of the curve (up to 9.5 kPa (70 mmHg) Pao_2), large amounts of oxygen can be released from haemoglobin with small changes in partial pressure of arterial oxygen (Pao_2); oxygen saturation is more sensitive than Pao_2 for monitoring patients.
- On the upper, flatter part of the curve, Pao_2 may change significantly, from 13–11 kPa (100–80 mmHg) for example, while haemoglobin saturation remains at around 95% and tissue hypoxia does not occur. As the change in Pao_2 is much greater than the change in oxygen saturation, Pao_2 may be the most accurate index of oxygenation. Obviously this is less practical than oximetry.
- Very little oxygen is carried in the blood dissolved in the plasma (1 mL oxygen/100 mL). One gram of haemoglobin, however, is capable of combining with 1.34 mL oxygen. As a result, 40–70 times more oxygen is carried by haemoglobin than by the plasma allowing the body to maintain a normal oxygen uptake provided cardiac output is reasonable. With a haemoglobin concentration of 15g/dL, 20.1 vol% (mL O_2 per 100 mL blood) of oxygen can be bound to haemoglobin.
- The oxygen content of the blood and therefore the theoretical maximum amount of oxygen available to tissues varies significantly with haemoglobin level. For example if Pao_2 is 70 mmHg and Sao_2 is 93% the oxygen content at haemoglobin of 5 g could be 6.3 vol%, and at 10 g 12.5 vol%, as opposed to 18.7 vol% at a haemoglobin level of 15 g.

Acidosis (decreased pH), increased temperature, or an increase in arterial carbon dioxide tension (Bohr effect) *or* an increase in 2,3-DPG shifts the curve to the right. This results in a decrease in affinity of haemoglobin for oxygen at low values of Pao_2 and therefore more oxygen is available to the tissues. The reverse process may occur in alkalosis, decreased arterial carbon dioxide tension, decreased temperature and decreased levels of 2,3-DPG.

Note that:

- 2,3 diphosphoglyceride (2,3-DPG) is bound to a lesser extent by HbF than HbA so that oxygen is released less readily from foetal oxyhaemoglobin than adult oxyhaemoglobin; conversely, oxygen is more avidly taken up by fetal blood at the low Pao_2 prevailing in the placenta.
- Prolonged hypoxaemia, for instance in chronic lung disease results in an increase in 2,3-DPG in red blood cells shifting the curve to the right. For a given Pao_2 the Sao_2 will therefore be lower.

The pulse oximeter

A pulse oximeter generally consists of two light emitting diodes at different wavelengths (one red wave length, one infrared) with a photo detector placed opposite (e.g. other side of the finger). The photo detector detects the ratio between red (R) and infrared (I) in the alternating current amplitude and a table relates oxygen saturation to the R:I ratio. This is calculated many times each cardiac cycle and averaged. Many things can interfere with the validity of this signal and hence the displayed value of Sao_2 (Table 21.1.) Three major limitations are worth mentioning in more detail.

Movement artefacts such as shivering, tremor and limb movements can have overwhelming effects on the signal. These are generally very obvious on a plethysmographic (pulse) trace if one is available. They can partly be overcome in modern machines that use ECG synchronization.

Malpositioning of the probe is a particular problem for sensors that are wrapped around small fingers or toes. If the red and infrared light emitting diodes are not exactly opposite the photo detector there maybe a large difference in the path length between each diode and detector resulting

Table 21.1: Potential problems with oxygen saturation monitors

- Mechanical artefacts, e.g. movement
- Electromagnetic interference, e.g. surgical diathermy
- Visible light, especially pulsatile visible light
- Malpositioning of probe (penumbra effect)
- Decreased pulse pressure
- Presence of carboxyhaemoglobin or methaemoglobin
- Physiological dyes, e.g. methylene blue
- Nail varnish
- Pulsatile veins
- Variation between instruments

in one pathway being overloaded and producing an erroneously low result. It is important to note that the plethysmographic signal may look normal but is generally coming from one wavelength signal only. This error can be picked up if there is a discrepancy between the heart rate displayed by the machine and the pulse rate taken by another means, and by a high index of suspicion if there is an unexpectedly low saturation result.

Pulse pressure is critical. Conditions that give either a decrease in pulse pressure (such as hypovolaemia or brachial artery occlusion) or an increase in venous pulsation (such as tricuspid incompetence) can affect the performance of an oxygen saturation monitor.

KEY POINTS IN PULSE OXIMETRY

- The oximeters are calibrated for adult haemoglobin.
- Do not use if patient has inhaled carbon monoxide – overestimated readings may be obtained.
- Pulse oximeters do not indicate the adequacy of ventilation especially if supplemental oxygen is being given; hypercapnia and acidosis should be assessed by means of arterial blood sampling if hypoventilation is suspected.
- Pulse oximeters are highly sensitive to movement artefact.

CLINICAL FEATURES OF HYPOXAEMIA

DEFINITIONS OF HYPOXIA AND HYPOXAEMIA

Hypoxaemia is defined as the reduction in the level of oxygen in arterial blood whereas hypoxia is the reduction in the amount of oxygen delivered to the tissues to meet the metabolic needs of the body.

There is limited normative data for blood gas levels and acid base balance. Cross-sectional data (aged 1 month to 24 years) taken using a standardized technique for arterialized capillary blood demonstrated that pH did not differ from adult levels but that Pa_{CO_2} was lower in infants (mean 34.9 mmHg, 4.7 kPa) and increased throughout childhood to adults levels (mean 40.5 mmHg, 5.4 kPa). Similarly Pa_{O_2} was lower in infants (mean 71.4 mmHg, 9.5 kPa) and increased to adult levels (mean 97.0 mmHg, 13 kPa) by age 7–12 years.[1]

1. Base-line hypoxaemia in a normal child is defined as an oxygen saturation less than 92%: this corresponds to a Pa_{O_2} of less than 8 kPa (60 mmHg).
2. Episodic hypoxaemia – the most common definition is a drop in oxygen saturation of 4% or more from base line.

SYMPTOMS AND SIGNS OF HYPOXIA

Hypoxia may result in a subtle change in a child's condition. Such changes may be difficult to separate from the physiological effects of the disease or disorder causing hypoxia.

Hypoxia stimulates the rate and depth of ventilation through stimulation of the aortic and carotid chemoreceptors. Acute hypoxia initially stimulates heart rate causing tachycardia. A Pa_{O_2} of less than 4 kPa (30 mmHg) (saturation less than 50%) may result in hypotension, shock, loss of consciousness, vasoconstriction and bronchoconstriction. Altered cerebral function manifested as restlessness, irritability, and headache or euphoria may occur with hypoxia. Delirium and coma may occur with progressive cerebral hypoxia. Severe hypoxia may result in bradycardia and cardiac arrest.

Cyanosis is a bluish discoloration of the skin and mucous membranes caused by an increase in the amount of reduced haemoglobin in tissue capillaries. Difficulties are encountered in attempting to correlate the degree of cyanosis with Sao_2. This may be related to the fact that clinically evident cyanosis is dependent on both the haemoglobin content and the rate of flow of blood. Cyanosis is less evident with a haemoglobin of 10 g/dL than a haemoglobin of 15 g/dL and may appear relatively later in children who can increase their blood flow in the presence of hypoxia.

WHY TO GIVE OXYGEN

Hypoxia can be secondary to inadequate oxygenation of the blood or inadequate delivery of blood to the tissues.

INADEQUATE OXYGENATION OF THE BLOOD (HYPOXAEMIA)

This may occur where there is low partial pressure of inspired oxygen, for example as seen at high altitude. Long-term exposure to high altitude results in compensatory mechanisms so that oxygen delivery to the cells is maintained by an increase in haemoglobin concentrations, a decrease in plasma volume and an increase in red blood cell mass. Lazano[2] found a mean oxygen saturation Sao_2 of 93% in 89 healthy children in Bogata which is 2640 meters above sea level.

There are four primary pulmonary causes of a reduced Pao_2 in arterial blood, which may occur singly or (more usually) in combination, in disease states.

Hypoventilation

If the volume of fresh gas to the alveoli per unit of time is decreased and if resting oxygen consumption is not correspondingly reduced hypoxaemia results. Hypoventilation also causes an increase in $PaCo_2$. Possible causes of hypoventilation are listed in Table 21.2.

Table 21.2: Causes of hypoventilation (with some clinical examples)

> **Central causes**
> Primary central hypoventilation (Ondine's curse)
> Depression of the respiratory centre secondary to drugs (morphine, barbiturates)
> Diseases of the medulla (encephalitis, trauma, neoplasm)
>
> **Peripheral nervous system**
> Abnormalities of the spinal conducting pathways (high cervical dislocation)
> Anterior horn cell disease (polio)
> Diseases of the nerve supply to the respiratory muscles (Guillain-Barré, diphtheria)
>
> **Muscle disorders**
> Disease in the myoneural junction (myasthenia)
> Disease of the respiratory muscles (progressive muscular dystrophy)
>
> **Mechanical problems**
> Thoracic cage abnormalities (stiff spine syndrome, scoliosis)
> Upper airway obstruction (obstructive sleep apnoea, inhaled foreign body)
> Severe pulmonary disease (airway obstruction, ARDS)

Illustrative respiratory patterns are shown in Figure 21.1. It is important to recognize hypoventilation and not to give oxygen indiscriminately. Oxygen therapy will promptly relieve hypoxaemia, but may abolish hypoxic drive to breathing and result in Co_2 narcosis.

Ventilation perfusion mismatch

Ventilation and perfusion mismatch which results in inefficient gas transfer, are the most common causes of hypoxaemia in children. It occurs in bronchiolitis, asthma and chronic obstructive lung disease. Ventilation perfusion mismatch will reduce the efficiency of transfer of all gases including CO_2 but generally, $Paco_2$ is much less severely affected than Pao_2. The normal response to hypoxaemia is to increase ventilation, which again will help clear CO_2 more than it improves oxygenation. Oxygen therapy will promptly relieve hypoxaemia in ventilation perfusion mismatch.

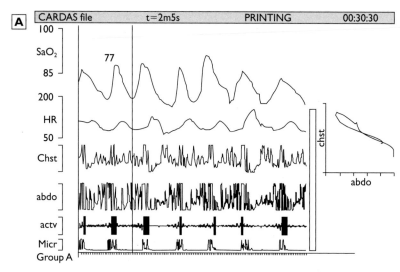

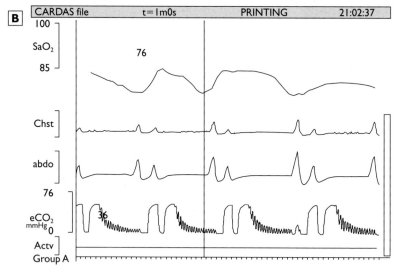

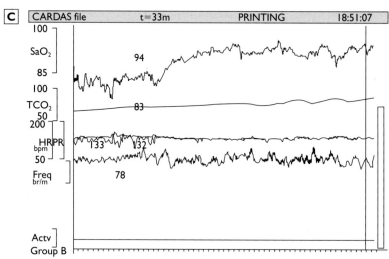

Figure 21.1: Polysomnographic recordings from children with hypoventilation. (A) Severe obstructive sleep apnoea. A 2-min recording demonstrating large dips in oxygen saturation. Each episode is terminated by an arousal indicated by gross body movement (actv) and loud respiratory noise (micro). Note that when chest movement is plotted against abdominal movement, they are completely out of phase (paradoxical). (B) Disordered central control of breathing A 1 min recording at a respiratory rate of eight breaths per minute, showing hypoxaemia secondary to hypoventilation. (C) Respiratory failure secondary to pulmonary hypoplasia and pulmonary hypertension. Note the gradual rise of transcutaneous CO_2 by approximately 20 mm Hg (2.7 kPa) over 33 minutes. Heart rate remains stable and breathing frequency is high with some variation. At the beginning of the recording, the child is awake and active, but is noted to have fallen asleep by a comment approximately a third of the time across this recording. The child was receiving low flow oxygen at the time of the recording. The low oxygen saturations recorded at the beginning of this recording are largely due to movement artefact confirmed by the pulse rate variability (from pulse oximeter signal compared with the heart rate from ECG). Note that once the child is asleep the signals are superimposed.

Key: Sao_2: oxygen saturation by oximetry; HR: heart rate; PR: pulse rate; chst: chest movement; abdo: abdominal movement; actv: activity; micr: sound; eCO_2: end-tidal CO_2; Tco_2: transcutaneous Pco_2; Freq: breathing frequency.

Shunt

A shunt is present when the blood reaches the arterial system without passing through ventilated regions of the lung. Shunts therefore can be:

- extra-pulmonary, as in congenital heart disease with right to left shunt;
- arterio-venous fistulae within the lung;
- intra-pulmonary shunts – when alveoli are not ventilated but are still being perfused as in pneumonia, atelectasis; this type of shunt can also be considered as a V/Q (ventilation-perfusion) ratio of 0.

In a normal lung a small amount of venous blood bypasses the ventilated lung and mixes with arterial blood resulting in a physiological shunt. Shunted blood in this situation comes from the bronchial veins and in part from the thebesian veins from the myocardium which drain into the left side of the heart. About 1–2% of the normal cardiac output constitutes the normal physiological shunt and results in a decrease in oxygen tension of 5 mmHg below alveolar Pa_{O_2} when room air is breathed.

Hypoxaemia resulting from V/Q abnormalities disappears with oxygen administration, but hypoxaemia caused by a true shunt does not, forming the basis of the 'alveolar arterial gradient test' described below. If hypoxaemia is such that it stimulates ventilation then Pa_{CO_2} may be lower than normal. Pa_{CO_2} is not normally raised if a pure shunt is the cause of hypoxaemia.

The 'alveolar arterial gradient test' has been recommended in the evaluation of cyanotic newborns. This involves breathing 100% oxygen for 15–20 minutes and then determining the Pa_{O_2}. With a low V/Q ratio, suggesting a pulmonary problem, all of the nitrogen is eventually washed out of alveoli and the pulmonary capillary blood reaches full oxygenation almost regardless of how poorly ventilated certain alveoli are in terms of bloodflow. This should result in a Pa_{O_2} of 75–80 kPa (550–600 mmHg). If venous blood is never exposed to alveolar oxygen, as in a cardiac right to left shunt, breathing 100% oxygen does not raise the Pa_{O_2} to this degree. The test can give a false result in the presence of pulmonary hypertension in infancy, where a reduction in pulmonary vascular resistance during the test, can profoundly affect right heart pressure and therefore intra-cardiac shunt.

Diffusion impairment

In diffusion impairment equilibration does not occur between the Pa_{O_2} in pulmonary capillary blood and alveolar gas because the blood–gas barrier is thickened; retention of CO_2 is not usually a problem in diffusion impairment because of the high solubility of CO_2. This is a rare cause of hypoxaemia in children, but can theoretically occur in conditions such as interstitial pneumonia, bird-fancier's lung, interstitial fibrosis and collagen diseases, although most hypoxia in these diseases is due to ventilation perfusion mismatch. It is worth remembering that any hypoxaemia secondary to diffusion impairment which occurs at rest will be exaggerated on exercise because of reduced contact time between the blood and the capillary and oxygen in the alveolus. As it can often be difficult or impossible to measure transfer factor in young children, oxygenation measured during an exercise test can be useful if diffusion impairment is suspected (the poor man's transfer factor).

INADEQUATE DELIVERY OF OXYGEN TO THE TISSUES (HYPOXIA)

Oxygen delivery depends on:

- the oxygen capacity of the blood, decreased for example in anaemia;
- cardiac output;
- distribution of blood flow to the periphery.

Diseases that cause hypoxaemia frequently occur simultaneously with other conditions that result in tissue hypoxia. For example a critically ill child with pneumonia may be febrile, anaemic and hypotensive and have a decreased cardiac output secondary to sepsis. Each of these factors may contribute to the child's hypoxia.

Oxygen alone is rarely a definitive treatment. It is supportive and must be used in conjunction with other strategies such as improving ventilation, treating infection, supporting blood pressure, restoring blood volume and blood transfusion.

HOW TO GIVE OXYGEN

HEAD BOX

Oxygen is delivered by the simple principle of increasing the concentration of oxygen in the ambient air. It is not easy to deliver Fio_2 over 0.6 in a head box.

Problems

SMALL BOX, LARGE BABY

When a small head box is used for a large baby there is little room for a leak around the neck. In this situation only a low flow of oxygen is required to maintain the oxygen concentration in the head box. However there is a possibility of CO_2 build up in the head box and a re-breathing situation being created. Adequate flow of air/oxygen mixture through the head box is necessary, rather than a trickle of pure oxygen.

LARGE BOX, SMALL BABY

In this situation there is a large leak and therefore a substantial flow of oxygen is required to maintain the oxygen concentration in the box above ambient. When oxygen is delivered from a wall oxygen source it is dry and cold and may cool the baby; humidification should be considered.

MEASUREMENT OF OXYGEN CONCENTRATION IN THE HEAD BOX

The oxygen concentration is not uniform within a head box. The oxygen sensor must therefore be placed near the infant's nose.

NASAL PRONGS

There are now a variety of sizes of nasal prongs suitable for both infants and children. They are generally soft and comfortable to wear (Figure 21.2). They deliver a continuous flow of 100% oxygen to the nares. The oxygen is diluted by the patient's peak inspiratory flow to provide an unknown concentration of oxygen. Inspiratory flow will differ from patient to patient and may vary within a patient. During episodes of breathlessness or exercise the patient inspiratory flow will increase and therefore decrease the oxygen concentration given. During

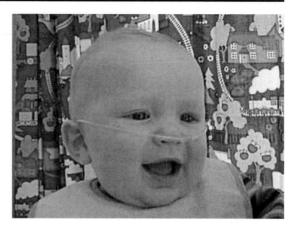

Figure 21.2: 9-month-old infant wearing nasal prongs.

sleep the patient's inspiratory flow will decrease and provide an increased oxygen concentration for a given oxygen flow.

Benefits

- Child can move, sit up, talk, eat and see what is happening, or even walk around.
- Comfortable.

Drawbacks

- Displaced easily and dependent on fixation.
- Flow limitation – small children can rarely tolerate more than 2 L/minute; therefore oxygen delivered by nasal prongs is unlikely to exceed 30–40% in a toddler.
- Unpredictable concentration; with nasal obstruction/mouth breathing, the contribution may be very small; severe upper respiratory tract infection is a problem.

NASOPHARYNGEAL CANNULA

A cheap, effective and relatively trouble-free method of oxygen delivery to the nasopharynx, beyond any nasal obstruction and unaffected by mouth breathing, was described several years ago.[3] It consists simply of an end-hole size 8 French suction catheter (or infant feeding tube with the tip removed), passed through one nostril to the nasopharynx to a depth equal to the distance from the side of the nose to the front of the ear. Oxygen flows of up to 1 L/minute can be provided. The cannula can be fixed to the cheek and neck with tape, in such a way that it is difficult for the child to remove it. The advantages are low cost, stability of oxygen supply and increased patient mobility. The cannula can become blocked by mucus.

MASKS

Low flow, close-fitting mask

A concentration up to 60% oxygen can be achieved with low/moderate flows (4–8 L/minute). At low oxygen flows (less than 5 L/minute) significant rebreathing may occur with mild CO_2 retention.

Close-fitting mask with reservoir bag (Figure 21.3)

Higher concentrations of oxygen can be delivered by using a large reservoir bag and a moderate oxygen flow. The patient may find a close-fitting mask hot and uncomfortable.

High flow fixed concentration masks (Venturi) (Figure 21.4)

These masks operate on a Venturi principle. As oxygen enters the mask through a narrow jet it entrains a constant flow of air through the surrounding hole. These masks will deliver an accurate concentration of oxygen providing the total gas flow delivered by the mask is equal to or greater than the peak inspiratory flow rate of the patient. Suggested flows are given by the manufacturer for each mask and are generally aimed at a peak tidal and inspiratory flow of 40–50 L/minute. These will be adequate for most children, but in a very breathless child may be less than the peak inspiratory flow. In these circumstances, the patient will feel uncomfortable and suffocated by the mask and for part of each inspiration the patient will be entraining air diluting the inspired oxygen. To combat this, the flow needs to be increased and with a set entrainment ratio this automatically increases the overall total flow available to the child (Figure 21.5). It is

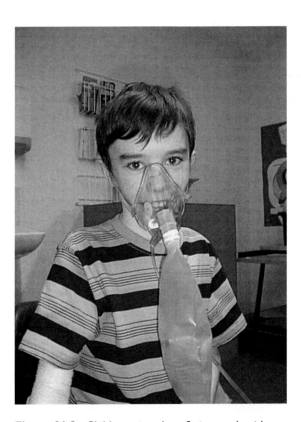

Figure 21.3: Child wearing close-fitting mask with reservoir bag.

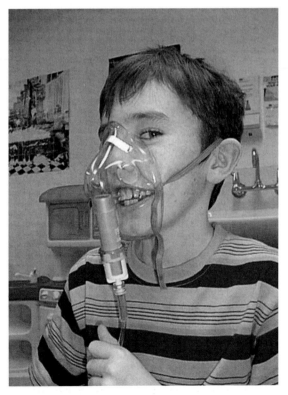

Figure 21.4: Child wearing high flow fixed concentration mask (Venturi).

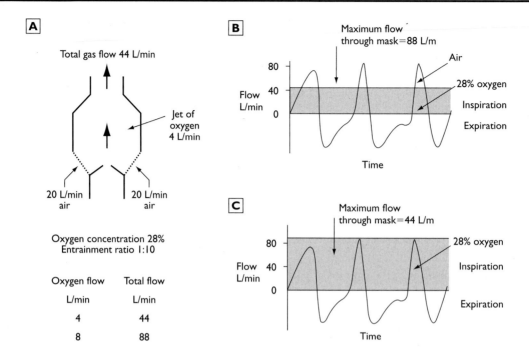

Figure 21.5: (A) Illustration of Venturi principle where to achieve an oxygen concentration of 28% there is a 1/10 entrainment ratio. For a jet of oxygen of 4 L/minute passing through the Venturi valve, 40 L of air will be entrained giving a total gas flow of 44 L/minute. Increasing the jet of oxygen to 8 litres per minute would result in an entrainment of 80 L/minute, hence delivering a total gas flow available to the patient of 88 L/minute. The oxygen concentration remains at 28%. (B) Representation of patient inspiratory flow profile versus time illustrating that with a maximum flow of 44 L/minute through the oxygen mask, the patient's peak inspiratory flow exceeds this resulting in an inspired mixture of less than 28% oxygen and air. (C) Representation of patient's inspiratory flow pattern versus time illustrating that when the peak flow rate of 28% oxygen available to the patient is 88 L/minute, this exceeds the patient's peak inspiratory flow rate hence the patient receives 28% oxygen throughout inspiration.

important to emphasize that increasing the flow will not alter the oxygen concentration delivered to the child, will do no harm, and may make the child comfortable and accept the mask. The disadvantage is that high flows are noisy and create quite a breeze that may also be cooling.

HUMIDIFICATION

Consideration must be given to both oxygen source and patient delivery device.

Oxygen sources

Oxygen from a piped source or a cylinder passes through a pressure regulator to bring the operating pressure to a safe level. The oxygen is cold and

dry and may dry the airway mucosa and decrease ciliary activity, particularly if delivered at high flows.

Oxygen from a concentrator is at a low pressure and flow and the oxygen is at room temperature and humidity – additional humidification is rarely necessary.

Patient delivery

Head box – oxygen is delivered at very low flows and humidification is rarely necessary.

Nasal prongs and cannulae – oxygen is delivered at low flows and can be humidified by a cold water bubble humidifier if needed, although at rates of flow of less than 1 L/minute, this is unnecessary.

Masks – at low flows less than 5 L/minute, a cold water bubble humidifier is adequate but humidification is increasingly important with high flow oxygen delivery. A heated humidifier is necessary to provide any humidity to the large volume of gas delivered at high flows.

OXYGEN IN THE HOME

In children who are stable but likely to require oxygen therapy for weeks or months, consideration should be given to providing oxygen at home (Tables 21.3 and 21.4). Oxygen can be provided either in cylinders or by an oxygen concentrator. Cylinders are large, cumbersome and expensive so for other than occasional use, concentrators are cost effective. The procedure for prescribing and supplying oxygen varies from country to country. In the UK, the GP prescribes the oxygen and contacts the supplying company contracted by the NHS for that region. Concentrators with a low flow meter are supplied along with tubing outlets to different rooms. All companies also provide a back-up cylinder in case of concentrator or electricity failure. It is important to remember that oxygen from a concentrator cannot exceed a flow rate of 5 L/minute and that the oxygen concentra-

Table 21.3: Conditions where home oxygen may be needed

- Chronic neonatal lung disease
- Cystic fibrosis
- Pulmonary hypertension
- Obliterative bronchiolitis
- Fibrosing alveolitis
- Alveolar proteinosis

Table 21.4: Criteria that must be fulfilled before discharge with home oxygen

- Oxygen responsive hypoxaemia
- Stable oxygen requirement
- Home conditions acceptable including a no smoking policy
- Telephone installed
- Community support organized
- Primary health care team accepts care plan
- Plan for emergency access to help
- Home insurers notified

tion is 92–95% up to 3 L/minute and drops at higher flows. Patients who require oxygen at high flows may need to use cylinder oxygen with a Venturi mask in order to achieve this.

For patients needing continuous oxygen, small portable cylinders are available, but are heavy and require frequent top ups from large cylinders (e.g. weight 5 kg; duration at 2 L/minute = 2.5 hours). An electronic (battery) oxygen-conserving device (Oxymatic) which delivers a pulse of oxygen during inspiration only, greatly extends the duration of oxygen supply in portable cylinders. This system uses light-weight aluminium cylinders (e.g. Oxylight 240 – weight 2.3 kg; duration of oxygen at 2 L/minute for approximately 14 hours). These are not prescribable in the UK and are expensive.

EVALUATION

HOW TO ASSESS/RE-ASSESS OXYGEN NEED

During therapy for acute illness in hospital, oximetry should be performed within 30 minutes of starting therapy and Fio_2 adjusted. A further oximetry check should be performed within 2 hours, and blood gas analysis performed if necessary (if the child's condition has deteriorated or if airway obstruction is the primary problem). For severely ill patients, continuous oximetry is indicated.

For patients on long-term oxygen therapy, assessment of need must take place in each physiological state; sleep, wakefulness, exercise and (for an infant) feeding. For domiciliary monitoring, a recording oximeter may be used. Records should cover several hours of sleep and wakefulness. An infant's representative sleep–wake cycle may be as short as 2–3 hours.

Sao_2 recording and playback permits analysis of baseline Sao_2 and desaturation episodes. For complex problems, additional channel recording e.g. chest and abdominal movement or airflow may be necessary. Miniature Sao_2 recording devices are now available for overnight recording in the patient's home and can then be delivered or even posted to the laboratory for analysis (Figure 21.6).

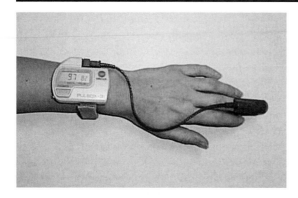

Figure 21.6: 'Wrist watch' oximetry recorder for overnight use (Minolta Pulsox).

WHEN TO STOP OXYGEN THERAPY

In an improving condition, maintenance of Sao_2 greater than 92% in air permits weaning from oxygen support in that physiological state (e.g. sleep). In infants with chronic neonatal lung disease, an Sao_2 greater than 92% after 40 minutes in room air predicted readiness for weaning from oxygen and such infants maintained growth over the next 6 months.[4]

BENEFITS OF LONG-TERM OXYGEN THERAPY

Hypoxaemia induces an increase in cardiac output and pulmonary vasoconstriction. In chronic neonatal lung disease, oxygen therapy reduces pulmonary hypertension, reduces reversible obstructive airways disease, improves growth and reduces the frequency of hypoxaemic/apnoeic episodes during sleep.[5, 6]

In children with cystic fibrosis, nocturnal low flow oxygen is effective in alleviating nocturnal hypoxaemia and permits continuation of school or work attendance but does not affect mortality rates or frequency of hospitalization.[6, 7]

In children with pulmonary vascular disease, long-term oxygen therapy may improve survival.[8]

HAZARDS OF OXYGEN THERAPY

There are recognized hazards of long-term oxygen therapy. For example, abolishing the hypoxaemic drive may lead to resulting CO_2 retention. In cystic fibrosis patients for example a small but clinically insignificant rise in CO_2 is noted after long-term nocturnal oxygen therapy is started. In the acute situation where high concentration oxygen therapy is used, there may be some toxicity to alveolar cells. In addition, small areas of atelectasis may occur if the patient is exposed to 100% oxygen for long periods. In the pre-term infant, retinopathy of prematurity is a recognized hazard. Saturation monitors do not recognize hyperoxia and their use therefore has to be very carefully regulated in this age group.[9] Finally, oxygen is a fire hazard.

EXTRA-CORPOREAL MEMBRANE OXYGENATION (ECMO)

Extra-corporeal life support with ECMO is achieved by diverting venous blood through an artificial lung for oxygenation and carbon dioxide removal (Figure 21.7). The blood is returned to either the arterial circulation (veno-arterial ECMO) or the venous circulation (veno-venous ECMO). During veno-arterial ECMO both the lungs and the heart can be supported. During veno-venous ECMO oxygenated blood is returned to the venous side where it is mixed with the venous blood returning from the tissues, thereby raising the oxygen content and lowering the carbon dioxide level in the right atrium. In either mode the lungs are allowed to 'rest and recover' without the stress of barotrauma and oxygen toxicity associated with prolonged conventional or high frequency therapy. ECMO may also permit reversal of pulmonary vasoconstriction and/or myocardial dysfunction related to hypoxia and acidosis.

PATIENT POPULATIONS BENEFITING FROM ECMO

Neonates

There is clear evidence of benefit in infants.[10] The most likely ECMO candidates are term or near term infants with respiratory failure secondary to: meconium aspiration syndrome, persistent pulmonary hypertension, neonatal sepsis/pneumonia, respiratory distress syndrome, congenital diaphragmatic hernia or severe cardiac or cardio-pulmonary failure.

The following guidelines have been used to determine eligibility for ECMO in the UK: gestational age >34 weeks, birth weight >2000g, reversible lung disease (mechanical ventilation <10 days), no major intra-cranial haemorrhage (grade 1 or less), no uncorrectable congenital cardiac lesions, no lethal congenital anomalies and no significant coagulopathy or uncontrolled bleeding complications.

Children and adults

Older patients that may benefit from treatment with ECMO include children with severe respiratory failure from the following diseases: pneumonia, bronchiolitis, pulmonary embolus, fat embolus, sepsis/septic shock, adult respiratory distress syndrome (ARDS), aspiration syndromes, intra-pulmonary haemorrhage, trauma, burns, poisoning or severe cardiac or cardio-pulmonary failure.

WHEN TO REFER

In most cases, deteriorating oxygenation will respond to increasing ventilatory support but the progression towards respiratory failure in criti-cally ill patients is often unpredictable, and may progress to refractory hypoxic cardiac arrest. To decrease the risk of death prior to transportation, the need for ECMO should be considered when certain criteria are met. There are no standard criteria for transfer; each case is unique. This is a *guide* to the need for ECMO in a patient who has received full and appropriate medical management:

- $Pa_{O_2} < 8$ kPa (60 mmHg).
- peak inspiratory pressure > 35 cm H_2O on conventional mechanical ventilation
- oxygenation index (OI) > 35 (except congenital diaphragmatic hernia where OI >30) for neonates, where

$$OI = [\text{mean airway pressure (cm } H_2O) \times Fi_{O_2}/Pa_{O_2} \text{ (mmHg)}].$$

- respiratory acidosis that is refractory to maximal medical therapy and not tolerated by the patient.

CLINICAL RESEARCH ISSUES

The development of secondary pulmonary hypertension significantly worsens the prognosis in children with chronic pulmonary disease. A major aim of long-term oxygen therapy is to prevent or ameliorate the progressive development of pulmonary hypertension. It is clear that there are a number of mechanisms involved in the adaptation of the pulmonary endothelium to hypoxia with endothelial nitric oxygen production playing a major role. Improved methods of non-invasive measurement of pulmonary vascular resistance are likely to guide oxygen therapy in the future and help establish a 'safe' level of oxygenation at different ages above which pulmonary hypertension is unlikely to develop.

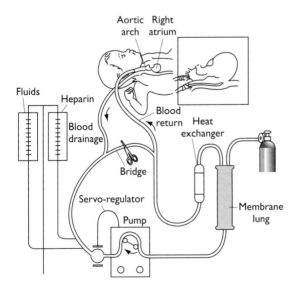

Figure 21.7: Diagram of a neonatal extra-corporeal membrane oxygenator (ECMO) circuit.

REFERENCES

1. Dong S-H, Lin H-M, Song G-W, Rong Z-P, Wu Y-P. Arterialised capillary blood gases and acid based studies in normal individuals from 29 days to 24 years of age. *Am J Dis Child* 1985; **139**: 1019–22.

2. Lozano JM, Duque OR, Buitrago T, Behaine S. Pulse oximetry reference values at high altitude. *Arch Dis Child* 1992; **67**: 299–330.

3. Shann F, Gatchalian S, Hutchinson R. Nasopharyngeal oxygen in children. *Lancet* 1988; **26**: 1238–40.

4. Simoes EA, Rosenberg AA, King SJ, Groothuis JR. Room air challenge: prediction for successful weaning of oxygen-dependent infants. *J Perinatol* 1997; **17**: 125–9.

5. Goodman G, Perkin RM, Anas NG, Sperling DR, Hicks DA, Rowen M. Pulmonary hypertension in infants with bronchopulmonary dysplasia. *J Pediat* 1988; **112**: 67–72.

6. Groothuis JR, Rosenberg AA. Home oxygen promotes weight gain in infants with bronchopulmonary dysplasia. *Am J Dis Child* 1987; **141**: 992–5.

7. Zinman R, Corey M, Coates AL, Canny GJ, Connolly J, Levison H, Beaudry PH. Nocturnal home oxygen in the treatment of hypoxemic cystic fibrosis patients. *J Pediat* 1989; **114**: 368–77.

8. Bowyer JJ, Busst CM, Denison DM, Shinebourne EA. Effect of long term oxygen treatment at home in children with pulmonary vascular disease. *Br Heart J* 1986; **55**: 385–90.

9. Cochran DP, Shaw NJ. The use of pulse oximetry in the prevention of hyperoxaemia in preterm infants. *Eur J Pediatr* 1995; **154**: 222–4.

10. UK collaborative randomised trial of neonatal extracorporeal membrane oxygenation: *Lancet* 1996; **348**: 75–82.

FURTHER READING

1. Moyle JTB. *Principles in practice series: Pulse oximetry.* London: BMJ Books, 1998.

2. Dodd ME, Haworth CS, Webb AK. A practical approach to oxygen therapy in cystic fibrosis. *J RSoc Med* 1998; **91(S34):** 30–9.

3. Bateman NT, Leach RM. ABC of oxygen: acute oxygen therapy. *BMJ* 1998; **317**: 798–801.

CHAPTER TWENTY TWO

COMPLIANCE *OR* ADHERENCE *TO* THERAPY

J. Paton

- Background
- Why do patients not comply?
- Measuring compliance
- Improving compliance – practical strategies

- The future: research
- References
- Further reading

BACKGROUND

Medical treatments of any kind are complicated by two major problems:

- the degree to which they are specific (the placebo problem);
- the extent to which they are taken by the patient (the compliance/adherence problem).[1]

Poor compliance is common. With drug treatments, it is estimated that one-third of patients comply adequately, one-third more or less adequately while one-third are non-compliant.[2,3] Studies have consistently shown that 40–50% of patients do not use medicines as prescribed.[4] Other aspects of medical care, such as appointment keeping, implementing preventive strategies or following a diet, are also affected. All such failures may lead to morbidity that would otherwise be avoidable and may waste scarce resources (Figure 22.1).

In children, failure to take treatment has been shown to occur in asthma, tuberculosis, cystic fibrosis, diabetes and antibiotic prophylaxis for sickle cell disease. Failure to take treatment has been noted even where the consequences may be life-threatening. It is thought to be an important cause of relapse in leukaemia[5] and of poor glycaemic control in brittle diabetes.[6] Even very

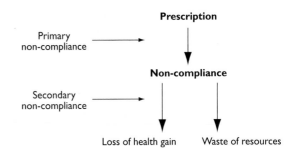

Figure 22.1: Classifying non-compliance and its consequences (adapted from Horne, RCP 1998).

young children may be affected, because their parents may not follow the prescription.[7]

Defining compliance is surprisingly difficult. Because compliance is not an all-or-nothing behaviour, simple definitions often fail to capture the complexity of the problem (Box 22.1). Virtually no-one follows doctors' prescriptions to the letter. In chronic diseases, the extent of non-compliance can vary over time. Further, how much non-compliance matters depends on the relation between compliance and clinical outcome. Ideally, non-compliance would be defined as the level below which a desired outcome was unlikely to be achieved. However, not all drugs rely on compliance to the same extent in producing effective responses. Some drug regimens are much more flexible than others. For example, oral penicillin

> **Box 22.1: Definition of compliance**
>
> The extent to which the patient's behaviour (in terms of taking medications, following diets or executing other life-style changes) coincides with the clinical prescription.
>
> Sackett DL. Introduction. In: Sackett DL, Haynes RB (eds). *Compliance with therapeutic regimens.* Baltimore and London: The John Hopkins University Press, 1976;1–6.

prophylaxis against rheumatic fever achieves adequate protection with compliance in excess of 33%. To date, little work has been done on defining 'sufficient' or 'good-enough' compliance for specific medicines[8].

Even the term compliance has been criticized because of its connotations of 'doctor knows best'. One common alternative, adherence, has similar overtones. Both convey an expectation that the patient will blindly but precisely follow doctor's orders. Nowadays, the idea that the doctor's rational and evidence-based prescription is superior to the patient's beliefs and wishes is increasingly questioned.

WHY DO PATIENTS NOT COMPLY?

Poor compliance is not a new problem. Hippocrates recommended that one should 'keep watch also on the faults of the patient, which often make them lie about the taking of things prescribed.' Indeed, non-compliance may have its origin in innate instinctive defences that help to protect animals from ingesting harmful or poisonous substances.[8]

Compliance behaviours have proved complicated to understand and difficult to improve. Patient, drug prescription and patient–therapist interaction, can each influence compliance.

PATIENT FACTORS

Poor compliance has not been closely associated with particular patient characteristics, such as age, sex, race, educational level, or personality traits,[9,4] or disease characteristics, such as diagnosis, duration. The most important factors to emerge have been either physical or social vulnerability, such as old age, or psychiatric illness, or failures of communication arising mainly from differences in health beliefs between doctors and patients. In general, neither demographic nor disease or symptom variables have provided convincing explanations of non-compliance.

In most circumstances, poor compliance is clearly not due to lack of knowledge or understanding. Sackett described this well:[10]

> 'This simplistic approach of many who wish to improve compliance (without necessarily understanding it) has been founded upon the perceived efficacy of the "information transfer" component of such messages with scant attention being paid to the "attitude change" component of the educational process. The resulting misapplication of misunderstood principles (the "cross-sterilization of disciplines") has led to a series of remarkably unsuccessful health information programmes and campaigns …'

Non-compliance has been divided into a number of categories. *Primary non-compliance* describes the situation when the patient fails even to have the medication dispensed. Surprisingly, up to one in five patients fail to have medication dispensed, even when the prescription has been actively sought.[11] *Secondary non-compliance* occurs when the prescription is dispensed but the patient does not take it as intended. Factors contributing to such non-compliance have been broadly classified as intentional or unintentional (Figure 22.2). Unintentional reasons include forgetting, lack of physical competence or misunderstanding between

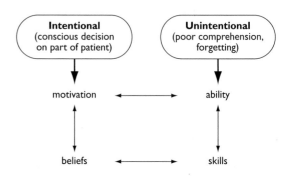

Figure 22.2: Understanding non-compliance – a framework (adapted from Horne, RCP 1998).

doctor and patient. Intentional non-compliance is thought to be commoner, and reflects active and rational choices by the patient based on their beliefs about both the illness and the medications (Case study 22.1).

Patients' beliefs

Behavioural scientists have used both psychological and sociological approaches in seeking to understand compliance behaviours. Psychological models have been developed to provide conceptual frameworks for understanding how a patient's beliefs influence and determine behaviour. For example, the Health Belief Model suggests that health behaviours are influenced by beliefs about:

- *perceived vulnerability* to the health threat
- *perceived seriousness* of the health threat
- *perceived benefit* associated with taking preventive action
- *perceived barriers* related to preventive action.

While the first two reflect the perceived threat to the individual from the health problem, the last two relate to the costs and benefits of a course of action. Good compliance would be predicted in those who perceive their problems as serious and who expect the benefits of treatment to be greater than the side effects.

Sociological research, based mainly on qualitative studies, has examined people's beliefs about treatments. A number of important common themes about medicines and medicine-taking have emerged[12,8]:

PERCEIVED EFFICACY AND BALANCING OF RISKS AND BENEFITS

Patients vary in their confidence in a drug's ability to help their symptoms and may attempt to balance their positive and negative views of a medicine. They may try a medication for a short period, stopping if it fails to deliver clear benefits. They may also set time limits for the achievement of specific outcomes. Not infrequently, patients will stop taking the drugs from time to time in an attempt to check they are still working.

DANGERS OF DEVELOPING IMMUNITY, TOLERANCE, ADDICTION AND DEPENDENCE

Worries about developing 'immunity' or 'tolerance', so that a drug might be ineffective when really needed, are common. Another frequent worry is that of addiction. Such concerns are closely related to ideas about loss of control and dependence associated with illness and medicine-taking. Manipulating medications may help a patient relieve a sense of dependence, and re-establish feelings of being in control.

ANTI-DRUG ATTITUDES

Drugs are often considered as poisons. The term 'drug' is associated with other 'drugs', such as cocaine and opiates, with all their anti-social and dangerous connotations. Furthermore, patients frequently view manufactured medicines as 'unnatural' and harmful, whereas naturally occurring substances such as plants or herbs are widely seen as 'safe' and 'natural'.

ADJUSTING TO EVERYDAY LIFE

Patients may alter their medication regime for reasons related to their daily lives. Such behaviour can reflect a wish to take control of their lives or to self-regulate to manage events in their daily routine.[13]

DISCREPANCIES BETWEEN THE DOCTOR'S AND PATIENT'S PERSPECTIVE

Discrepancies between the doctor's view of the diagnosis and treatment and the patient's or parent's may also be important. Parents may not

---

Case study 22.1: No bronchodilator before activities

Christine knew that her terbutaline Turbohaler could help prevent wheezing during games – the doctor had often told her this at the clinic. Usually she did not bother with it, except when she knew she was likely to be very wheezy. Occasionally she forgot to bring it to school. More often she did not take it because she preferred not to let her friends see that she needed medicine. At her clinic appointment, the problem was discussed. Christine knew about using her inhaler before games and agreed she would think about using it more often.

agree with the doctor's diagnosis and may then be reluctant to use medicines, especially if these are perceived as dangerous. Professional advice must be carefully phrased if it is not, inadvertently, to act as a deterrent. Parents have reported that professionals' attempts to persuade them that the risks of vaccine damage were minimal actually deterred them from having their child vaccinated.[14]

Although often unspoken, such patients' beliefs about illness and medicines appear to be among the most important determinants of compliance behaviours. Accordingly, understanding these beliefs can provide important insights into why patients act in a particular way. Finally, beliefs are particularly important because once understood they may be alterable. Doctors, therefore, require strategies that actively explore their patients' beliefs, worries and fears. Such understanding can then form the basis of a therapeutic concordance which takes account of both the patient's and the doctor's goals.

DRUG AND PRESCRIPTION FACTORS AFFECTING COMPLIANCE

There are a number of drug-related factors that can influence compliance[12]:

Efficacy

Medications that are inappropriately prescribed and consequently ineffective are likely to be poorly complied with.

Side effects

Obvious and unpleasant side effects, such as vomiting, will make patients much less likely to take a drug. The relationship between less obtrusive side effects and compliance is less clear.

Number of drugs and dosage regimens

The more drugs prescribed, the less likely they are to be taken as recommended. Dosing frequency also affects compliance. Twice-a-day regimes are followed better than three or four times a day.[15]

There is little evidence, however, that once a day is better. If a dose is then missed, levels will remain low for 18–24 hours, unless the drug has a long half-life. A more important underlying factor may be the degree of behaviour change a regimen requires. Passive co-operation may be easily attained, but breaking a personal habit, such as smoking, may be difficult or impossible.

Drug formulation and route

In adults, most modern oral drug formulations should not influence adherence. In children, the formulation may be more important. Young children may not be able to swallow tablets or may refuse to take unpleasant liquids. While compliance with oral medication is thought superior, there is surprisingly little work comparing compliance with the oral route with compliance with other routes.

Duration of therapy

Compliance generally deteriorates in the long term. It also declines between clinic visits.[16] Clinic non-attendance may pinpoint a group where non-compliance is likely and, conversely, regular follow-up may encourage good compliance.

PATIENT–THERAPIST INTERACTIONS

Research has also shown that features of the patient–doctor interaction can improve compliance.

Supervision and compliance

Increased patient supervision improves compliance. Thus hospitalized patients are generally more compliant than day patients. Increasing the frequency of clinic visits, arranging home visits, or recruiting a family member to supervise the taking of medication can all help to improve compliance.

Patient satisfaction

Patient satisfaction, and a sense that the doctor has met with expectations, has been positively associated with compliance.[17]

PROBLEMS SPECIFIC TO CHILDHOOD

Children have special problems with compliance. As noted, they may not be able to swallow tablets and they do not like unpleasant tastes.

A child's developmental stage may also affect his ability to take a medicine. For example, most children are unable to use a metered dose inhaler properly, while small children may not have sufficient inspiratory capacity to open a spacer valve or to suck a dry powder inhaler. Depending on age and intelligence, a child may not have the capacity to remember to take a medicine every day at a certain time, nor the concentration to sit quietly throughout administration. Consequently, in young children it is the carer who will determine adherence and the carer whom the doctor will need to convince and educate about medication benefits. However, even very young children may recognize that medication relieves symptoms, and may bring the medicine to the carer for administration.

As children get older, they will increasingly determine their medication use. Asthmatic children begin to have full responsibility for their medication from as early as 10 years.[18]

MEASURING COMPLIANCE

Ideal methods of measuring of compliance have been defined as ones that are usable over a prolonged period of time; are unobtrusive, non-invasive, practicable, and cheap; yield immediate results; and are not susceptible to manipulation.[19] In practice, most current compliance measures are far from that ideal.[20] The methods used can be broadly classified into several categories.

TECHNIQUES OF MEASUREMENT

Listening to patients

The simplest approach is to ask the patient what medications they have taken. This can be done retrospectively using questioning, or prospectively using a patient-completed diary. Unfortunately, comparison of patient estimates with simultaneous objective measurements from electronic monitoring or measuring metabolite concentrations has shown that patients consistently overestimate their actual medication use by between 30–50%. However, patients' self-reports of *non-compliance* may be more accurate. Appropriately phrased questions ('most people don't manage to take their medicines all the times – how often does that happen to you?') may then produce useful information, particularly if the question is directed at the child and not the parents.

If patients' self-reports are unreliable, doctors' assessments are no better. Studies have shown that doctors tend to overestimate compliance and are poor at predicting which patients are not complying. Indeed, doctors' predictions of compliance behaviours have been found to be no more accurate than chance, even with patients whom they have known for years.

Counting tablets, canister weighing and checking prescriptions

A second common approach is some variation of pill counting. Returned pills or other used formulations, such as dry powder discs, are counted and compared with the use that would have been expected in the period. Weighing returned aerosol canisters to determine the number of puffs used is another variation. Some dry powder inhaler devices now include a dose counter within the device (Figure 22.3).

While these approaches provide an integrated estimate of compliance over time, they also have been shown to overestimate adherence. For example, the common practice of test firing an inhaler

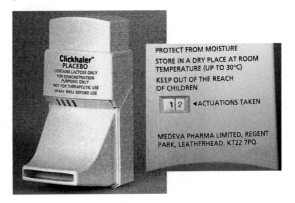

Figure 22.3: A dry powder inhaler showing the built-in dose counter.

Case study 22.2: 'Difficult asthma'

Jonathan, an 11-year-old boy attending a hospital asthma clinic, had been prescribed increasing inhaled corticosteroids because of poor asthma control. Electronic monitoring showed that he was not taking any medication for days at a time. However, he used ('dumped') approximately 70 doses in a few minutes just before his clinic visit. The situation improved when he was seen independently of his parents and was able to negotiate his own management plan.

will result in the weight of returned aerosol canisters overestimating use. Perhaps more importantly, similar counts may be obtained from widely differing patterns of compliance. Thus a patient who has taken no medication but 'dumped' doses before a clinic visit (Case study 22.2) and someone who has followed instructions precisely may appear identical.

With computerization of GP prescribing, prescription uptake records have increasingly been used as an indirect compliance measure. Again these are likely to overestimate patients' true medication use, particularly in the light of evidence that prescriptions are often not presented for dispensing. In the future, prescription records may become more useful if they are routinely linked with dispensing.

Electronic pill counters or inhaler timer devices (Figure 22.4) have been developed over the last 15 years. These techniques give much more detailed information. They have provided important insights into drug usage including 'drug holidays', 'white coat adherence' (the tendency to use medicines regularly in the days before a clinic appointment) and 'canister dumping' (multiple actuations within a short period of time before a clinic visit) (Figure 22.4). The ethical aspects of covert electronic monitoring have been considered in detail.[21] Surprisingly, compliance is frequently poor even when the patient knows they are being monitored.

Virtually all of these approaches rely on a key assumption – that drugs taken are reliably delivered to the site of action. So, for example, if a child's anti-tuberculosis prescriptions are collected at appropriate intervals, then it is assumed that the child is receiving the medication appropriately. Similarly if an inhaler has been used, then it

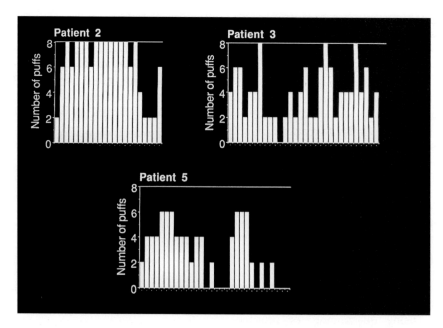

Figure 22.4: An inhaler timer (Chronolog) was attached to a large volume spacer (Nebuhaler) to obtain these data from 3 subjects. The bar charts show the number of puffs used each day over various periods of time.

is assumed that each actuation has been correctly and has delivered an equivalent, effective drug dose to the site of action. Such assumptions are not always valid.

Measuring drug metabolites and other markers

The third common approach is to measure a drug metabolite or marker in blood, urine, saliva or faeces. These methods are often technically complicated, expensive and slow. Blood sampling is particularly unpopular with children. Even when available, blood levels can be complicated to interpret especially if drug interactions change metabolism.

Urine staining of a nappy (diaper) orange can be used to monitor rifampicin therapy for tuberculosis. Rifampicin is easily identified because it turns urine and other body fluids red-orange. Colouring of the urine may then indicate that the patient is taking the medicine. However, there may be a positive result even if the drug has not been taken regularly. Unfortunately, children may not always be willing to provide a urine sample on demand.

Clinical outcomes as markers of drug effects have proved of little value. Even compliance with a placebo can confer benefit! Some clinical pointers may point to patients more likely to be non-compliant (Box 22.2).

RECENT DEVELOPMENTS

Although most currently available compliance measures are not ideal, newer developments are coming closer. Home CPAP machines are now available with built-in monitors that measure duration of therapy and pressures delivered. A recently developed nebulizer not only delivers medication in response to a correct inspiration, but also includes electronic monitoring to provide detailed information subsequently about the patient's medication use.

Until such technology becomes widely available, no single method of measuring compliance can be regarded as ideal. Multiple measures will often be required in order to obtain the best overall picture. The method adopted will also depend on whether measurement is being carried out for

Box 22.2: Spotting non-compliance – some clinical clues

- **Patients admitting to missing medication doses on questioning**
  Developing good interviewing skills and a non-judgemental approach are essential. 'Allowing' the patient to admit to non-compliance helps ('How often do you forget your .....?').

- **Loss of responsiveness to a usually or previously adequate regime**
  (see Case study 22.2).

- **Clinic non-attendance**
  Failure to attend for appointments has been associated with worse compliance. In TB failure to attend is common and should be an indication for rapid community intervention with review of prescription uptake and a TB liaison health visitor visit (see Case study 22.3).

research purposes or as part of a treatment programme. For certain treatments, such as anti-tuberculous therapy, where maximal compliance is important the aim may be to detect as many non-compliers as possible, and to render non-compliance less risky (in terms of drug resistance) by prescribing only combination drug therapy.

IMPROVING COMPLIANCE – PRACTICAL STRATEGIES

Since doctors cannot reliably predict who will and who will not take their treatment, strategies to improve compliance have to be applied to all. In general, it is increasingly clear that success requires a shift away from a narrow focus on medicine taking to a broader emphasis on negotiation and mutual agreement between the patient and doctor about treatment goals as well as precise treatment plans. Fink has highlighted some important principles[22]:

- there is no such thing as a standard regime;
- health decisions and behaviours are carried out in the real world; regimes that take account of patient and family settings are more likely to be effective;

- individual health problems are constantly changing. Most are managed without recourse to a doctor; an important goal is to enhance a patient's ability to be self-sufficient in solving health problems;
- the doctor–patient relationship should be one of mutual participation with the goal of achieving objectives that are patient or child focused as well as doctor focused.

In practice, choosing the best approach will depend upon the nature of the disease. For a chronic variable disease such as asthma, the most effective approach appears to depend on helping patients to control their own disease in order to achieve their personal goals.[23] For other diseases, particularly TB, ensuring maximal compliance may be important and strategies such as directly observed therapy more useful (Case study 22.3). Whatever the circumstances, it is important to remember that good compliance is not an end in itself – it is merely a step on the path to a desired therapeutic outcome. There are several approaches to improve compliance:

HEALTH CARE TEAM EDUCATION / TRAINING

Strategies have been identified to help improve doctor–patient communication and empathy consultations (Table 22.1). Training can help.[24] A recent study found that training improved physicians' communications behaviour and prescribing, led to more favourable patient responses and reduced health care utilization.[23] Significantly, for hard-pressed clinicians, such training resulted in briefer consultations.

Nowadays, patients often see other members of the health care team such as nurses or physiotherapists. They also will need training if consistent messages are to be delivered.

SIMPLIFYING REGIMES

The most effective simplification is to stop treatments that are not working. Other important steps include:

- Always using the least medication necessary to treat the symptoms.
- Reducing dose frequency to once or twice daily regimens where possible.
- Avoiding poly-pharmacy.
- Ensuring that each member of the clinical team uses simple and consistent labels for medications (e.g. 'relievers' and 'preventers') and that each delivers consistent messages.

To date, combining drugs has not been particularly helpful. However, there are some circumstances where it can be valuable particularly in TB where drug combinations of rifampicin and isoniazid may help minimize the development of drug resistance.

PARENT / CHILD TRAINING THROUGH EDUCATION AND COUNSELLING

Approaches to encourage active patient participation and promote adherence are given in Table 22.2. The emphasis is now on negotiating a *concordance* between the 'client', child or parent, and the doctor about the therapeutic plan. The challenge is to create an open and honest relationship, so that both sides can proceed on the basis of 'reality and not of misunderstanding, distrust or concealment'.[8] (See also Chapter 15.)

Case study 22.3: Tuberculosis with worsening X-ray changes

Douglas was 2 years old. He presented with culture-positive pulmonary tuberculosis. He was started on treatment with standard triple therapy with daily rifampicin, isoniazid and pyrazinamide. He regularly failed to attend for follow-up. When he finally came, his CXR appearances were deteriorating. Follow-up cultures remained positive and showed that the organism had become isoniazid resistant. Further investigation revealed social chaos: his parents were separated; the child was shuttled between them, with some of his medicines often remaining behind. Once this was discovered, he was treated with directly observed therapy with four anti-tuberculous drugs administered three times a week by a nurse for a year. He made a complete recovery.

Table 22.1: Strategies to improve doctor–patient communication (adapted from Refs 23 and 25)

	Technique	Effect
Treatment plan strategy focus	Tailor medication regimes by eliciting information and addressing potential problems in timing, dosage or side-effects.	
	Reach agreement on short-term goals that both doctor and patient will strive for that is important to the patient.	
	Review the physician's long-term therapeutic plan with the patient knowing what to expect over time.	
	Help patient develop and use criteria for management decisions.	
Congenial demeanour	Maintain an interactive conversation through the use of open-ended questions ('Tell me about it?'), simple language, analogies to teach important concepts.	Dialogue that is interactive produces richer information.
	Listen attentively, e.g. use eye contact, sit at same level rather than stand, lean slightly forward.	
	Give encouragement by using non-verbal communication, e.g nodding, smiling.	
	Give verbal praise for things done well.	
Reassuring communication	Elicit patient's underlying concerns and worries.	
	Give specific reassuring information in response.	Reduces fear as a distractant allowing the patient to focus on the message.
	Address immediate concerns.	Enables family to refocus their attention on the information being provided.

THE FUTURE: RESEARCH

It is clear that poor compliance remains a largely unrecognized and unacknowledged problem. A recent report justifiably highlighted the need for nationally co-ordinated programmes of research, development and training combined with a strategy for raising public awareness.

Particular research issues concern the recognition of non-compliance (where computer technology may help), its origins (health psychology is largely neglected in basic and continuing professional training) and its impact (at both personal and public health levels).

The emphasis on evidence-based medicine has highlighted the gulf between the tightly controlled conditions of the randomized controlled trial and 'real life' conditions that apply to individual sick children in their homes and schools. There is still much to do.

Table 22.2: Strategies to enhance patient adherence

Provide targeted information about treatment and disease
- elicit and answer the patient's specific questions
- investigate and address patient's beliefs
- teach how to use any devices
- give clear written instructions including specific advice on how to vary the medication

Modify and individualise the administration schedule
- keep the prescription as simple as possible
- reduce dosage frequency
- provide cues for action ('take the medication in the morning and evening before you brush your teeth')

Increase motivation
- by using verbal encouragement and praise to reinforce good behaviours
- by persuasion
- by helping to resolve practical problems

Collect information for future planning
- focus on patient's specific problems
- plan to collect information using a daily log or diary
- telephone before next appointment

Change contingencies
- shorten waiting times
- provide appointment reminders
- pay attention to side effects
- stress importance of compliance and discuss compliance failures
- help to remove blocks to medication use
- use formal contracts with the patient
- schedule more frequent reviews if compliance is poor

Enlist additional help if required
- provide assistance to solve social or financial problems
- use a second opinion to provide reassurance and support
- involve the parent and other siblings.

Adapted from:
1. Cramer JA, Spilker B (eds). Patient compliance in medical practice and clinical trials. New York: Raven Press, 1991.
2. Haynes RB et al. A critical review of interventions to improve compliance with prescribed medications. *Patient Educ and Counsel* 1987;**10**: 155–66.

REFERENCES

1. Anonymous. Keep on taking the tablets. *BMJ* 1977; **1**: 793.

2. Gordis L, Markowitz M, Lilienfeld AM. Why patients don't follow medical advice: a study of children on long-term antistreptococcal prophylaxis. *J Pediat* 1969; **75**: 957–68.

3. Wright EC. Non-compliance – or how many aunts has Matilda? *Lancet* 1993; **342**: 909–13.

4. Mellins RB, Evans D, Zimmerman B, Clark NM. Patient compliance. Are we wasting our time and don't know it? *Am Rev Respir Dis* 1992; **146**: 1376–7.

5. Lilleyman JS, Lennard L. Non-compliance with oral chemotherapy in childhood leukaemia. An overlooked and costly cause of relapse. *BMJ* 1996; **313**: 1219–20.

6. Morris AD, Boyle DI, McMahon AD, Greene SA, MacDonald TM, Newton RW. Adherence to insulin treatment, glycaemic control, and ketoacidosis in insulin-dependent diabetes mellitus. *Lancet* 1997; **350**: 1505–10.

7. Northfield M, Patel RK, Richardson A, Taylor MD, Richardson PD. Lifestyle changes in mild asthma during intermittent symptom-related use of terbutaline inhaled via 'Turbohaler'. *Curr Med Res Opin* 1991; **12**: 441–9.

8. Royal Pharmaceutical Society of Great Britain. *From compliance to concordance: towards shared goals in medicine taking*. London: RPS, 1997.

9. Haynes RB. A critical review of the 'Determinants' of patient compliance with therapeutic regimens. In: Sackett DL, Haynes RB, (eds). *Compliance with therapeutic regimens*. Baltimore and London: The John Hopkins University Press, 1976; 26–39.

10. Sackett DL. The magnitude of compliance and non-compliance. In: Sackett DL, Haynes RB, (eds). *Compliance with therapeutic regimens*. London and Baltimore: The John Hopkins University Press, 1976; 9–25.

11. Beardon PH, McGilchrist MM, McKendrick AD, McDevitt DG, MacDonald TM. Primary non-compliance with prescribed medication in primary care. *BMJ* 1993; **307**: 846–8.

12. McGavock H, Britten N, Weinman J. *A review of the literature on drug adherence*. Royal Pharmaceutical Society of Great Britain and Merck Sharp and Dohme, 1996.

13. Conrad P. The meaning of medications: another look at compliance. *Soc Sci Med* 1985; **20**: 29–37.

14. New SJ, Senior ML. 'I don't believe in needles': qualitative aspects of a study into the uptake of infant immunisation in two English authorities. *Soc Sci Med* 1991; **33**: 509–18.

15. Coutts JA, Gibson NA, Paton JY. Measuring compliance with inhaled medication in asthma. *Arch Dis Child* 1992; **67**: 332–3.

16. Cramer JA, Scheyer RD, Mattson RH. Compliance declines between clinic visits. *Arch Intern Med* 1990; **150**: 1509–10.

17. Francis V, Korsch BM, Morris MJ. Gaps in doctor–patient communication. Patients' response to medical advice. *N Engl J Med* 1969; **280**: 535–40.

18. Osman LM, Roberston R, Calder C, *et al.* Parents' perceptions of responsibility for asthma medication management among 10 to 16 year olds. *Am J Respir Crit Care Med* 1997; **155**: A722.

19. Pullar T, Feely M. Problems of compliance with drug treatment: new solutions? *Pharm J* 1990; **245**: 213–15.

20. Horn CR. The assessment of therapeutic compliance by asthmatic patients. *Eur Respir J* 1992; **5**: 126–7.

21. Levine RJ. Monitoring for adherence: ethical considerations. *Am J Respir Crit Care Med* 1994; **149**: 287–8.

22. Fink DL. Tailoring the consensual regimen. In: Sackett DL, Haynes RB (eds). *Compliance with therapeutic regimens*. Baltimore and London: The John Hopkins University Press, 1976; 110–18.

23. Clark NM, Gong M, Schork MA, *et al.* Impact of education for physicians on patient outcomes. *Pediatrics* 1998; **101**: 831–6.

24. Neuwirth ZE. Physician empathy – should we care? *Lancet* 1997; **350**: 606.

25. Clark NM, Gong M, Schork MA, *et al.* A scale for assessing Health Care Providers' teaching and communication behavior regarding asthma. *Health Educ Behav* 1997; **24**: 245–56.

FURTHER READING

1. Sackett DL, Haynes RB. *Compliance with therapeutic regimens*. Baltimore and London: John Hopkins University Press, 1976.

2. Royal Pharmaceutical Society of Great Britain. *From compliance to concordance: towards shared goals in medicine taking*. London: RPS, 1997.

3. Wright EC. Non-compliance – or how many aunts has Matilda? *Lancet* 1993; **342**: 909–13.

4. Compliance issues in asthma. *Eur Respir Rev* 1998, No. 56.

CHAPTER TWENTY THREE

PHYSIOTHERAPY

S. Pike and G. Phillips

- Background
- Techniques and applications
- Evaluating outcome

- Planning the future management
- Clinical research issues
- References

BACKGROUND

The paediatric physiotherapist has an important role in the management of infants and children with respiratory disorders. Physiotherapy for every child involves an initial assessment at each new contact, and constant re-evaluation of the outcome and of the changing needs of individual patients. Performance of treatment techniques must always be assessed. Supporting and encouraging both child and carers is an essential part of the management especially where it is necessary that treatment is carried out at home. Regular reviews by the physiotherapist can take place in the community or at the outpatient clinic.

This chapter briefly describes the objectives of physiotherapy and outlines the techniques available to the physiotherapist.

AIMS OF PHYSIOTHERAPY

Once the need for physiotherapy has been identified (Box 23.1), any contra-indications to treatment should be determined and precautions established. It is important to note that in some respiratory conditions, for example the acute phase of bronchiolitis in a non-ventilated infant, hands-on chest physiotherapy may actually exacerbate symptoms.[1] However, the physiotherapist can still advise on positioning to decrease the work of breathing. Through regular review, assessment may identify when a change in condition may indicate the need for treatment, for

Box 23.1: The aims of physiotherapy

- Clearance of bronchopulmonary secretions
- Re-inflation of lung collapse/atelectasis
- Improvement in ventilation/perfusion matching
- Relief of breathlessness
- Reduction in airway obstruction
- Increase exercise tolerance
- Postural maintenance/advice
- Education
- Thoracic mobility
- Pain relief

example if the infant develops lobar atelectasis. Therefore, the approach the physiotherapist should take is one of treating the child and not the condition.

Effective physiotherapy management often involves a combination of different techniques. Considering the patient as a whole, various factors may also come into play and techniques may be adapted to suit the individual. For example where gravity-assisted positioning would enhance clearance of bronchial secretions, in a child who is very breathless, the head tipped downwards position could cause distress and therefore modified positioning is indicated. The age of the child is an important consideration and will influence the techniques that can be used. A one-year-old infant can play no active part in their treatment and this affects the techniques available to the physiotherapist. Conditions that present with an acute, focal problem will require intensive and specific physiotherapy. In contrast long-term stable conditions (e.g. cystic fibrosis) will need a different approach. This will incorporate a rotating programme to cover all areas of the lungs and guidance on when and how to increase this, as well as exercise, postural advice and so forth.

As well as assessing the severity and nature of the problem, co-existing medical conditions can influence the choice of treatment. A child with a congenital heart defect will be compromised by certain gravity-assisted positions. Another situation is asthma: appropriate bronchodilators should be administered prior to physiotherapy.

TECHNIQUES AND APPLICATIONS

There are a variety of techniques available to the physiotherapist, as well as adjuncts to assist in the optimization of care.

POSTURAL DRAINAGE/GRAVITY-ASSISTED POSITIONING

Gravity-assisted positions are used to aid in the clearance of bronchial secretions.[2] Each position is specific for drainage of a lobe or segment and is used in conjunction with other techniques (Figure 23.1).

CHEST CLAPPING/PERCUSSION

Chest clapping is performed using a cupped hand or fingers, depending on the size of the child. It is a rhythmical movement using one or two hands, and loosens secretions from the bronchial wall.[3] Chest clapping is most effective in combination with 3–4 thoracic expansion exercises (deep breathing), and this also prevents hypoxaemia.[4] It is performed throughout the respiratory cycle. In infants who are unable to take voluntary deep breaths, short sessions (30 seconds) of clapping with rest periods in-between are recommended.

CHEST SHAKING/VIBRATIONS

Chest shaking is carried out with thoracic expansion exercises but only during expiration. The vibratory action is in the direction of rib movement and aids the clearance of secretions from the periphery.[5] Care is taken to ensure the vibration is not continued into the functional residual capacity, as this may cause airway collapse. For this reason it is not advised in self-ventilating infants, where the rate and depth of respiration cannot be controlled.

ACTIVE CYCLE OF BREATHING TECHNIQUES (ACBT)

ACBT consists of thoracic expansion exercises in conjunction with breathing control and the forced expiratory technique (FET). ACBT can be performed independently or with an assistant. It can be used in gravity-assisted position and chest clapping and/or shaking may be used depending upon individual assessment. ACBT can be introduced at an early age (2–3 years) with blowing games.[6] This technique is the most extensively researched and has been shown to improve lung function[7] and effectively clear secretions,[8] without causing hypoxia or airflow obstruction[4] (Figure 23.2).

Breathing control involves normal tidal breathing using lower chest and diaphragm, with the upper chest relaxed. This component prevents any increase in airflow obstruction and is used between the active parts of the cycle. In such conditions as asthma, it is an important technique to help decrease the work of breathing and reduce breathlessness, thus helping the child control their breathing.

Thoracic expansion exercises involve 3–4 deep breaths with the emphasis on inspiration. Expiration is passive and relaxed. They may be used in conjunction with chest clapping or shaking. The aim of thoracic expansion exercises is to increase lung volume thus assisting in the mobilization of secretions and the re-expansion of lung atelectasis.

In the *forced expiration technique* a combination of one or two forced expirations (huffs) alternates with periods of breathing control. A huff is a forced expiration against an open glottis. The huff is performed from mid to low lung volumes which causes dynamic compression at points along the airways. This point moves from bronchial level to the proximal airways and therefore assists in the movement of secretions.[9]

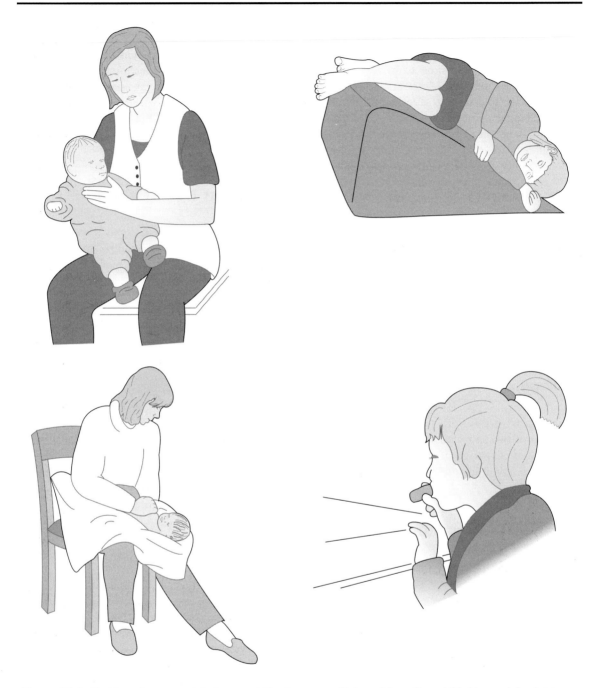

Figure 23.1: Positions for postural drainage and blowing games. (Adapted from Prasad SA, Hussey J. *Paediatric Respiratory Care*. Chapman & Hall, London, 1995.).

POSITIVE EXPIRATORY PRESSURE (PEP)

PEP can be applied using a facemask or mouth-piece and delivers a resistive pressure of 10–20 cmH$_2$O during expiration. The aim is to increase collateral ventilation[10] and thus the mobilizations of secretions. It is often combined with breathing control and huffing.

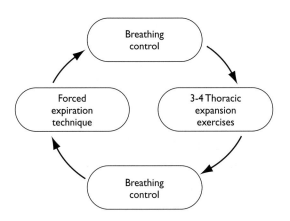

Figure 23.2: Active cycle of breathing techniques (ACBT).

FLUTTER

The flutter is a pipe-shaped device containing a ball-bearing resting in a small cone. The child breathes out into the device and the ball moves up and down the cone setting up varying levels of positive pressure, and creating an oscillatory effect in the airways. Periods of breathing control and huffing will improve clearance of secretions.[11,12]

AUTOGENIC DRAINAGE (AD)

AD was conceived in Belgium and is a technique combining controlled breathing during three phases, at different lung volumes. Inspiration includes a hold to allow equal filling of lung segments. Expiration is through the mouth, with high but not forced expiratory flow rates. The first phase begins at low lung volumes to mobilize secretions, the next at a tidal volume to collect, and the final phase at high volume to expectorate.[13] The treatment time can be up to 45 minutes.

POSITIONING

It is possible to use positioning to optimize lung function, maximize V/Q (ventilation-perfusion) matching and relieve breathlessness. The prone position improves lung compliance, tidal volume and oxygenation[14] compared with the supine position. Monitoring during prone positioning is advisable because of its association with sudden infant deaths. Side lying assists in drainage of secretions from the uppermost lung, can adversely affect the distribution of ventilation/-perfusion (and hence oxygenation) in infants. Forward lean sitting supports the diaphragm to facilitate its contraction during inspiration. This position also stabilizes the upper body, and in a breathless child (e.g. asthmatic) it can help to relieve dyspnoea.

ASSISTED COUGH

In children who have a marked muscular weakness (e.g. muscular dystrophy or spinal cord injuries) assisted coughing can aid clearance of secretions. The aim is to create an upward and inward force against the thorax thus replacing the abdominal muscle work.[15] Positioning of the hands and forearms is vital and this technique can be more effective with intermittent positive pressure breathing, where an increase in tidal volume is achieved prior to the manoeuvre.

EXERCISE

Exercise is very important for children with respiratory disease. It has many benefits:

- aids sputum clearance
- increases lung function
- improves cardio-respiratory fitness
- muscle strengthening
- posture maintenance
- increases self-esteem/well-being.

The choice of exercise depends on the nature of the disease, but should be fun. It may be useful to perform exercise testing to assess fitness levels or oxygen requirements. There are various tests available, such as, shuttle walking test,[16] 6-minute walk and 3-minute step tests.[17] However, these tests have been validated and performed predominately in children with cystic fibrosis, and which test is appropriate, is dependent on the desired objective.

ADJUNCTS

Intermittent positive pressure breathing (IPPB)

IPPB uses positive pressure during inspiration to increase tidal volume and therefore helps in the mobilization of secretions.[18] This is important in children who are too tired or weak to perform deep breaths effectively. IPPB machines can be used simultaneously to administer bronchodilators, and if used correctly can also relieve the work of breathing, which can be beneficial in the acute asthmatic patient.

Continuous positive airway pressure (CPAP)

CPAP maintains a positive pressure (5–15 cmH$_2$O) throughout inspiration and expiration. The main aim of CPAP is to increase FRC and reduce the work of breathing, thus improving oxygenation.[19] Although effective in type I respiratory failure, administering CPAP to young children and infants is difficult as it involves a tight-fitting mask. In some cases intermittent use in conjunction with other techniques will re-inflate areas of lung collapse, although the large dead space created by some masks can increase PaCO_2.

Non-invasive ventilation (NIV)

NIV is respiratory support using negative or positive pressure ventilators. In recent years a variety of positive pressure machines have been available for children with chronic respiratory failure resulting in hypoventilation and hypercapnia. The choice of ventilator and length of use is assessed on an individual basis. The physiotherapist may use the ventilator to facilitate deep breaths as part of the treatment of a child. Negative pressure jackets set up to create vibrations on the chest wall have yet to prove effective as an adjunct to physiotherapy.[20]

EVALUATING OUTCOME

When any physiotherapy technique is used it is important the child is assessed prior, during and following every treatment. Physiotherapy should never be considered a routine and the physiotherapist must always assess the effects.

In clinical practice, outcome measures include; expectoration of sputum, changes in sputum colour, quantity, consistency and smell; changes in signs (for example auscultation) and symptoms. In the acute setting, continuous monitoring of arterial oxygen saturation gives a readily available objective measure of the effects of treatment. Other measures used for objective recording are: spirometry, peak expiratory flow, full laboratory lung function reporting, sputum weight (wet/dry), blood gas chemistry and exercise tolerance, and subjectively: visual analogue scores/report scores measuring, for example, breathlessness.

Research in chest physiotherapy frequently involves the comparison of different treatment methods. As stated previously, techniques are rarely used in isolation and as a result care must be taken when interpreting outcome reports. For example chest clapping in isolation can cause bronchospasm or desaturation, but when combined with deep breathes or rest periods this is avoided.[4] Many studies have reported on airway clearance techniques and results are conflicting.[21] ACBT is considered the gold standard treatment as no other modality has been shown to be more effective.[22] Since the evolution of the forced expiratory technique, most physiotherapists incorporate it into their treatment regimens. Of key importance, however, with planning any treatment and evaluating outcomes is patient adherence especially with respiratory disorders requiring long-term physiotherapy management. Compliance is a major component to be considered, for no matter how effective the outcomes of a singular, supervised and closely monitored treatment appear to be, if the child doesn't like the regimen it will not be done. In addition such issues as time involved, cost of equipment and availability of space must also be considered. Again this highlights the importance of regular and constant assessment of the child and their carers and the need to be flexible. Continuous evaluation ensures the most effective outcome.

PLANNING THE FUTURE MANAGEMENT

The future management of any child is dependent on the effectiveness of the physiotherapy and the indication for its continuance. In the acute situation, for example a baby with right upper lobe collapse, positioning and intermittent chest clapping would have been instigated prior to feeds. Once observations and chest X-ray confirm re-inflation of the lung, no further physiotherapy is indicated. A child diagnosed with bronchiectasis will need a daily routine of physiotherapy. For an infant, parents provide this input, but by the age of two or three the child can join in with blowing games. Older children can treat themselves independently. Throughout this time the physiotherapist must support and review the programme, changing and adjusting to maximize the benefit. In addition to factors previously mentioned concerning effectiveness, time, availability, feedback from the child is important and their concerns should be addressed. Where possible, planning must ensure children can lead a normal, active life, and they realise that regular physiotherapy can help to maintain this.

CLINICAL RESEARCH ISSUES

Chest physiotherapy is often difficult to assess with many component parts and often no direct outcome measures. Individual experience shows the benefits of physiotherapy and in some conditions it is the main prophylactic treatment. An example of conflicting opinions is found with postural drainage and gastro-oesophageal reflux (GOR) in cystic fibrosis. Button et al. (1997)[23] showed an increase in GOR in infants during tipped positions, compared to modified, but this was not found by another study by Phillips et al. (1998),[24] where sitting was found to be twice as likely to cause reflux, a result supported by research on positioning infants with gastro-oesophageal reflux. Whatever the outcome, more questions need answering, for example is gastro-oesophageal reflux associated with aspiration? Are modified positions detrimental to an infant

with cystic fibrosis? These are just a couple of examples of the difficulties physiotherapists face when assessing effectiveness. It is clear more work must be done in all areas, but in particular specific outcome measures must be found to support personal experience.

REFERENCES

1. Webb MSC, Martin JA, Cartlidge PH, Ng YK, Wright NA. Chest physiotherapy in acute bronchiolitis. *Arch Dis Child* 1985; **60**: 1078–9.

2. Nelson HP. Postural drainage of the lungs. *Br Med J* 1934; **2**: 251–5.

3. Sutton PP, Lopez-Vidriero MT, Pavia D, *et al.* Assessment of percussion, vibratory-shaking and breathing exercises in chest physiotherapy. *Eur J Respir Dis* 1985; **66**: 147–52.

4. Pryor JA, Webber BA, Hodson ME. Effect of chest physiotherapy on oxygen saturation in patients with cystic fibrosis. *Thorax* 1990; **45**: 77.

5. Stiller K, Geake T, Taylor J, *et al.* Acute lobar atelectasis. A comparison of two chest physiotherapy regimens. *Chest* 1990; **98**: 1336–40.

6. Thompson B. *Asthma and your child*, 5th edn. Christchurch, New Zealand: Pegasus Press. 1978.

7. Webber BA, Hofmeyer JL, Morgan MD, Hodson ME. Effects of postural drainage, incorporating the forced expiration technique, on pulmonary function in cystic fibrosis. *Br J Dis Chest* 1986; **80**: 353–9.

8. Pryor JA, Webber BA, Hodson ME, Batten JC. Evaluation of the forced expiration technique as an adjunct to postural drainage in treatment of cystic fibrosis. *Br Med J* 1979; **2**: 417–18.

9. West JB. *Pulmonary pathophysiology*, 4th edn. Baltimore:. Williams and Wilkins, 1992, 8–11.

10. Falk M, Kelstrup M, Andersen JB, *et al.* Improving the ketchup bottle method with positive expiratory pressure, PEP, in cystic fibrosis. *Eur J Respir Dis* 1984; **65**: 423–32.

11. Schibbler A, Casaulta C, Kraemer R. Rationale of oscillatory breathing as chest physiotherapy performed by the flutter in patients with cystic fibrosis. *Pediat Pulmonol* 1982; **4** (Suppl. 8): 301.

12. Pike SE, Machin AC, Dix KJ, Pryor JA, Hodson ME. Comparison of flutter VRP1 and forced expirations

(FE) with active cycle of breathing techniques (ACBT) in subjects with cystic fibrosis (CF). *Netherlands J Med* 1999; **54**: S55:125.

13. Chevaillier J. *Die Autogene Drainage*. Unpublished manual of the Belgian autogenic drainage method. Zeeprevatorium De Haan, Belgium, 1986.

14. Wagaman MJ, Shutack JG, Moomjian AS, *et al.* Improved oxygenation and lung compliance with prone positioning of neonates. *J Pediat* 1979; **94**: 787–91.

15. Brownlee S, Williams S. Physiotherapy in the respiratory care of patients with high spinal injury. *Physiotherapy* 1987; **73**: 148–52.

16. Singh SJ, Morgan MD, Scott S, *et al.* Development of a shuttle walking test of disability in patients with chronic airways obstruction. *Thorax* 1992; **47**: 1019–24.

17. Balfour-Lynn IM, Prasad SA, Laverty A, Whitehead BF, Dinwiddie R. A step in the right direction: assessing exercise tolerance in cystic fibrosis. *Pediat Pulmonol* 1998; **25**: 278–84.

18. Sukumalchantra Y, Park SS, Williams MH Jr. The effect of intermittent positive pressure breathing (IPPB) in acute ventilatory failure. *Am Rev Respir Dis* 1965; **92**: 885–93.

19. Lindner KH, Lotz P, Annefeld FW. Continuous positive airway pressure effect on functional residual capacity, vital capacity and its subdivisions. *Chest* 1987; **92**: 66–70.

20. Phillips GE, Pike SE, Jaffe A, Bush A. Active cycle of breathing techniques versus high frequency oscillations in cystic fibrosis. *Respir Crit Care Med* 1999; **159**: 3: A687.

21. Prasad SA, Main E. Finding evidence to support airway clearance techniques in cystic fibrosis. *Disabil Rehabil* 1998; **6**: 235–46.

22. Pryor JA, Webber BA. *Physiotherapy for respiratory and cardiac problems*, 2nd edn. Edinburgh: Churchill Livingstone, 1998.

23. Button BM, Heine RG, Catto-Smith AG, Phelan PD, Olinsky A. Postural drainage and gastro-oesophageal reflux in infants with cystic fibrosis. *Arch Dis Child* 1997; **76**: 148–50.

24. Phillips GE, Pike SE, Rosenthal M, Bush A. Holding the baby: head downwards positioning for physiotherapy does not cause gastro-oesophageal reflux. *Eur Respir J* 1998; **12**: 954–7.

CHAPTER TWENTY FOUR

GUIDED SELF-MANAGEMENT

H. Dunbar and D. Wensley

- Introduction
- Background information
- Advantages and disadvantages
- Types of plan available
- References
- Further reading

INTRODUCTION

Chronic disease management focuses on control by active intervention. Clinicians manipulate treatment to minimize symptoms, improve objective measures of disease state and to enhance patients' quality of life. Frequent treatment changes mean that visits to the doctor and hospital attendance are commonplace for children with chronic disease. Often these changes may be minor and the ability to 'fine tune' prescribed treatment at home with guidance, to maintain health, is preferable to recurrent consultations. This is guided self-management.

> 'Guided self-management involves the patient or parent having appropriate knowledge and training, so that when faced with a variety of circumstances they know when to seek medical attention and how and when to adjust treatments according to a plan worked out in advance with a health professional.'[1]

This chapter will discuss the origins of self-management and the evidence for and against its use in clinical practice; advantages of self-management plans and problems with their use; the implementation and evaluation of their effects; and finally areas for future research in self-management.

BACKGROUND INFORMATION

Self-management has its origins in psychology and involves interplay between health education and social learning theory.[2] Its use has increased in recent years, possibly in response to the increase in the overall burden of chronic disease and an emphasis on community care embodied in the UK in the 1989 Government White Paper. Keeping patients at home and laying the responsibility for care with the patient/carers has become an important aspect of management and policy.[3] Self-management has long been used in the field of diabetes where patients need to make frequent decisions during the day. Over the last 20 years greater consideration has been given in respiratory medicine, mainly asthma, to the importance of patient education and self-management.[2] Both national and international guidelines in asthma management now stress the importance of patient education.[4–7]

Self-management is not simply handing over control to the child or family, but a recognition that the patient too is responsible for his/her disease management. Introducing self-management is of little use without comprehensive training and education.[8] Research in this area has demonstrated the benefits of self-management, although it is difficult to know which parts of the process are responsible for these benefits.[5] Responsibility for prescribing remains with the health professional whilst compliance rests with the patient. Compliance with medication is often questioned and different studies have suggested reasons why people fail to comply such as forgetfulness, lack of understanding, depression, fear of side effects and failure by health professionals to realize the goals of the individual patient when initiating guidelines[9,10] (Chapter 22) If patients are given appropriate information about why they need treatment, and training in its use, they may feel more in control and more inclined to comply.[8,11,12]

> 'The two principal components of guided self-management are compliance with medication and adherence to self-treatment guidelines'.[13]

Almost all the relevant development work and research has been conducted in the field of asthma. Guidelines vary from simple instructions through to much more complex written information with varying pathways dependent on changes in condition. Guided self-management has been used in adults with asthma with success in some instances but failure in others.[5,14] Studies using children are fewer in number and more research needs to be carried out in this area.

Children with chronic respiratory conditions other than asthma are managed at home despite limited recognition of self-management as a formal process. In cystic fibrosis the chronic and deteriorating nature of the condition means that patients and their families are actively involved in daily care; at the simplest level patients and families carry out basic daily practices of medication administration, physiotherapy and dietary supplements. This has been the case for many years but formal self-management, allowing families some discretion in their actions, is new in this area.[15] In chronic lung disease of prematurity, parents may make changes in domiciliary oxygen therapy as well as inhaled and oral medication, in response to changes in their child's condition.

ADVANTAGES AND DISADVANTAGES OF GUIDED SELF-MANAGEMENT

ADVANTAGES

There are benefits from self-management to the child and family, the health service and outside carers (e.g. school).

Child and family

By minimizing medical contacts, guided self-management should improve family dynamics by keeping the child at home and school more consistently (Case study 24.1). Increased patient understanding, confidence and satisfaction has the potential to enhance compliance,[8,11,12] although this has yet to be proved. Patient/carers' responsibility for, and involvement in, treatment is increased, thus creating a real partnership in care, not one which is doctor-dominated. A better relationship with professionals may develop, through enhanced communication.[16] Improved quality of life can result from self-management of asthma (although this is not always accompanied by

---

Case study 24.1: Chronic lung disease of prematurity

Tim is 3 years old and has chronic lung disease as a result of prematurity. His prescribed medication includes continuous oxygen therapy at a flow rate of 0.1 L/min, inhaled corticosteroids and bronchodilators. Tim is in the process of being weaned off oxygen during the day. His parents have already worked through the process of weaning and Tim can have up to 6 hours in a day out of his oxygen when he is well. Over the last two days Tim has developed a mild URTI. He has become increasingly short of breath, is coughing, and is more tired than usual. His parents are aware of these signs of respiratory distress and with the help of his individualized self-management plan they commence bronchodilator therapy, and decrease the amount of time out of oxygen to 3 hours once a day until he is well. They then return to his regular medications and gradually extend his time out of oxygen to 6 hours once again. During this time phone advice is available. Throughout his cold Tim is managed at home. However his parents, aware of previous episodes, may alter their management and seek medical help at any time. The general practitioner is aware of the weaning programme and has a copy of Tim's management plan.

Box 24.1: Oxygen management in chronic lung disease of prematurity

When instructed to, begin process of weaning, (child normally receiving 0.2 L/min or lower of oxygen via nasal prongs).

- 15 min off oxygen twice a day
- 30 min off oxygen twice a day
- 1 h off oxygen twice a day
- 2 h off oxygen once a day, then twice a day
- 3 h off oxygen once a day, then twice a day
- 6 h off oxygen once a day
- 8 h off oxygen once a day
- off oxygen all day
- overnight oxygen saturation recordings
- off oxygen day and night
- overnight oxygen saturations checked at intervals of one week, one and two months later.

If at any time child develops a cold then go back two steps; if no improvement put back onto continuous oxygen at 0.2 L/min and seek medical help.

objective improvement). Reduction in time lost from school by the child[18] and from work by the parents[19] have both been demonstrated in self-management for asthma.

Health services

Decreased costs to NHS as a result of fewer hospital admissions and shorter lengths of stay have been demonstrated for asthma self-management.[18–20] Emergency visits may be fewer.[21] Increase in the provision of community care with the child remaining at home, may involve extra work for community paediatric nurses, dealing with oxygen-dependent ex-

preterm infants, for example. Increase in communication and liaison between primary and secondary sectors,[22] and between doctors and nurses in community and primary care are essential to consistent guidance. Everyone involved in the child's care must become aware of management and treatment issues and follow the same plan.

School and outside carers

Where non-parental carers are co-operative, the advantage of their involvement is that continuity of education and social contacts at school are less likely to be disrupted. Teachers become more familiar with the needs of children with chronic respiratory illness and better informed (Case study 24.2).

DISADVANTAGES

Communication, education and organization of care are central to the process of guided self-management.[8,23] Once a plan is agreed however, self-management is the work of the child and/or parent. They must be motivated and happy to take on this role. Despite these factors problems with self-management may exist for the child, family, health professionals and others involved in care.

Problems for the child and family

Compliance with treatment may vary with the age of the child. Infants and recalcitrant toddlers present problems of drug administration. Time must be spent with the child and parent encouraging drug administration as part of play, using diversion techniques such as songs or nursery rhymes, or surrogates such as teddy bears (Chapter 15). Expectations of greater compliance with parental responsibility for drug administration may be

Case study 24.2: Exercise-induced asthma at school

Claire is 7 years old with asthma. She becomes wheezy and breathless with exercise. Claire enjoys taking part in games and her teachers are aware of the importance of allowing her to do so. At school Claire has her reliever medication (β_2 agonist inhaler) available for use. Claire's teachers have had an asthma education session from the school nurse and the school has implemented an asthma policy (ref NAC). Claire is permitted to carry her inhaler at all times, in a small pouch. With the help of her self-management plan both Claire and her teachers know that she is to have four puffs of her reliever medication before PE, which can be repeated again, if she becomes wheezy.

misplaced.[24] Adolescents may be unwilling to learn or reluctant to accept the need for continual therapy and negotiation is important. Focusing on patient-selected goals and allowing choice may be valuable tools with this group.

Language and literacy may be limiting with some families. Written information without verbal education and practical training to reinforce it is of little use for those parents whose first language is not English or who are unable to read. Provision of information needs to be patient-led and given in small quantities, with regular reinforcement.[8]

Access to appropriate information should be provided. Vast amounts of information are available, much of it overwhelming, and mostly provided by major pharmaceutical companies. It is vital that all health professionals involved in the care of the child agree with the self-management plan adopted and tailor information and education given around this. Where possible self-management plans used should be based on published guidelines, and free of (subliminal) advertising to the parent or professional.

Parents and child must be motivated to learn and have an idea of their own goals. Asking what the child or parent wants to achieve for themselves may provide a means of focusing the treatment and improving motivation.[25]

Problems for professionals

The initial consultation for self-management requires time and follow-up is important.[23] Since many appointments are time-limited, education may be hurried. In both primary and secondary care, professionals other than doctors, are increasingly involved in the process of development of management plans and of health education.

Standardization of treatment among all professionals involved in the child's care may be difficult to achieve if a variety of plans is available. The types of plan to be used should be agreed by everyone within the locality. This should limit the number of plans in circulation. Regular review is needed to audit their effectiveness and determine whether changes should be made. Despite national guidelines, there are often differences in treatments preferred by different health professionals. It may be useful to standardize treatments for certain conditions and ages, again on a locality-wide basis. In the USA, Health Maintenance Organizations (HMOs) and in the UK, Primary Care Groups (PCGs) and National Health Service Trusts can facilitate standardization.

Costs of medications are a concern, in a climate of increased drug spending. Effective use of medication through guided self-management should decrease the need for rescue medications and hospitalizations and hence reduce costs, albeit at greater overall drug expenditure.[26]

Focus on the traditional medical model of care (drug treatment and cure) is not possible with many chronic diseases. Control is the issue and a recognition that the patient's perception is far from the medical model. Theirs is the major role in management. There is limited research in paediatrics in the use of guided self-management. The research available varies widely and outcomes are difficult to compare.[5]

Problems for schools and playgroups

Where children are at playgroup or school, the role of playleaders or teachers in the child's management must be agreed. This may mean creating a policy or procedure at the educational establishment, providing training for staff and providing written guidelines for each child (together with appropriate medication). The legal position of non-parental carers may be an issue for some. This applies especially to teachers on school trips.

Despite these problems most clinicians are already using self-management in the care of asthma, and increasingly in other chronic respiratory diseases in children. A variety of plans are available but need to be adapted according to individual circumstances. The next section will demonstrate how plans can be developed using examples and clinical cases for different conditions.

TYPES OF PLAN AVAILABLE

In both primary and secondary care allied professionals work as part of a team in the education process. Co-ordination and communication between specialist respiratory nurses, practice nurses, physiotherapists and medical practitioners is very important for successful self-management.[22]

Sharing of information ensures that the same information is given by and available to all involved in patient care thereby avoiding confusion. Referral guidelines for secondary care should be developed locally to prevent time delay by the patient and GP and allow appropriate referral to a specialist centre where necessary.

Where possible self-management plans should be based on national guidelines, locally adapted by a properly constituted team representing primary care, secondary care, public health and community health. These basic outline plans should be tailored to individual use, with the expectation of enhanced compliance.[11] The level of complexity of an individual plan will be dependent on factors such as parent and child's level of understanding, previous experiences and prior knowledge, who gives the information, age of child and disease severity.

Simple plans involve basic didactic advice, reinforced with written information (Box 24.2). Advice can be tailored to individual need and dependent on the condition. Limited (information only) education is ineffective.[27] in comparison with a written self-management plan.[28]

When patients are more experienced with their treatments, self-management plans can include information which allows parent and child to make *changes in their regular treatment* in response to changes in their condition (Case study 24.3).

Self-management plans like this take more time and resources from health professionals to assess and improve parent and child confidence. They usually need several appointments to reinforce information and offer support. Parents should have a point of contact for information, support or advice and emergency care should be accessed in the usual way.

A variety of tools are available which can form part of self-management and may be a useful addition for some patients or carers and boost confidence. In asthma, self-management protocols have been developed incorporating traffic light (Figure 24.1) and peak flow monitoring. Peak flow monitoring offers 'objective' information. Self-management plans backed up by home recording of PEF are widely used to improve well being and reduce the need for hospital admission in adults.[29–30] Whether or not PEF monitoring enhances outcome in children is a subject of research.

Box 24.2: Simple, didactic advice

Condition	Problem	Action
Asthma	If you/ your child are coughing/ wheezy	Take 2 puffs of blue inhaler
Cystic fibrosis	Increased sputum production/ discoloured	Commence antibiotics and increase physiotherapy
Oxygen dependency	Showing signs of a cold/ runny nose	Increase oxygen to ....L/min
Tracheostomy	Showing signs of cold/ noisy breathing	Administer suction

---

Case study 24.3: Brittle asthma

John, aged 8 years, has had repeated admissions to hospital because of brittle asthma. Through past experiences both John and his parents are now able to recognize in advance when he is becoming unwell. He becomes irritable with a tickly dry cough and an odd sensation in his throat. At home they have available to them John's regular bronchodilator, inhaled steroids and also a short course of oral steroids.

Over the past few hours, John has developed his premonitory symptoms.

Following his self-management plan, John increases his bronchodilator to 3–4 hourly and his mother administers the first dose of oral prednisolone. The next morning, John's mother telephones the surgery to inform the GP that she has commenced steroids. The GP is aware of the management plan and agrees that in John's case, early oral prednisolone is important. She is told to bring John for assessment if his condition deteriorates, or if he has not recovered at the end of 3 days of prednisolone therapy.

(a)

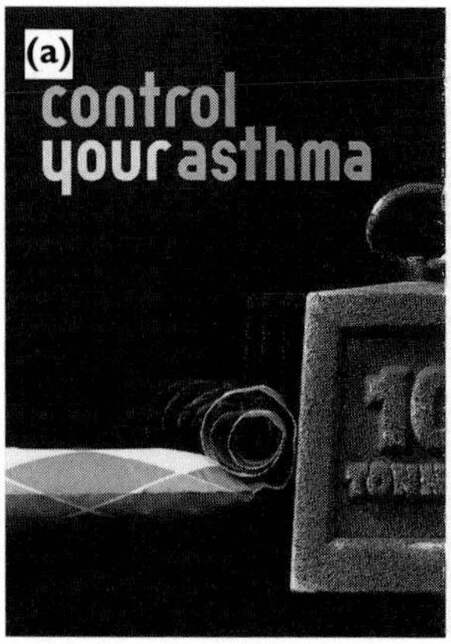

control your asthma

Your name

Family doctor

Doctor's telephone

Asthma is a common condition. It can be easily controlled with modern treatments. However, in order to look after your asthma properly you need to know a little about your medicines, and you need to know the signs that might suggest your asthma is worsening.

Preventer inhalers
(usually brown, red or orange)

These are the most important medicines. They help prevent the symptoms of asthma from appearing – coughing, wheezing, tight chest and shortness of breath. Preventers will not work unless they are taken every day, as advised by your doctor or nurse.

Your preventer is

which you should take in a daily dose of

with a (specific device)

Reliever inhalers
(usually blue)

These rescue you from asthma symptoms as they happen. You should take your reliever, as advised by your doctor or nurse.

Your reliever is

which you should take with a (specific device)

Other treatments are

What to do on a usual day if...

(b)

...YOU FEEL FINE

- not waking more than 1 night per week
- not wheezy when you wake up in the morning more than once a week
- needing **RELIEVER** for exercise up to three times in the last week

- take your regular preventer treatment:
  ....
- use your **RELIEVER** if needed up to:
  ....

...ASTHMA GETTING WORSE

- wheezy in morning or waking up with asthma at night 2 or more times in the last week
- wheezy in the day (e.g. with exercise) more than 3 times in the last week
- taking extra **RELIEVER most** days in the last week

- Increase your **PREVENTER**
  .... to ....
  until you have been back to normal for
  ....
- Take **RELIEVER** as needed
  ....

ASTHMA MUCH WORSE THAN USUAL

- waking up every night for last 2-3 nights
- needing **RELIEVER** every 3-4 hours or **RELIEVER** not lasting 3 hours
- too wheezy to run or hurry
- tight chest all the time with annoying cough

- Take the whole course of prednisolone tablets daily for .... days
- Take extra **RELIEVER** as needed
- If your **RELIEVER** lasts for at least 3-4 hours, **CALL YOUR DOCTOR NEXT MORNING**
- If it does not last 3-4 hours **CALL YOUR DOCTOR AT ONCE.**

What to do if your asthma is getting worse with a COLD, FEVER or INFECTION

ASTHMA ATTACK STARTING

Although you have a cold you

- don't wake up with a cough and wheeze at night
- can run easily and wheeze is relieved by **RELIEVER**
- get full relief from **RELIEVER** taken up to four times a day

- Take your regular **PREVENTER**
  ....
- Use your reliever if needed up to
  .... times a day

ASTHMA GETTING WORSE

- waking at night for last 2 nights
- coughing and wheezing with exercise even after **RELIEVER**
- **RELIEVER** lasts less than 4 hours or needed more than 4 times daily

- Take the whole course of prednisolone tablets daily for .... days
- Continue your regular **PREVENTER**
- Take your **RELIEVER** and if you do not go back to your normal level for at least 3 hours then:
  CALL A DOCTOR AT ONCE. In any case call your doctor next day at the latest.

SEVERE ASTHMA

Feel worse with

- little sleep
- wheezy and tight all the time
- too breathless to walk about
- **RELIEVER** works for one hour or less

- Take extra **RELIEVER** as often as you need and
  CALL A DOCTOR AT ONCE or GO STRAIGHT TO HOSPITAL

IF YOU ARE GETTING A BAD ATTACK .... *turn over page*

Figure 24.1: Self-management plan with PEF. (a) Simple plan. (b) Symptom-based plan with 'traffic lights' (green on the left, yellow in the centre and red to the right).

Self-management plans can be used with diseases other than asthma, but there are no standard national guidelines and local versions abound.

For instance, for patients with a new tracheostomy, through intensive education, parents are taught and assessed in a range of skills prior to discharge (Chapter 19, Table 19.2, p.215). These are the skills necessary to respond to specific situations (Box 24.3). Assessment of competence and confidence in carrying out these procedures unsupervised is followed by the preparation, together with parents of the individualized self-management plan, before discharge home with a contact number for advice (Case study 24.4).

Another example concerns the locally developed weaning programme for a child with chronic lung disease of prematurity receiving domiciliary oxygen. The family work through a staged process of weaning with the support of, for example, a community paediatric nurse or specialist respiratory nurse. Decisions to move from stage to stage are based on oxygen saturation monitoring, clinical presentation and symptom reporting. Parents are taught that if a deterioration in condition occurs they must go back to the previous stage and contact their named doctor or specialist nurse to inform them of the situation. Moving from stage to stage is highly individualized although the general plan remains the same.

These are examples of self-management plans for a variety of conditions. General self-management advice is often simple, but the specific information for individuals needs to be regularly revised and reiterated because:

- Parents/children (or even professionals) frequently mislay information.
- Plans should be altered with every change of medication or intervention in order to maintain continuity and updates copied to other professionals involved in the child's care; where a plan is in place from another professional this needs to be developed not replaced.
- The condition may change, for better or worse, rendering the existing plan outdated.

- Children or parents may be unable/unwilling to learn; time is required to develop a rapport between patient and health professional in order to impart knowledge and advice and to motivate the patient/carer.
- As parents/children become more competent, more complex procedures can be added to the plan.

As well as regular updating, the outcome needs to be assessed. The process (adherence to the plan) and the health outcome should be evaluated at each contact.

EVALUATING OUTCOMES

Comparison between studies is difficult because of the many measures of outcome used, differences in patient populations and differences in trial design. A broad perspective is necessary when considering outcomes as they may be subjective or objective, and both short-term (e.g exercise tolerance) or integrated over a longer period of time (e.g. re-admission rate) (Box 24.4).

In clinical practice however, to access this depth of information for each patient would be impractical and patient self-reporting is the most common method of gathering information.

Box 24.3: Tracheostomy care		
Problem	**If problem persists**	**With no improvement**
Increased secretions	Secretions thicker than	No change in condition despite
Rise in respiratory rate	normal	regular suctioning
and effort	Increasing respiratory distress	Pale and clammy
	Irritable	Obvious distress
	Attempting to vocalize	
Action:	**Action:**	**Action:**
Suction as required	Suction using 0.5 mL saline	Change tracheostomy tube
	down the tracheostomy tube	immediately
	Seek advice if worried	Observe child after and inform
		community nurse/GP/hospital
		of increased secretions and need
		to change tube
		Specialist review if appropriate.

Case study 24.4: Tracheostomy care

Mark is now 6 months old; he had a tracheostomy performed 4 months ago for congenital subglottic stenosis. He has been well since he was discharged from hospital 10 weeks ago. Both parents, although extremely competent in the care of his tracheostomy, have continued to want the supervision of the specialist respiratory nurse when changing his tracheostomy tube at home on a 2-weekly basis. Mark is due to have a routine change of his tube in 2 days' time.

Over the last 2 days Mark's secretions, particularly in the morning, have been thicker than usual. There has not been any colour or odour change. Today however after suctioning first thing in the morning, Mark's mother has noticed that his secretions are thick and green in colour. At the same time Mark appears irritable, has a high temperature and his respiratory effort seems to be more than normal. His mother suctions him once more; there is little secretion removed within the suction catheter and there continues to be no change in his clinical condition.

As previously taught, Mark's mother decides to use some saline down his tracheostomy tube. She instils three to four drops of saline down the tube and repeats suctioning. Again the result is minimal. At this point Mark is becoming very clammy and his respiratory rate has increased dramatically as he becomes more irritable and appears to be attempting to vocalize.

Applying the education she has received, Mark's mother decides that at this point she must change his tracheostomy tube on her own. Parents are taught to always have a spare tube ready and without wasting any time Mark's mother changes his tracheostomy tube. Immediately Mark appears much more settled and after a cuddle, examination of the old tracheostomy tube reveals a hard green mucus plug which is occluding the end of the tube.

Mark's mother rings the respiratory nurse to inform her of what has happened, and as Mark's condition appears to have improved and his mother is happy, the nurse arranges to visit that afternoon to review Mark and obtain some secretions to send for analysis in the laboratory. Mark's mother has successfully performed her first emergency tracheostomy tube change.

FURTHER RESEARCH

It is difficult to know which aspects of self-management affect outcome, because of the interplay between education, organization of care, guidelines and compliance. Research protocols should supplement patient reports with objective data. It is difficult to compare studies because of lack of standardization of plans, lack of formal measures and use of a variety of outcome measures.

- The respective roles of children and parents in the process of self-management should be explored.

Box 24.4: Outcome measures in asthma self-management

Objective or measurable clinical outcomes

Physical examination
- chest signs
- lung function

Medical records/information systems
- A&E attendance
- emergency GP attendance
- hospital admission
- use of rescue medication

School attendance
- school records

Subjective outcomes which impact on the individual

Daily recordings
- sleep disturbance
- daytime symptoms
- exercise tolerance
- β_2 agonist use

Questionnaires
- quality of life

- Which part of the process of self-management (education, information, support or the written plan itself) is the most important and improves outcome?
- Can self-management be effectively standardized for use across primary and secondary care levels?
- Does self-management improve compliance?
- The role of self-management in schools is contentious; operational research in educational settings could be valuable.
- The role of monitoring such as peak flow in asthma and oxygen saturation recording in self-management of chronic lung disease of prematurity, should be proved.
- National guidelines based on adequate evidence, should be created for diseases other than asthma. Advice such as 'double your preventer at the first signs of an attack' have been based on tradition rather than science,[31] and have recently been questioned in a formal clinical trial in children.[32]

REFERENCES

1. Partridge MR. Self-management plans: uses and limitations. *Br J Hosp Med* 1996; **55**: 120–2.

2. Creer TL, Holroyd KA. *Self management for chronic disease*. London: Academic Press, 1986.

3. The Health Committee. *Health services for children and young people in the community: home and school*. 1997; **3**: (Abstract).

4. British Thoracic Society. The British guidelines on asthma management. *Thorax* 1997; **52**: suppl.1.

5. Meijer RJ, Kerstjens HA, Postma DS. Comparison of guidelines and self-management plans in asthma. *Eur Respir J* 1997; **10**: 1163–72.

6. National Heart and Lung Institute NI. International Consensus report on diagnosis and management of asthma. *Eur Respir J* 1992; **5(5)**: 601–41.

7. Warner JO, Gotz M, Landau LI, *et al.* Asthma: a follow-up statement from an international consensus group. *Arch Dis Child* 1992; **67(2)**:240–48.

8. Partridge MR. Delivering optimal care to the person with asthma: what are the key components and what do we mean by patient education? *Eur Respir J* 1995; **8**: 298–305.

9. Cochrane GM. Compliance and outcomes in patients with asthma. *Drugs* 1996; **52**: (Suppl 6): 12–19.

10. Cochrane GM. Assessment of compliance. In: Thomson NC, O'Byrne P (eds). *Manual of asthma management*. Cambridge: University Press, 1995.

11. Osman L. Guided self-management and patient education in asthma. *Br J Nurs* 1996; **5**: 785–9.

12. Taggart VS, Zuckerman AE, Lucas S, Acty-Lindsey A, Bellanti JA. Adapting a self-management education program for asthma for use in an outpatient clinic. *Ann Allergy* 1987; **58**: 173–8.

13. van der Palen J, Klein JJ, Rovers MM. Compliance with inhaled medication and self-treatment guidelines following a self-management programme in adult asthmatics. *Eur Respir J* 1997; **10**: 652–7.

14. Anonymous. Peak flow meter use in asthma management. Thoracic Society of Australia and New Zealand. *Med J Aust* 1996; **164**: 727–30.

15. Cottrell CK, Young GA, Creer TL, Holroyd KA, Kotses H. The development and evaluation of a self-management program for cystic fibrosis. *Pediat Asthma All Immunol* 1996; **10**: 109–18.

16. Clark NM, Evans D, Zimmerman BJ, Levison MJ, Mellins RB. Patient and family management of asthma: theory-based techniques for the clinician. *J Asthma* 1994; **31**: 427–35.

17. Boulet LP, Boutin H, Cote J, Leblanc P, Laviolette M. Evaluation of an asthma self-management education program. *J Asthma* 1995; **32**: 199–206.

18. Wesseldine L, McCarthy P, Silverman M. Structured discharge procedure for children admitted to hospital with acute asthma: a randomised controlled trial of nursing practice. *Arch Dis Child* 1999; **80**: 110–14.

19. Taitel MS, Kotses H, Bernstein IL, Bernstein DI, Creer TL. A self-management program for adult asthma. Part II: Cost-benefit analysis. *J Allergy Clin Immunol* 1995; **95**: 672–6.

20. Sorrells VD, Chung W, Schlumpberger JM. The impact of a summer asthma camp experience on asthma education and morbidity in children. *J Fam Pract* 1995; **41**: 465–8.

21. Ronchetti R, Indinnimeo L, Bonci E, *et al.* Asthma self-management programmes in a population of Italian children: a multicentre study. Italian Study Group on Asthma Self-Management Programmes. *Eur Respir J* 1997; **10**: 1248–53.

22. Charlton I, Antoniou AG, Atkinson J, *et al.* Asthma at the interface: bridging the gap between general prac-

tice and a district general hospital. *Arch Dis Child* 1994; **70**: 313–18.

23. Charlton I, Charlton GF. Caring for patients with asthma. Teaching self management takes time. *BMJ* 1994; **308**: 1370–1.

24. Gibson NA, Ferguson AE, Aitchison TC, Paton JY. Compliance with inhaled asthma medication in preschool children. *Thorax* 1995; **50**: 1274–9.

25. Clark NM, Starr-Schneidkraut NJ. Management of asthma by patients and families. *Am J Respir Crit Care Med* 1994; **149**: Pt 2: S54–66.

26. Liljas B, Lahdensuo A. Is asthma self-management cost effective? *Patient Educ Couns* 1997; **32**: S97–S104.

27. Gibson PG, Coughlan J, Wilson AJ, *et al.* Limited (information only) patient education programs for adults with asthma (Cochrane Review). *The Cochrane Library*, Issue 1, 2000. Oxford Update Software.

28. Gibson PG, Coughlan J, Wilson AJ, *et al.* Self-management education and regular practitioner review for adults with asthma (Cochrane Review). *The Cochrane Library*, Issue 1, 2000. Oxford Update Software.

29. Charlton I, Charlton G, Broomfield J, Mullee MA. Evaluation of peak flow and symptoms only: self management plans for control of asthma in general practice. *BMJ* 1990; **301**: 1355–9.

30. Lahdensuo A, Haahtela T, Herrala J, *et al.* Randomised comparison of guided self management and traditional treatment of asthma over one year. *BMJ* 1996; **312**: 748–52.

31. Beasley R, Cushley M, Holgate ST. A self management plan in the treatment of adult asthma. *Thorax* 1989; 200–4.

32. Garrett J, Williams S, Wong C, Holdaway D. Treatment of acute asthmatic exacerbations with increased dose of inhaled steroid. *Arch Dis Child* 1998; **79**: 12–17.

FURTHER READING

1. Lahdensuo A. Guided self management of asthma – how to do it. *BMJ* 1999; **319**: 759–60.

2. Wolf FM, Grum CM, Clark NM. Educational interventions for asthma in children (Cochrane Review). In: *The Cochrane Library*, 4, 1999. Oxford: Update Software.

3. Haby M, Waters E, Robertson C. Interventions for educating children who have attended the emergency room for asthma (Cochrane Review). In: *The Cochrane Library*, 4, 1999. Oxford: Update Software.

CHAPTER TWENTY FIVE

AVOIDING ENVIRONMENTAL TRIGGERS

A. Custovic and A. Woodcock

- Background
- Methods to reduce allergen exposure in homes
- Evidence

- Conclusions
- References

BACKGROUND

Outdoor air pollution has received a lot of scientific interest as a possible cause of respiratory symptoms and a contributory factor in the increase of asthma. However, the majority of people in the developed world spend most of their time inside one type of building or another, and the indoor environment has begun to attract deserved attention over the last several years.[1] We are beginning to appreciate that living in a damp house may have more adverse effects on respiratory health than living next to a busy motorway. The indoor environment of modern homes contains many substances that can cause or exacerbate allergic disease in susceptible individuals. The major biological sources of allergens are acarids (e.g. house-dust mites), insects (e.g. cockroaches), domestic animals (cats and dogs) and fungi, but also such sources as rodents and pollens derived from outside. In addition, environmental tobacco smoke (ETS), indoor air pollution (e.g. NO_2 and ozone) and endotoxin may have potential roles as the enhancers of allergic sensitization.

ALLERGENS

Exposure to allergens has a profound effect on the development of IgE-mediated sensitization (primary sensitization), progression from sensitization to allergic disease (secondary exposure) and the severity of symptoms in the established disease (tertiary exposure) (Figure 25.1).[2-5] This chapter will deal specifically with the role of allergen avoidance in the management of established disease.[5-6]

LESSONS FROM HIGH ALTITUDE STUDIES

In Europe, mite allergen levels are very low at high altitude where the ambient humidity is insufficient to support mite populations. Long-term residence at high altitude can be beneficial for dust-mite-sensitive asthmatic children with a progressive reduction in non-specific airway reactivity after a one-year period spent in Davos (Figure 25.2).[7] Other observational studies have reported a reduction in asthma symptoms and significant decreases in mite allergen-induced basophil histamine release, mite-specific serum IgE level and methacholine and allergen-induced airway reactivity.[8] However, further studies also observed reversal of this trend towards improvement 15 days after returning to sea level. The results of high-altitude studies suggest that mite allergen avoidance leads to an improvement in specific and non-specific airway reactivity and symptoms and that re-exposure results in a rapid relapse. These studies were not controlled, and there is a

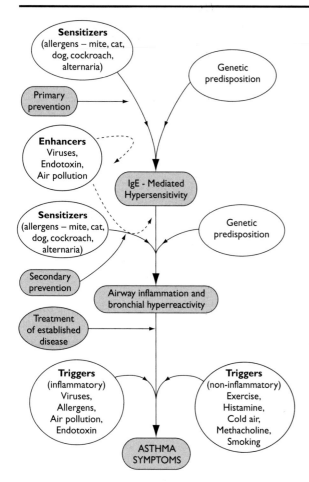

Figure 25.1: The potential benefits of allergen avoidance: (1) Prevention of allergic sensitization (primary prevention by allergen avoidance). (2) Prevention of atopic disease in sensitized individuals (secondary avoidance). (3) Treatment of the established disease.

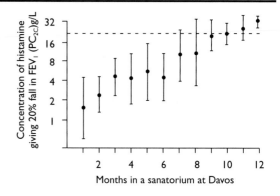

Figure 25.2: Progressive reduction in non-specific bronchial hyperreactivity (histamine) in 10 mite allergic children with asthma who moved from home to a mite-free environment of a sanatorium in Davos, Switzerland. (From Platts Mills TAE, Chapman MD. Dust mites: immunology, allergic disease, and environmental control. *J Allergy Clin Immunol* 1987; **80**: 755–75; Original data: Kerrebijn KF. Endogenous factors in childhood CNSLD: methodological aspects in population studies. In: *Bronchitis III*. Orie NGM, Van der Lende R (eds), Royal Van Gorcum Assen, The Netherlands, 1970: 38–48; with permission.)

immunological parameters to become fully apparent.

High altitude studies also provide an important proof of a principle: a substantial reduction in allergen exposure over a long period of time may result in clinical improvement in allergic asthmatic patients. However, the real challenge for practising physicians is to create a low allergen environment in patients' homes.

METHODS TO REDUCE ALLERGEN EXPOSURE IN HOMES

Although not easy, it is possible to achieve substantial reductions in allergen exposure.[9] Effective control strategies should be tailored to individual allergens, flexible to suit individual needs and cost-effective. Many different avoidance measures for dust mite allergens have been suggested (sometimes with widely exaggerated claims by the manufacturers), but only a few have been subjected to controlled trials.[8,10]

possibility that other domestic factors (e.g. exposure to pets, environmental tobacco smoke, etc.) contributed to the observed improvement in asthma control. Nevertheless, mite avoidance is the most plausible reason for clinical success.

The high altitude studies suggest that:

- to get clinical effect, it is essential to achieve and maintain a major reduction in allergen levels; and
- even with such a reduction in exposure, it may take many months for the effect on symptoms, medication use, pulmonary function, non-specific and specific airway reactivity and

HOUSE-DUST MITES AND MITE ALLERGENS

Practical measures

Mite allergens are predominately carried on larger particles, which become airborne only during vigorous artificial disturbance and settle quickly. The majority of exposure to mites probably occurs in bed, where we spend on average one third of our lives in close contact with mattresses, pillows and duvets. These facts have to be taken into account when planning the avoidance strategies.

BED AND BEDDING

Covers. The most effective and probably most important avoidance measure is to cover the bed (mattress, pillows and duvet) with covers that are impermeable to mite allergens.[7,9,12] Bed covers were initially made of plastic and uncomfortable to sleep on, but water vapour-permeable fabrics, which are both mite allergen impermeable and comfortable, have considerably increased compliance. The covers should be robust, easily fitted and easily cleaned, as their effectiveness is reduced if they are damaged. Allergen levels are dramatically reduced after covering the bed (Figure 25.3). As mite allergen can accumulate on the covers, it is important that they are wiped at each change of bedding.

Washing. The ordinary cycle of laundry washing (~30°C) reduces allergen levels, but most of the mites survive. All exposed bedding should be washed at 55°C, as this is the temperature that kills mites. Additives for the detergents (e.g. 0.03% benzyl benzoate, dilute solutions of essential oils) in normal and low temperature washing may provide alternative methods of mite control, but these are not widely available in the UK.

Feather vs. synthetic. Advice to asthmatic patients to avoid using feather pillows and to replace them with those filled with synthetic fibres has been challenged recently with the finding that

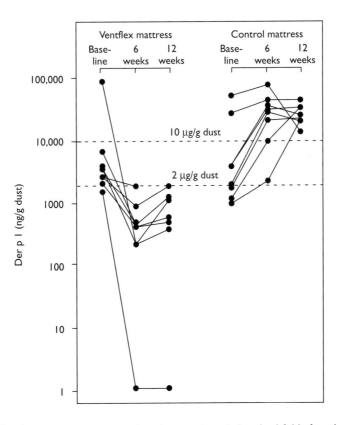

Figure 25.3: Allergen levels on mattresses are reduced approximately hundred-fold after the introduction of covers that are impermeable to mite allergens. (Based on the data from: Owen S, Morgenstern M, Hepworth J, Woodcock A. Control of house dust mite in bedding. *Lancet* 1990; **335**: 396–7; with permission.)

the use of synthetic pillows was a risk factor for severe asthma and for the increase in the prevalence of wheeze.[11,12] Polyester-filled pillows contain substantially more allergens (dust mite, cat and dog) then those filled with feathers.[13,14] So, what advice should we be giving to mite-sensitive patients: feather or synthetic? At present, don't spend a fortune on new 'hypoallergenic' synthetic pillows and quilts – because they are not hypoallergenic. Irrespective of the pillow filling, allergen impermeable covers are the best way to achieve substantial reduction in exposure.[12]

CARPETS AND UPHOLSTERED FURNITURE

Vacuum cleaning. Wall-to-wall fitted carpets and vacuum cleaners are part of modern life and provide expanded reservoirs for dust mite growth. Ideally, fitted carpets should be replaced with polished wood or vinyl flooring. Intensive vacuum cleaning may remove large amounts of dust from carpets, reducing the size of allergen reservoir. Older vacuum cleaners (with inadequate exhaust filtration) are one of the very few ways of producing an aerosol of mite allergens for direct inhalation. Atopic asthmatic patients should use HEPA (high efficiency particulate air) filter vacuum cleaners with double thickness vacuum cleaner bags, although the benefits have not been established in a clinical trial. Nevertheless, they probably make the process of cleaning safer.

In certain climatic zones (e.g. Australia) exposing carpets to direct strong sunlight has been shown to kill mites. This simple and effective treatment may be used in loosely fitted carpets and rugs. High temperature–high pressure steam cleaning may be used as a method of killing mites and reducing allergen levels in carpets.

Acaricides, liquid nitrogen and tannic acid. A number of different chemicals that kill mites (acaricides) have been identified, and shown to be effective under laboratory conditions.[15] However, data on whether these chemicals can be successfully applied to carpets and upholstered furniture is still conflicting. The method of application of the benzyl-benzoate moist powder on carpets is very important. Allowing the powder to remain on carpet for 12 to 18 hours with repeated brushing, followed by vigorous vacuum cleaning is probably the optimal way of applying the chemical, but is not very practical, particularly as the procedure needs to be repeated every 8–12 weeks. Thus, the main problem of chemical treatment is not its ability to kill mites, but getting the chemicals to penetrate deep into carpet and soft furnishing, the persistence of mite allergen until re-colonization occurs, and the nuisance of frequent reapplication. Freezing with liquid nitrogen can kill mites. However, the technique can only be carried out by a trained operator, which limits its use, especially since treatment needs to be repeated regularly. When used, both acaricides and liquid nitrogen should be combined with intensive vacuum cleaning following administration.

Tannic acid does not kill mites, but denatures allergens, and due to this property has been recommended for the reduction of allergen levels in house dust. However, high levels of proteins in dust (e.g. pet allergens in homes with pets) blocks its effect. Aggressive vacuum cleaning should be carried out before the treatment.

HUMIDITY CONTROL

High levels of humidity are essential for mite population growth, and reducing humidity may be an effective control method. However, detailed models of the humidity profile of domestic microclimates (e.g. in relation to humans in bed) are not yet available. Reducing central humidity alone may be ineffective in reducing humidity in mite microhabitats (e.g. in the middle of a mattress).

Several studies from Scandinavian countries have reported successful control of dust mites within domestic dwellings by the use of mechanical ventilation units, which replace humid indoor air with dry outdoor air. This approach to controlling mite population has the greatest chance of succeeding in areas with dry cold winters. However, in regions where outdoor humidity is high throughout the year such as the UK, neither mechanical ventilation nor portable dehumidifiers reduce indoor humidity sufficiently to control mite population growth.[16] Thus, allergen avoidance measures should not only be allergen-specific, but also specific to a particular geographic area, with housing and climatic conditions being taken into account.

AIR FILTRATION AND IONIZERS

Due to the aerodynamic characteristics of mite allergens, it makes little sense to use air filtration units and ionizers as the only way of reducing personal exposure.

INTEGRATED APPROACH TO HOUSE-DUST MITE ALLERGEN AVOIDANCE

A large number of proprietary mite allergen control products are currently available on the market, with claims of clinical efficacy, which have not been adequately tested. Mites live in different sites throughout the house and it is unlikely that a single measure can solve the problem of exposure. An integrated approach (e.g. including barrier methods, dust removal and removal of mite microhabitats) is needed for a comprehensive reduction in mite allergen exposure (Table 25.1). Even in the same geographic area there is a marked difference in mite allergen levels between houses, and the design of houses has a profound effect on mite allergen levels. These issues need to be addressed in designing and building 'low-allergen houses'.

PET ALLERGEN AVOIDANCE

The background

Asthma is often severe and difficult to control in pet sensitized asthmatics who keep the pet in their homes. Complete avoidance of pet allergens in the UK is probably impossible, as sensitized patients can be exposed to pet allergens not only in homes with pets, but also in those without pets and in public buildings and public transport (Figures 25.4 and 25.5).[17–19]

Major cat allergen Fel d 1 is produced under hormonal control primarily in the sebaceous glands and in the basal squamous epithelial cells of the skin. Castration of male cats results in a 3 to 5-fold reduction of Fel d 1 concentration in skin washing. Fel d 1 production is higher in male than in female cats, but the observed gender difference in Fel d 1 secretion is too low to suggest that patients allergic to cats could benefit by getting a female rather than male cat, or by castrating their male cats.

Practical measures

REMOVAL OF THE ANIMAL FROM HOME

The best way to reduce exposure to cat or dog allergen is to remove the animal from the home. However, even after permanent removal of the animal, it can take many months before allergen levels in the house dust decrease. It is therefore important to inform patients that it may take some time for the improvement in asthma symptoms to become apparent.[20]

CONTROL OF PET ALLERGENS WITH A PET IN HOME

Unfortunately, despite continued symptoms many cat and/or dog allergic patients insist on keeping their pet. Every effort should be made to reduce exposure to pet allergens in homes where pets may coexist with a sensitized individual. Airborne pet allergen levels increase by ~5-fold when the pet is in the room, indicating that the immediate presence of a pet contributes to airborne allergen levels.[17,18] When it is not possible to remove the animal, the pet should be kept out of the bedroom, and preferably outdoors or in a well ventilated area (e.g. kitchen).

Cat and dog washing. Washing the animal reduces allergen concentration in hair and dander.[21] However, the level of allergen increases by 3 days after washing. This would suggest that the washing needs to be done a minimum of twice a week to be effective. Twice weekly washing could decrease the build-up of allergen in the dust reservoirs within the home. In addition, washing the pet regularly may reduce the level of airborne allergen in homes with pets. However, it is unlikely that the short-term and modest reduction in the airborne allergen achieved by washing can significantly improve asthma control in sensitized individuals.

Air cleaners. Pet allergens in homes with pets can be substantially reduced by the use of HEPA air cleaners (Figure 25.6).[18,22] In our recent study, the absolute allergen level in rooms with dogs during active air filtration was similar to the

Table 25.1: Actions for avoiding exposure to mite allergens in relation to asthma in Britain

Do help	May help	Do not help
Special bed covers (with or without cleaning)	Acaricides	Air filters or ionizers
Removal of habitat (e.g. carpet)	Liquid nitrogen	Ventilation systems
Moving to Switzerland!	Tannic acid	Dehumidifiers

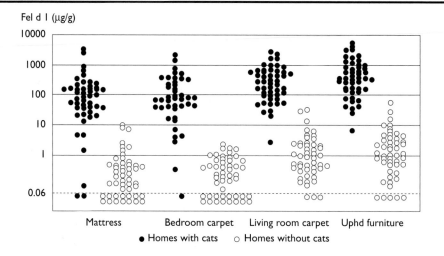

Figure 25.4: Cat allergen levels in homes with and without cats. (From: Custovic A, Smith A, Pahdi H, Green RM, Chapman MD, Woodcock A. Distribution, aerodynamic characteristics and removal of the major cat allergen Fel d I in British homes. *Thorax* 1998; **53**: 33–8; with permission.)

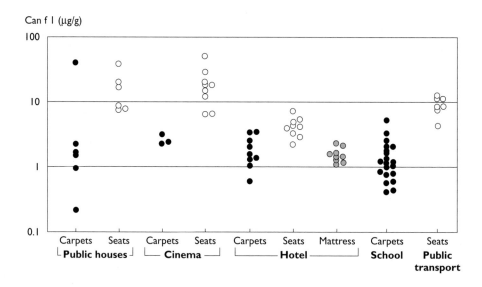

Figure 25.5: Dog allergen levels in public buildings and transport. (Based on the data from: Custovic A, Green R, Taggart SCO, *et al.* Domestic allergens in public places II: dog (Can f I) and cockroach (Bella g 2) allergens in dust and mite, cat, dog and cockroach allergens in air in public buildings. *Clin Exp Allergy* 1996; **26**: 1246–52; with permission.)

baseline level in the same rooms without active air filtration, but with the dog elsewhere in the house.[22] This emphasizes the need to keep pets outside sleeping and living areas, since they are a continual source of allergen.

Vacuum cleaners

We have recently investigated the effectiveness of different types of vacuum cleaners in preventing

the leakage of dog allergen into the air. None of the vacuum cleaners which contained integral HEPA filters and double thickness bags leaked Can f 1 when tested in the experimental room when brand new and after 6 months of domestic use, but vacuum cleaners without integral HEPA filters leaked allergen into the air.[23]

Since getting rid of the family pet is rarely a viable option, we currently advise a set of measures

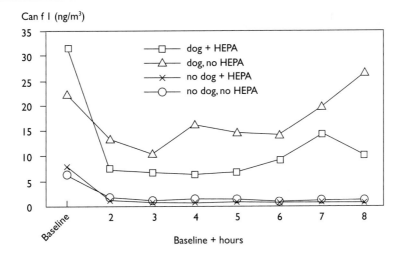

Figure 25.6: The effect of high efficiency particulate air (HEPA) filtration unit on airborne Can f 1 in homes with dogs (From: Green R, Simpson A, Custovic A, Faragher B, Chapman MD, Woodcock A. The effect of air filtration on airborne dog allergen. *Allergy* 1999; **54**: 484–8, with permission.)

listed in Table 25.2 to patients who are allergic to cats or dogs and persist in keeping their pet.[9] The clinical benefit afforded by the proposed avoidance measures has not yet been established.

AVOIDANCE OF COCKROACH ALLERGENS

Sensitization to cockroach allergens is an important risk factor for asthma in the US, where cockroach infestation is common in sub-standard housing apartment complexes. Cockroach asthma occurs primarily among lower socio-economic groups and minority populations. This patient population has the highest asthma mortality and morbidity and is also the least compliant with any form of asthma treatment. Cockroaches have also been reported to be an important cause of asthma in the Far East (Taiwan, Japan) and France. In the colder climate of the UK, cockroach allergens are not routinely used in the evaluation of allergic disease, though there have been recent case-reports of cockroach infestation associated with asthma.

Both physical and chemical methods can control cockroach populations in houses. Reducing access to food and water is critical. Waste food should be removed and reducing leakage through faulty taps and pipe-work should contain surface water. Caulking and sealing cracks and holes in the plasterwork and flooring may restrict cockroach access. Several chemicals are marketed in the US and elsewhere for controlling cockroach infestation, including diazinon, chlorpyrifos and boric acid. The most useful for patients with allergic disease are bait stations, where the chemical is retained within a plastic housing. These stations may contain hydramethylonon (marketed

Table 25.2: Avoiding cat and dog allergens

	Reduce airborne allergen	Gives clinical benefit
Removal of pet	✓	✓
Pet *in situ*		
Wash pet	✓	?
Remove carpets	✓	?
High efficiency particulate air filter	✓	?
Castrate male or get a female (cat)	✓	?

as COMBAT) or avermectin (AVERT). A paste formulation of hydramethylonon (SIEGE) is also marketed for use on cockroach runways and underneath counters etc.

Bait stations are generally effective at reducing cockroach levels for 2–3 months. The effect of cockroach control measures on allergen levels in houses has not been extensively studied, though a number of trials are underway. Cockroaches in apartment complexes are especially difficult to treat because of re-infestation from adjacent apartments. Asthma is the only disease unequivocally associated with cockroach infestation of houses and it an important public health problem in towns and cities across the US, where housing conditions sustain large cockroach populations. Many patients are unaware that cockroaches may cause asthma. Thus attempts to reduce cockroach allergen exposure rely on improving patient education and concerted attempts by pest control companies and public health departments to reduce cockroach infestation.

THE EVIDENCE

Background

Before considering the science behind allergen avoidance strategies, the important question is whether allergen avoidance in homes improves asthma control in sensitized patients. This is an area of controversy, mainly because of the inadequacies of the clinical studies on allergen avoidance. It is very difficult to conduct a placebo-controlled trial in this area: the combination of skin wheal and home visit is a potent stimulus for a change in behaviour, resulting in increased cleaning, removal of mite habitats and reduction in allergen levels even in a non-intervention group. Virtually every controlled study has observed a significant reduction in mite allergen levels and sometimes improved clinical symptoms in both the control group as well as the active group. Furthermore, as stressed previously, a successful trial would need to achieve and maintain a major reduction in allergen levels, be sufficiently long (i.e. probably not less than a year, with at least 6 weeks run-in period) and have adequate power.

The majority of studies on allergen avoidance in patients' homes have been small, poorly controlled and have often used measures that we now realize do not reduce mite allergen exposure. Consequently, many fail to show clinical benefits. We have recently reviewed 31 trials of mite allergen avoidance regimens in asthma in the literature.[8] Of the 31 studies, only six showed significant reduction in mite counts and/or mite allergen levels, together with an adequate treatment period. All used bed covers. Although these six studies had different endpoints, they all showed some evidence of clinical benefit.

In a recently published meta-analysis on the effectiveness of mite allergen avoidance,[24] only three of 23 studies met our criteria. These three studies (one in adults, two in children, total randomized subjects 123), although small and with diverse end-points, suggest some clinical benefit. Whilst all trials of bed coverings suggest they are clinically effective, the impact of their widespread use by asthmatics has not been determined in a public health context. Which patients benefit and whether treatment is cost-effective is unknown. Large-scale trials are underway to answer these questions.

Clinical trial of pet allergen avoidance

A recent study investigated the effectiveness of environmental allergen control using high efficiency particulate arrest (HEPA) air cleaners in the management of asthma and rhinitis in cat allergic patients who were sharing their home with one or more cats.[25] Although a small reduction in airborne Fel d 1 was observed in the active (but not in the control) group, there was no difference between the groups in any of the outcome measures during the 3 months of the study. The reduction in cat allergen exposure afforded by the measures used in this trial was modest (~50%). It seems likely that a much more complex series of measures are needed if substantial reduction in exposure to airborne cat allergen is to be achieved, including keeping the pet out of the bedrooms and main living areas, installing HEPA air filtration units in the main living areas and bedrooms, washing the pet twice a week, thorough cleaning of the upholstered furniture (or replacing it with leather furniture), replacing carpets with linoleum or wood flooring and using a vacuum cleaner with integral HEPA filter and double thickness bags. Although such an integrated approach may have the desired clinical effect, it has not been validated in a clinical trial.

Environmental tobacco smoke (ETS)

Approximately 50% of children in the UK are exposed to smoking from one or more parent/carer. ETS exposure is associated with an increase in prevalence of respiratory symptoms in cross sectional studies and worsening of symptoms in children with pre-existing conditions such as asthma.[26,27] There is a clear dose-response relationship, with children both of whose parents smoke suffering more than those where the mother alone smokes, with less respiratory symptoms in those children from families with no ETS exposure. Maternal smoking increases the severity and frequency of asthma symptoms in children. The presence of one or more smokers in the household of asthmatic children has been shown to increase the number of emergency room visits. Furthermore, ETS may act as an adjuvant for the effects of allergen exposure or endotoxin exposure, but this has not been studied in the epidemiological studies. However, whilst there are very large numbers of studies conducted to demonstrate the harm caused by parental smoking, very few interventions have tested the potential beneficial effects of reducing parental smoking.[5] The effect of smoking cessation interventions up until now has been relatively modest.

CONCLUSIONS

Minimizing the impact of identified environmental risk factors is a first step to reduce the severity of asthma.[28] Although environmental control is difficult, we predict that it will be an integral part of the overall management of allergen-sensitized patients. As a recommendation for the future trials, the Third International Workshop on Indoor Allergens and Asthma concluded:

'There is an urgent need to develop adequately powered, randomized, controlled studies to investigate the potential benefits of low-allergen domestic environments in patients with allergic disease. Such studies

need to address compliance, cost-effectiveness, be of adequate length (e.g. 12 months), and be tailored for different socio-economic groups and age groups'.[29]

The 1995 revision of the British Thoracic Society Asthma Guidelines states:

'Support for house dust mite avoidance measures reflects a change to the 1993 Guidelines, but further research into methodology and duration of action of these measures is needed'.

If the benefits attributable to allergen avoidance were instead attributed to a new drug, that drug would be the subject of trials involving thousands of patients. It is unfortunate that the perceived lack of commercial benefit has discouraged large-scale population-based trials.

The results of ongoing large-scale trials of the widespread applicability of mite allergen avoidance and the effect on patient symptoms, exacerbation rate, use of medication and overall health costs study will conclusively show whether a simple intervention designed to reduce domestic mite allergen exposure can improve the clinical control of asthma, which subgroups of patients benefit, and whether the intervention is cost-effective. There are little data on benefits of primary and secondary prevention by environmental control, and several prospective studies are currently under way. Furthermore, it is essential to devise new interventions to address the problem of ETS exposure in a more positive and helpful way.

REFERENCES

1. Pope AM, Patterson R, Burge H (eds). *Indoor allergens – Assessing and controlling adverse health effects.* Washington DC: National Academy Press, 1993.

2. Custovic A, Smith A, Woodcock A. Indoor allergens are the major cause of asthma. *Eur Respir Rev* 1998; **8**: 155–8.

3. Custovic A, Simpson A, Woodcock A. Importance of indoor allergens in the induction of allergy and elicitation of allergic disease. *Allergy* 1998; **53** (Suppl. 48): 115–20.

4. Custovic A, Chapman M. Risk levels for mite allergens. Are they meaningful? *Allergy* 1998; **53** (Suppl. 48): 71–6.

5. Peat JK, Li J. Reversing the trend: reducing the prevalence of asthma. *J Allergy Clin Immunol* 1999; **103**: 1–10.

6. Tovey ER, Marks G. Methods and effectiveness of environmental control. *J Allergy Clin Immunol* 1999; **103**: 179–91.

7. Platts-Mills TAE, Hayden ML, Woodfolk JA, Call RS, Sporik R. House dust mite avoidance regimens for the treatment of asthma. In: David TJ (ed). *Recent advances in paediatrics 13*. Edinburgh: Churchill Livingstone; 1995: 45–58.

8. Custovic A, Simpson A, Chapman MD, Woodcock A. Allergen avoidance in the treatment of asthma and atopic disorders. *Thorax* 1998; **53**: 63–72.

9. Woodcock A, Custovic A. ABC of Allergies Avoiding exposure to indoor allergens. *BMJ* 1998; **316**: 1075–8.

10. Colloff MJ, Ayres J, Carswell F, *et al*. The control of allergens of dust mites and domestic pets: a position paper. *Clin Exp Allergy* 1992; **22** (Suppl. 2): 1–28.

11. Butland BK, Strachan DP, Anderson HR. The home environment and asthma symptoms in childhood: two population-based case–control studies 13 years apart. *Thorax* 1997; **52**: 618–24.

12. Custovic A, Woodcock A. Feather or synthetic? That is the question. *Clin Exp Allergy* 1999; **29**: 144–7.

13. Rains N, Siebers RW, Crane J, Fitzharris P. House dust mite allergen (Der p 1) accumulation on new synthetic and feather pillows. *Clin Exp Allergy* 1999; **29**: 182–5.

14. Hallam C, Custovic A, Simpson B, Houghton N, Simpson A, Woodcock A. Mite allergens in feather and synthetic pillows. *Allergy* 1999; **54**: 407–8.

15. Colloff MJ. Practical and theoretical aspects of the ecology of house dust mites (Acari: Pyroglyphidae) in relation to the study of mite-mediated allergy. *Rev Med Vet Entomol* 1991; **79**: 611–29.

16. Colloff MJ. Dust mite control and mechanical ventilation: when the climate is right. *Clin Exp Allergy* 1994; **24**: 94–6.

17. Custovic A, Green R, Fletcher A, *et al*. Aerodynamic properties of the major dog allergen, Can f 1: distribution in homes, concentration and particle size of allergen in the air. *Am J Respir Crit Care Med* 1997; **155**: 94–8.

18. Custovic A, Smith A, Pahdi H, Green RM, Chapman MD, Woodcock A. Distribution, aerodynamic characteristics and removal of the major cat allergen Fel d 1 in British homes. *Thorax* 1998; **53**: 33–8.

19. Custovic A, Fletcher A, Pickering CA, *et al*. Domestic allergens in public places III. House dust mite, cat, dog and cockroach allergen in British hospitals. *Clin Exp Allergy* 1998; **28**: 53–9.

20. Wood RA. Indoor allergens: thrill of victory or agony of defeat. *J Allergy Clin Immunol* 1997; **100**: 290–2.

21. Hodson T, Custovic A, Simpson A, Chapman MD, Woodcock A, Green R. Washing the dog reduces dog allergen levels but the dog needs to be washed twice a week. *J Allergy Clin Immunol* 1999; **103**: 581–5.

22. Green R, Simpson A, Custovic A, Faragher B, Chapman M, Woodcock A. The effect of air filtration on airborne dog allergen. *Allergy* 1999; **54**: 484–8.

23. Green R, Simpson A, Custovic A, Woodcock A. Vacuum cleaners and airborne dog allergen. *Allergy* 1999; **54**: 403–5.

24. Gotzsche PC, Hammarquist C, Burr M. House dust mite control measures in the management of asthma: meta analysis. *BMJ* 1998: **317**: 1105–10.

25. Wood RA, Johnson EF, Van Natta ML, Chen PH, Eggleston PA. A placebo controlled trial of a HEPA air cleaner in the treatment of cat allergy. *Am J Respir Crit Care Med* 1998; **158**: 115–20.

26. Working Party of the Royal College of Physicians. *Smoking and the young*. London: Royal College of Physicians, 1992.

27. Strachan D, Cook D. Summary of effects of parental smoking on the respiratory health of children and implications for research. *Thorax* 1999; **54**: 357–66.

28. Woodcock A, Custovic A. Role of indoor environment in determining the severity of asthma. *Thorax* 1998; **53** (Suppl. 2): S47–S51.

29. Platts Mills TA, Vervloet D, Thomas WR, Aalberse RC, Chapman MD. Indoor Allergens and Asthma: Report of the Third International Workshop. *J Allergy Clin Immunol* 1997; **100** (6): S1–S21.

INDEX